ADVANCES IN Pediatrics

Editor-in-Chief
Carol D. Berkowitz, MD, FAAP, FACEP

Chief,
Division of General Pediatrics,
Department of Pediatrics,
Harbor-UCLA Medical Center,
Distinguished Professor of Pediatrics,
David Geffen School of Medicine at UCLA,
Torrance, CA

ELSEVIER

PHILADELPHIA LONDON TORONTO MONTREAL SYDNEY TOKYO

ADVANCES IN
Pediatrics

VOLUMES 1 THROUGH 71 (OUT OF PRINT)

VOLUME 72

Ethical Issues in Pediatric Endocrinology: A Primer for the Practitioner, *by Jennifer M. Ladd and Rohan K. Henry*

Artificial Intelligence in Pediatric Endocrinology, *by Sabitha Sasidharan Pillai and Ambika P. Ashraf*

Pharmacology in Pediatric Renal Solid Organ Transplantation, *by Christine Tabulov, Kelly McGee, and Beatriz Fabiola Marin Ruiz*

A Practical Approach to Functional Abdominal Pain and Irritable Bowel Syndrome in Children and Adolescents, *by Biren J. Desai and Hannibal Person*

A Review of Wolff-Parkinson-White for the General Practitioner, *by Ismael Corral and Cherlyn Angela Perez-Corral*

Editor: Kerry Holland
Developmental Editor: Malvika Shah

Printed by Sheridan at 450 Fame Avenue, Hanover, PA 17331.

Publishing Office:
Elsevier Inc.
1818 Market Street,
Suite 3323
Philadelphia, PA 19103-2899
United States

International Standard Serial Number: 0065-3101
International Standard Book Number: 13: 978-0-443-43188-3

CONTRIBUTORS

SASHA-JANE ABI-AAD, MD, MSc, Postdoctoral Research Fellow, Department of Pediatrics, Division of Gastroenterology, Hepatology and Nutrition, University of South Florida Morsani College of Medicine, Tampa, Florida

NAJIBE ABOU-ANTOUN, MS, Researcher, Department of Pediatrics, David Geffen School of Medicine at UCLA Harbor UCLA Medical Center, Laboratory Operations Manager, Lundquist Institute for Biomedical Innovation at Harbor UCLA Medical Center, Torrance, California

KRISTINA ADACHI, MD, Associate Clinical Professor, Department of Pediatrics, Division of Infectious Diseases, University of Californian Los Angeles, Los Angeles, California

DENISE AL ALAM, PhD, Associate Professor, Department of Pediatrics, David Geffen School of Medicine at UCLA, Harbor UCLA Medical Center, Investigator, Lundquist Institute for Biomedical Innovation at Harbor UCLA Medical Center, Torrance, California

DEAN ANSELMO, MD, FACS, FAAP, Associate Professor of Clinical Surgery, Division of Pediatric Surgery, Department of Surgery, Children's Hospital Los Angeles, Los Angeles, California

MARY T. AUSTIN, MD, MPH, Professor, Division of Pediatric General Surgery, Department of Surgery, University of Washington Medicine, Seattle, Washington

ANDREW P. BAIN, MD, Resident, Department of Surgery, University of Texas Southwestern Medical Center, Dallas, Texas

CHAITHANYA REDDY BANDI V, MD, Assistant Professor, Department of Pediatrics, Division of Pediatric Neurology, University of South Florida Morsani School of Medicine, Tampa, Florida

MUSTAFA BARBOUR, MD, Professor, Department of Pediatrics, Division of Pediatric Hematology-Oncology and Stem Cell Transplant, University of Louisville School of Medicine, Louisville, Kentucky

NANCY L. BECK, MD, Assistant Professor, Department of Pediatrics, Texas Tech University Health Sciences Center, Lubbock, Texas

SIMONE M. CHANG, MBBS, Assistant Professor, Department of Pediatrics, Division of Pediatric Hematology-Oncology, University of South Florida Morsani School of Medicine, Tampa, Florida

JESSICA CLARION, MD, Pediatric Pulmonary Fellow, Division of Pulmonary and Sleep Medicine, Seattle Children's Hospital, University of Washington, Seattle, Washington

SOULA DANOPOULOS, PhD, Assistant Professor, Department of Pediatrics, David Geffen School of Medicine at UCLA, Harbor UCLA Medical Center, Investigator, Lundquist Institute for Biomedical Innovation at Harbor UCLA Medical Center, Torrance, California

SONEET DHILLON, MD, MHA, Resident, Department of Internal Medicine, Harbor UCLA Medical Center, Torrance, California

CLAUDIA M. DOUGLAS, MD, MS, Faculty Scientist, Department of Pediatrics, Seattle Children's Hospital and Research Institute, University of Washington, Seattle, Washington

CATHERINE M. GORDON, MD, MS, Senior Investigator, Adolescent Bone and Body Composition Laboratory, Clinical Director and Chief, Eunice Kennedy Shriver National Institute of Child Health and Human Development, National Institutes of Health, Bethesda, Maryland

MORAN GOTESMAN, MD, Assistant Clinical Professor, Department of Pediatrics, Director of the Sickle Cell Disease Specialty Care Center, David Geffen School of Medicine at UCLA, Pediatric Hematologist-Oncologist, The Lundquist Institute of Biomedical Innovation at Harbor UCLA Medical Center, Torrance, California

DESMOND L. GREEN, MD, MPH, Post-Pediatric Portal Fellow, Department of Child and Adolescent Psychiatry and Behavioral Sciences, Children's Hospital of Philadelphia, Philadelphia, Pennsylvania

H. MOLLIE GROW, MD, MPH, Professor, Department of Pediatrics, University of Washington School of Medicine, Seattle, Washington

ALEXANDRA HA, DO, Physician, Department of Pediatrics, Harbor-UCLA Medical Center, Torrance, Department of Allergy and Immunology, David Geffen School of Medicine at UCLA, Los Angeles, California

NADINE HORNECK, MD, Resident, Department of Internal Medicine, St Mary Medical Center, Long Beach, California

MICHELLE HOUGH, MD, Surgical Resident and Research Fellow, Division of Pediatric Surgery, Department of Surgery, Children's Hospital Los Angeles, Los Angeles, California

MICHAEL ANGELO C. HUANG, MD, MS, Associate Professor of Pediatrics, Division of Hematology and Oncology, Mid Campus Center, Washington University in St. Louis, St Louis, Missouri

PETER HUYNH, MD, Assistant Clinical Professor, Department of Anesthesiology, Anesthesiologist, Pain Management Specialist, Harbor UCLA Medical Center, David Geffen School of Medicine at UCLA, Torrance, California

RAMIN JAMSHIDI, MD, FACS, FICS, Associate Professor, Departments of Surgery and Child Health, Creighton University School of Medicine, Omaha, Nebraska; Assistant Professor, Department of Surgery, University of Arizona College of Medicine, Tucson, Arizona; Assistant Professor, Departments of Surgery and Pediatrics, Mayo Clinic, Phoenix, Arizona; Director of Endocrine Surgery, Phoenix Children's Hospital, Phoenix, Arizona

FERESHTEH SALIMI JAZI, MD, Pediatric Surgical Critical Care Fellow, Department of Surgery, University of California San Diego, Rady Children's Hospital, San Diego, California

RACHA T. KHALAF, MD, MSCS, Associate Professor, Department of Pediatrics, Division of Gastroenterology, Hepatology and Nutrition, University of South Florida Morsani College of Medicine, Tampa, Florida

MAGGIE KOZMAN, MD, FAAP, FACP, Assistant Clinical Professor of Pediatrics, David Geffen School of Medicine at UCLA, Los Angeles, Internal Medicine, Pediatrics, Harbor-UCLA Medical Center, Torrance, California

SHONA LOWE, MD, MPH, FASAM, Assistant Medical Director, Los Angeles General Primary Care West Clinic, Los Angeles, California

CAROLYN MADDEN, APRN, Faculty Instructor, Department of Pediatrics, University of South Florida Morsani College of Medicine, Tampa, Florida

MEGHAN McGARRY, MD, MAS, Associate Professor, Division of Pulmonary and Sleep Medicine, Seattle Children's Hospital, Center for Respiratory Biology and Therapeutics, University of Washington, Seattle, Washington

BINDI NAIK-MATHURIA, MD, MPH, FACS, FAAP, Professor of Surgery and Pediatrics, University of Texas Medical Branch, Galveston, Texas

SAGARIKA NALLU, MD, FAAN, FAAP, FAASM, Associate Professor of Pediatrics, Associate Program Director of Sleep Medicine Fellowship, Chief of Pediatric Neurology, Director of Pediatric Sleep Medicine at Tampa General Hospital, University of South Florida Morsani College of Medicine, Tampa, Florida

SRIDEVI NARAYANAN, DO, Resident Physician, Department of Pediatrics, University of South Florida Morsani College of Medicine, Tampa, Florida

THERESA NEVAREZ, MD, Associate Professor of Family Medicine, David Geffen School of Medicine at UCLA, Faculty, Harbor UCLA Family Medicine, Torrance, California

KARIN NIELSEN-SAINES, MD, MPH, Professor, Department of Pediatrics, Division of Infectious Diseases, University of California Los Angeles, Los Angeles, California

KAREN OLMOS, MD, MPH, Assistant Professor of Family Medicine, David Geffen School of Medicine at UCLA, Program Director, Harbor UCLA Family Medicine, Torrance, California

KINSA THI OO, MD, Resident, Department of Pediatrics, David Geffen School of Medicine at UCLA, Harbor UCLA Medical Center, Lundquist Institute for Biomedical Innovation at Harbor UCLA Medical Center, Torrance, California

MCKENNA F. PARNES, PhD, MSEd, Assistant Professor, Department of Pediatrics, University of Washington School of Medicine, Investigator, Treuman Katz Center for Pediatric Bioethics and Palliative Care, Seattle Children's Research Institute, Seattle, Washington

NEEMA PITHIA, MD, Fellow, Department of Pediatrics, Division of Infectious Diseases, David Geffen School of Medicine at UCLA, Los Angeles, California; Attending Physician, Kaiser Pernanente, Department of Neonatology, Oakland, California

HARINDER DOSANJH RAIPURIA, DNP, Consultant, Pediatric Endocrinology, Eunice Kennedy Shriver National Institute of Child Health and Human Development, National Institutes of Health, Bethesda, Maryland

MARISSA RAY, MD, MS, General Surgery Resident, Department of Surgery, University of Cincinnati Medical Center, Research Fellow, Cincinnati Children's Hospital Medical Center, Cincinnati, Ohio

MICHAEL ROGERS, DO, MPH, Assistant Professor, Department of Pediatrics, Physician, Division of Gastroenterology, Hepatology, and Nutrition, University of Cincinnati, Cincinnati, Ohio

GLORIA SANCHEZ, MD, FASAM, Physician, Director of Addiction Medicine, Associate Clinical Professor, Department of Family Medicine, David Geffen School of Medicine at UCLA, Director, Medications Addiction Treatment, Harbor UCLA Medical Center, Torrance, California

JANIS L. SETHNESS, MD, MPH, Department of Pediatrics, Seattle Children's Hospital and Research Institute, University of Washington, Seattle, Washington

MARNI SHEAR, DO, MPH, Pediatric Hospitalist, Assistant Clinical Professor, Department of Pediatrics, Harbor UCLA Medical Center, The Lundquist Institute of Biomedical Innovation, David Geffen School of Medicine at UCLA, Torrance, California

JAN SMOGORZEWSKI, MD, Associate Program Director and Director of Inpatient Dermatology Education, Division of Dermatology, Department of Internal Medicine, Harbor UCLA, Torrance, California

CHARLES SONG, MD, Chief, Department of Allergy and Immunology, David Geffen School of Medicine at UCLA, Los Angeles, California; Department of Pediatrics, Harbor-UCLA Medical Center, Torrance, California

ALYSSA STETSON, MD, MPH, MMSc, Research Fellow, Boston Children's Hospital, General Surgery Resident, Bringham and Women's Hospital, Boston, Massachusetts

GREGORY M. TIAO, MD, Professor, Department of Surgery, Division of Gastroenterology, Hepatology, and Nutrition, Division Director, Pediatric General and Thoracic Surgery, Surgical Director, Liver Transplant Program, Cincinnati Children's Hospital Medical Center, Cincinnati, Ohio

KATIE TRIBULS, DO, Fellow, Department of Pulmonary, Critical Care and Sleep Medicine, University of South Florida Morsani School of Medicine, Tampa, Florida

NEIL G. USPAL, MD, Professor, Division of Pediatric Emergency Medicine, Department of Pediatrics, University of Washington, Seattle, Washington

ELLIOTT M. WEISS, MD, MSME, Associate Professor, Department of Pediatrics, University of Washington School of Medicine, Treuman Katz Center for Pediatric Bioethics and Palliative Care, Seattle Children's Research Institute, Seattle, Washington

MACKENZIE L. WYATT, MD, Pediatric Pulmonary Fellow, Division of Pulmonary and Sleep Medicine, Seattle Children's Hospital, Center for Respiratory Biology and Therapeutics, University of Washington, Seattle, Washington

AMI TAKEI YUEN, MD, Physician, Department of Pediatrics, Harbor-UCLA Medical Center, Torrance, California; Department of Allergy and Immunology, David Geffen School of Medicine at UCLA, Los Angeles, California

CONTENTS

VOLUME 73 • 2026

Opioids and Adolescents: How to Prevent and Treat Addictions Early 25

Gloria Sanchez, Shona Lowe, Theresa Nevarez, and Karen Olmos

Addiction is a treatable, chronic condition of pediatric onset. Providers will learn how to use evidence-based methods for prevention , screening, and treatment of substance use among adolescents. Treating adolescents who use substances can be an opportunity to provide life-saving harm reduction resources including naloxone and start medications for opioid use disorder such as buprenoprhine. Identifying early, at-risk substance use is increasingly critical given the risk of lethal overdose due to fentanyl contamination.

Updates in Adolescent Contraception 41

Claudia M. Douglas and Janis L. Sethness

Adolescent contraceptive care is rapidly evolving, shaped by updated clinical guidance, an expanding range of contraceptive options, and a growing emphasis on reproductive justice and equity. This review summarizes recent trends in adolescent sexual activity and birth rates, examines current guidance from the American Academy of Pediatrics and American College of Obstetricians and Gynecologists, and highlights clinically relevant updates to the US Medical Eligibility Criteria and Selected Practice Recommendations. Key topics include confidentiality, shared decision-making, expanding access across diverse clinical settings, and the role of digital platforms in adolescent sexual and reproductive health education.

Sickle cell pain is a complex and multifaceted condition that varies widely across individuals, necessitating a personalized approach informed by a comprehensive history and careful consideration of the biopsychosocial context. Although opioids remain the mainstay of pain management for individuals experiencing acute pain during a vaso-occlusive episode (VOE), multiple disease-modifying therapies have emerged and are demonstrating promise in helping to reduce the frequency and duration of VOEs. In addition, nonopioid analgesics and nonpharmacologic interventions show potential as adjunct therapies that can further support children and adolescents presenting with sickle cell VOE.

In this article, we will describe pharmacologic interventions and physical restraints use in children with agitation in the prehospital and hospital setting, disparities that exist in their use, evidence-based practices surrounding appropriate restraint use, techniques for de-escalation to reduce the need for restraint, specific techniques and medications for restraint when indicated, regulations surrounding the use of restraints, and effort to reduce the use of restraints.

Built on the foundation of trauma-informed care, screening and intervention for trauma, adverse childhood experiences, and resilience in the *inpatient* medical setting is a burgeoning field that has predominantly been pioneered in pediatric subpopulations. Several studies have shown that screening during medical hospitalization is feasible and uncovers high levels of adversity in patients and caregivers that correlate to poorer outcomes. Further study is needed for screening all-comers in pediatric medical/surgical units admitted for any reason, with the goal of supporting patients' resilience factors by efficiently mobilizing desired multidisciplinary resources in the hospital to buffer their adversity.

Type 1 diabetes is an autoimmune-mediated disease affecting persons with a genetic predisposition. Screening for the presence of pancreatic autoantibodies has enabled identification of persons who can benefit from immunomodulatory therapies, with one anti-CD3 monoclonal antibody therapy now in clinical use. Other therapies under investigation include those related to β-cell replacement and regeneration. Diabetes device technology has progressed rapidly, with continuous glucose monitoring and automated insulin delivery via closed-loop systems providing for improved glycemic control and enhanced quality of life.

Advances in Down Syndrome 145

Kinsa Thi Oo, Najibe Abou-Antoun, Soula Danopoulos, and Denise Al Alam

Trisomy 21 (T21) is the most common chromosomal disorder worldwide and the leading cause of intellectual disability. Individuals with T21 present with unique facial features, developmental challenges, and multiorgan system defects including cardiovascular, pulmonary, gastrointestinal, endocrine, neurologic, hematological, immunologic diseases, and other systems. We reviewed the latest changes and advances in T21 management over the last 10 years, focusing on new findings and improvements in diagnosing, preventing, and treating complications across different organ systems, which have led to a longer lifespan and better quality of life for children with T21.

Paradigm Shifts in Cystic Fibrosis Newborn Screening and Care in Infancy 161

MacKenzie L. Wyatt, Jessica Clarion, and Meghan McGarry

There have been advances in the care of children with cystic fibrosis (CF) that allow for early disease identification and intervention in early childhood. Universal and the rise of modulator therapy have revolutionized CF care, so the life expectancy in children with CF has improved. With the changing landscape in advances in CF care, there is uncertainty in interpretation of tests and clinical phenotypes that are indeterminate for CF diagnosis.

Gastrointestinal and Pancreatic Manifestations of Cystic Fibrosis in the Era of Highly Effective Modulators 179

Sasha-Jane Abi-Aad, Sridevi Narayanan, and Racha T. Khalaf

This review synthesizes emerging evidence on gastrointestinal (GI) disorders, specifically luminal and pancreatic function in the era of triple cystic fibrosis transmembrane conductance regulator (CFTR) modulator therapy. Elexacaftor–tezacaftor–ivacaftor has been associated with mild improvements in GI symptoms and disease burden in patients' reported outcomes and has shown a significant increase in growth and body mass index reflecting improved nutritional status, even among individuals who remain pancreatic insufficient. Long-term data on triple CFTR modulators remain limited, highlighting the need to understand their long-term impact on GI manifestations, as survival improves and chronic intestinal inflammation persists.

Adolescents with malignant and nonmalignant diagnoses can require hematopoietic stem cell transplantation (HSCT), with the volume increasing 5% to 10% per annum in the United States. HSCT is an established therapy for malignancies, hemoglobinopathies, bone marrow failure, inborn errors of metabolism, and immunodeficiency. Gonadotoxic-conditioning regimens, immunosuppressive agents, and glucocorticoids are essential therapies required for a successful transplant course. Secondary endocrine sequelae can occur, however, including iatrogenic adrenal insufficiency, reduced bone mineral density, medication-induced hyperglycemia, and premature ovarian insufficiency. With broader indications for HSCT use, at-risk endocrinopathies in the post-transplant period require prompt recognition and assessment, monitoring, and medical management.

Parathyroid glands regulate calcium and phosphate homeostasis through the production of parathyroid hormone. Pediatric parathyroid disease is uncommon but can have severe physiologic consequences. This is true of both hyperparathyroidism and hypoparathyroidism. Robust understanding of these disorders is supported by knowledge of underlying physiology, relevant laboratory analyses, imaging, and pharmacology. Technological advancements in intraoperative visualization/identification and parathyroid imaging may significantly influence future care. As these are quite uncommon disorders in the pediatric population, physicians or centers with limited experience may benefit from consultation and collaboration with larger pediatric centers where multidisciplinary approaches are undertaken and greater experience can be shared.

Maternal-fetal surgery has advanced rapidly, offering targeted prenatal interventions that can improve outcomes for conditions such as myelomeningocele, sacrococcygeal teratoma, congenital diaphragmatic hernia, lung lesions, lower urinary tract obstruction, and twin-twin transfusion syndrome. This review summarizes current fetal therapies, patient selection, contraindications, and maternal risks, emphasizing the need for multidisciplinary evaluation. Emerging innovations, including fetoscopic repair techniques, stem cell and gene-based therapies, and tissue engineering, highlight the expanding potential of fetal intervention. Ethical frameworks remain essential to ensure that maternal autonomy and safety are prioritized while pursuing fetal benefit.

genotype-driven therapy, biomarker development, and long-term outcomes will further refine care for this complex and heterogeneous disease.

Pediatric brain tumors are the most common solid malignancy in childhood, and they remain the leading cause of cancer-related mortality. Presentation varies by age, tumor type, and location, often including persistent headaches, vomiting, or focal neurologic deficits. Advances in molecular diagnostics have refined classification and have revolutionized the role for targeted therapies. Successful management requires a multidisciplinary team consisting of neurosurgery, oncology, radiation, and supportive care. Long-term follow-up is essential to monitor for recurrence and manage treatment-related sequelae, underscoring the importance of coordinated survivorship programs.

Current Management of Food Allergies in Pediatric Patients 283

Alexandra Ha, Ami Takei Yuen, and Charles Song

Food allergy is a growing public health concern affecting up to 8% of children. The underlying pathophysiology involves a complex interplay of genetic predisposition, microbiome dysbiosis, and environmental factors disrupting epithelial barrier integrity, leading to a spectrum of immune reactions. Diagnosis is a clinical process integrating a detailed patient history with sensitization tests, with the oral food challenge serving as the definitive tool. While strict avoidance and emergency epinephrine form the foundation of management, the paradigm is shifting toward proactive immunomodulatory therapies, including oral immunotherapy.

Pediatric hidradenitis suppurativa is a chronic relapsing skin disease that peaks in adolescence and is often misdiagnosed. Clinical diagnosis is made by identifying recurrent, painful nodules in flexural sites that have risk of tunneling and scarring. Initiate education, gentle skin care, and topical therapy while adding age-appropriate oral antibiotics when indicated. Screen for comorbidities and refer early to dermatology for medical management as well as procedural and biological treatments.

Sleep is essential for healthy growth and neurocognitive development in children, however, sleep disturbances in the pediatric population are still largely undiagnosed. Children with craniofacial abnormalities are at particular risk for developing sleep disturbances, which can have long-lasting neurodevelopmental, cardiovascular, and respiratory consequences. This article seeks to fill knowledge gaps in screening, evaluation, and management of common sleep disorders in children with craniofacial abnormalities. With early identification and treatment, clinicians can significantly improve the overall health, developmental outcomes, and quality of life in children with craniofacial syndromes.

under 5 years of age. This article provides a comprehensive overview of the epidemiology, diagnosis, and management of ingested objects, including magnets, button batteries, sharp and blunt items, and water beads. It highlights the unique risks, complications, and decision-making algorithms associated with each type, integrating evidence-based recommendations from recent literature and the North American Society for Pediatric Gastroenterology, Hepatology and Nutrition. Special attention is given to radiolucent materials, such as water beads, which present diagnostic challenges and may require advanced imaging or surgical intervention.

Advances in Pediatrics 73 (2026) xxxiii–xxxvi

ADVANCES IN PEDIATRICS

PREFACE

Navigating Stormy Seas, in Turbulent Times, and Moving Ahead

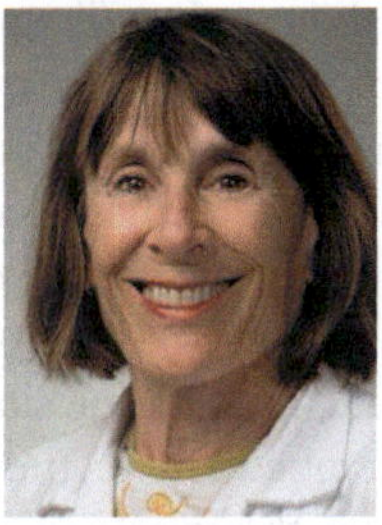

Carol D. Berkowitz, MD, FAAP, FACEP
Editor

We are traveling on stormy seas with tall waves that may capsize our boat and jettison our cargo. Yet despite the storm, we continue to advance forward, better understanding the ills that affect our patients and better defining treatments to address these ills. The stormy seas represent the attack we as physicians have witnessed in an anti-science environment and the disregard for evidence-based preventive strategies, such as immunizations with their proven track-record of disease prevention and saving countless lives.

It is almost paradoxical that many of our articles in this year's edition of *Advances in Pediatrics* on "Turning the Rising Tide" specifically as it relates to certain conditions, such as congenital syphilis, which over the past decade has been declared a public health crisis in the United States (in Pithia and colleagues, "The congenital syphilis surge: clinician lessons to turn the rising tide"). In a like mode, the opioid epidemic has taken an increasingly large toll on adolescents, especially since the introduction of fentanyl (in Sanchez and colleagues, "Opioid and adolescents: how to address and treat addictions early"). It is important to recognize MOUD (medications opioid use disorder) to be able to effectively manage the condition through early recognition and intervention. Likewise, there have been notable advances in adolescent reproductive health and reproductive justice. The move has been toward care with

https://doi.org/10.1016/j.yapd.2026.04.001
0065-3101/26/© 2026 Published by Elsevier Inc.

developmentally appropriate counseling and prioritizing adolescent autonomy (in Douglas and Sethness, "Updates in adolescent contraception").

While some youth misuse opioids, others, particularly those with sickle cell disease, are relieved by these medications (in Shear and colleagues, "Pain management in pediatric patients with sickle cell disease"). But it is important to promote newer agents, such as buprenorphine and nonpharmacologics, so as to wholistically manage patients with sickle cell disease. Besides sickle cell disease, other genetic diseases have also experienced a swell of new information that can positively affect the management of these conditions. Just like it is critical to select the most appropriate medications when treating patients with sickle cell disease, it is important to be able to manage the agitated pediatric patient (in Green and Uspal, "Reducing restraint use in the pediatric agitated patient: a review of approaches and best practices"). The focus is on evidence-based approaches to de-escalation and to minimize the use of physical restraints. Many of these youngsters are dealing with challenging home situations and backgrounds. Trauma-informed screening, well-embedded in the outpatient setting, is equally helpful in caring for patients on the inpatient unit (in Kozman, "Trauma-informed screening and intervention for trauma, ACEs, and resilience in the pediatric inpatient setting").

The world of genetics continues to advance despite misinformation that floods social media sites. We recognize that type 1 diabetes is an autoimmune disease, and there is on-going research into the use of monoclonal antibodies to delay the onset of the disease and B-cell replacement to obviate insulin (in Beck, "Recent advances in the management of type I diabetes in children").

Management of Down syndrome has also progressed with advances in cardiac surgery, and the use of endocrine and metabolic surveillance (in Thi Oo and colleagues, "Advances in Down syndrome"). Likewise, there have been advances in the care of infants and children with cystic fibrosis, through universal newborn screening (in Wyatt and colleagues, "Paradigm shifts in cystic fibrosis newborn screening and care in infancy"). The rise of modulator therapy has revolutionized cystic fibrosis care. CFTR (cystic fibrosis transmembrane conductance regulator) moderators may help reduce the amount of enzyme replacement therapy needed. These modulators may also affect the microbiome (in Abi-Aad and colleagues, "Gastrointestinal and pancreatic manifestations of cystic fibrosis in the era of highly effective modulators").

There is a link between genetics and endocrinopathies. Adolescents who have undergone hemopoietic stem cell transplantation are at risk for endocrinopathies related to their need for immunosuppression (in Raipuria and Gordon, "The hidden burden: endocrinopathies in adolescents after hemopoietic stem cell transplantation"). They risk iatrogenic adrenal insufficiency as well as premature ovarian failure. Disorders of the parathyroid gland are rare in children, but diagnoses of these disorders have been assisted by technical advances in imaging, localization of lesions, and intraoperative identification (in Jamshidi, "Parathyroid disorders in children: physiology, pharmacology, and practical management").

Advances in pediatric surgery continue to be in the forefront. Fetal surgery can alter the natural history of select congenital anomalies, improving long-term survival and quality of life (in Bain and Austin, "Fetal surgery today: indications, outcomes, and future innovations"). In a like mode, early diagnosis of biliary atresia using serum testing for matrix mettalloproteinase-7 and genetic testing with jaundice chip microarrays can diagnosis biliary atresia, which can best be managed with a Kasai portoenterostomy, and if needed, liver transplantation (in Stetson and colleagues, "Infant jaundice: updates in biliary atresia").

Lymphatic malformations (previously called lymphangiomas or cystic hygromas) are now categorized as vascular anomalies and managed surgically as well as medically by multidisciplinary teams (in Hough and Anselmo, "Updates on lymphatic malformations: medical therapies, sclerotherapy, and surgery"). Multidisciplinary teams also provide care to children with brain tumors, which are the most common solid tumor of childhood with an incidence of 6.05 per 100,000 in the United States (in Chang and ccolleagues, "Pediatric brain tmors"). More common but equally challenging is the problem of food allergies, which affect 8% of children. The pathophysiology of food allergies involves an interplay of genetics, microbiome, dysbiosis, and environmental factors. In 2024, a new era of FDA-approved therapies, including anti-IgE biologic omalizumab, has been realized (in Ha and colleagues, "Current management of food allergies in pediatric patients").

Unlike food allergies, hiradenitis supprativa is rare in children and tends to appear between 15 and 17 years of age, though then persists as a chronic inflammatory skin condition treated with antibiotics and affecting quality of life (in Dhillon and colleagues, "Hiradenitis in pediatrics"). The condition leads to permanent scarring.

Sleep disturbances are common in children but are particularly problematic in children with craniofacial anomalies (in Tribuls and colleagues, "Sleep disturbances in pediatric craniofacial syndromes"). It is important to proactively assess children with craniofacial anomalies for sleep-disordered breathing, which includes primary snoring, upper airway resistance syndrome, obstructive sleep apnea, and hypoventilation. There are lists of chromosomal, syndromic craniosynostotic, and microsomic conditions and others associated with sleep-disordered breathing.

Diagnosing the cause of gait disturbances is challenging (in Bandi and Nallu, "Approach to a child with gait disturbances"). Most children are misdiagnosed as experiencing dizziness. Gait evolves as children grow older, and the pediatrician should recognize when a gait is not appropriate for the child's age. Some disordered gait is on a neurologic basis.

Another challenging area is related to the ingestion of nonfood items, such as multiple magnets, button batteries, and water beads (in Naik-Mathuria and Jazi, "Management of foreign bodies: beads, coins, and magnets"). Expediated removal of these objects is paramount lest they lead to obstruction or perforation. Parental education is integral to help prevent these events.

This preface began with an analogy between stormy seas and the stormy scientific climate of the times. But our real climate and climate change are pressing issues (in Parnes and colleagues, "Climate stewardship in the clinical setting"). Pediatricians have a key role in monitoring children's health and sharing evidence-based findings with the medical community through reports and peer-reviewed papers and articles. This is how we move forward, recognizing the ill effects that climate change is responsible for, diagnosing, and managing these emerging conditions.

Disclosures

The author has no conflicts of interest to disclose.

Carol D. Berkowitz, MD, FAAP, FACEP
Division of General Pediatrics
Department of Pediatrics
Harbor–UCLA Medical Center
David Geffen School of Medicine at UCLA
Torrance, CA, USA

E-mail address: cberkowitz52@gmail.com

Advances in Pediatrics 73 (2026) 1–23

ADVANCES IN PEDIATRICS

The Congenital Syphilis Surge

Clinician Lessons to Turn the Rising Tide

Neema Pithia, MD[a,b], Karin Nielsen-Saines, MD, MPH[a], Kristina Adachi, MD[a,*]

[a]Department of Pediatrics, Division of Infectious Diseases, UCLA, Los Angeles, CA, USA; [b]Kaiser Department of Neonatology

Keywords

• Congenital syphilis • In utero syphilis • Nontreponemal and treponemal tests

Key points

- Congenital syphilis (CS) is an important cause of preventable fetal and infant morbidity and mortality around the world.
- CS can be prevented by timely syphilis screening and treatment of pregnant women and their partners.
- Over the past decade, CS has become a US public health crisis.
- Many states and professional societies now recommend testing for syphilis 3 times in pregnancy (first trimester, third trimester, and delivery).
- Most infants do well if diagnosed and treated early for CS.

BACKGROUND AND HISTORICAL SIGNIFICANCE

Syphilis is an infection caused by *Treponema pallidum* subspecies *pallidum*, a motile, microaerophilic spirochete bacteria [1,2]. Its name *Treponema* derives from the Greek words for "turning (trepo) the thread (nema)," alluding to its helical shape [1–3].

An ancient and feared disease, syphilis has been detailed in history for over 500 years. Characteristic syphilitic periosteal reactions have been identified in New World skeletal remains at the time of Columbus' arrival in 1492 [4]. At the end of the fifteenth century, syphilis was considered an emerging infectious disease in Europe and colloquially referred to as the "Italian disease," the "French disease," and the "Great pox." [2] Its name is believed to originate

*Corresponding author. 10833 Le Conte Avenue, 22-340 MDCC, Los Angeles, CA 90095-1752. *E-mail address:* kadachi@mednet.ucla.edu

https://doi.org/10.1016/j.yapd.2025.12.005

Abbreviations

AAP	American Academy of Pediatrics
CBC	complete blood cell
CDC	Centers for Disease Control and Prevention
CDPH	California Department of Public Health
CNS	central nervous system
CS	congenital syphilis
CSF	cerebral spinal fluid
CXR	chest x-ray
FTA-ABS	fluorescent treponemal antibody-absorption
HIV	human immunodeficiency virus
ID	infectious diseases
IM	intramuscular
IV	intravenous
NNPTC	National Network of STD Clinical Prevention Training Centers
PCR	polymerase chain reaction
RPR	rapid plasma reagin
STD	sexually transmitted disease
TP-PA	*Treponema pallidum* particle agglutination
VDRL	Venereal Disease Research Laboratory
WHO	World Health Organization

from the 1530 story of the shepherd "Syphilus," who insulted the Sun God and was in turn punished with a devastating disease [4].

In the United States, the history of syphilis has been indelibly marked by the Tuskegee study with its haunting legacy of systemic racism and medical injustice. This infamous US Public Health Service syphilis study spanned 4 decades (1932–1972). Six hundred Black men from rural Alabama were recruited as participants to understand the natural history of syphilis; treatment of syphilis was withheld even after penicillin was found to be effective. The study only ended after a whistleblower reported these ethical concerns to the press [5–7]. Of the 400 men with syphilis, 28 died of syphilis and 100 died of syphilis-related complications. In addition, 40 wives were infected, resulting in 19 children born with congenital syphilis (CS) [6]. These disturbing human research subject violations ultimately led to the Belmont report and the establishment of the Office of Human Subjects Research Protections. However, the Tuskegee study has left vestiges of medical mistrust in its wake, which continue in many communities to this day.

EPIDEMIOLOGY

CS remains a major cause of preventable global fetal morbidity and mortality. Syphilis and thus CS disproportionately affect the most vulnerable populations in wealthy and poor countries. The global CS surge has been fueled by societal inequities, especially impacting disenfranchised, undocumented, indigenous, racial/ethnic minorities, and socioeconomic disadvantaged populations. Pregnancy compounds these issues of inequality in many places around the world [8–10].

Syphilis is one of the most common sexually transmitted infections worldwide. In 2007, the World Health Organization (WHO) created the WHO Global Health Initiative to eliminate syphilis mother to child transmission with the goal of decreasing CS to 50 cases per 100,000 livebirths [8,11]. Although there has been some improvement in certain geographic areas, CS case numbers remain unacceptably high [12]. In 2022, the WHO estimated there are 700,000 global CS cases with 390,000 adverse birth outcomes including 150,000 early fetal deaths and stillbirths, 70,000 neonatal deaths, 55,000 preterm or low-birth weight births, and 115,000 infants with a CS clinical diagnosis [13]. Globally, CS remains the second leading cause of preventable stillbirth. Among infants with documented adverse outcomes, 21% of mothers did not receive prenatal care, 53% of women were not tested for syphilis despite receiving prenatal care, 16% tested positive for syphilis but received inadequate or no treatment, and 9% tested positive despite appropriate treatment [13].

The CS global burden is not equally distributed around the world. The WHO African Region accounts for 62% of global CS cases (400,000 cases; rate of 1119 cases per 100,000 live births) followed by the Eastern Mediterranean Region with 17.1% (113,000 cases; rate of 635 cases per 100,000 live births) [9,14]. Over the past decade, the region of the Americas has also seen a skyrocketing number of cases. Countries like Brazil now account for 85% of all CS cases in the Pan American Health Organization with 51,000 CS cases (650 cases per 100,000 live births) reported [11,15]. The true burden of global CS is likely underestimated given variability in prenatal screening practices, access to prenatal/postnatal syphilis testing, treatment, and surveillance data quality [11,16] (Fig. 1).

In recent years, CS cases have also increased dramatically in many high-income countries around the world. US CS cases have increased 700% to 1000% over the past decade [17] (Fig. 2). Since 2012, the number of US cases increased from 335 to 3941 in 2024. States such as New Mexico (355.3), South Dakota (351.8), Arizona (281), Texas (246.8), Oklahoma (227.2), Mississippi (207.6), and Nevada (193) have some of the highest CS incidence rates per 100,000 live births in the country in contrast to overall US rates in 2018 (33.1) and in 2024 (109.6) [18,19] (Fig. 3A, B).

The US increase in CS was observed across all ages and racial/ethnic groups, although the largest increases have been seen in American Indian/Alaska Natives, Native Hawaiian/Pacific Islanders, and Black/African Americans, where case rates have been approximately 12, 7, and 4 times higher than US White populations [18,20]. US racial/ethnic minorities have faced the "brunt" of the CS epidemic with the main risk factor being living in communities with high rates of syphilis. These disparities are believed to "stem from decades of deeply entrenched social determinants of health" and underscore differences in access to health care, levels of poverty, housing instability, and other factors that have disproportionately impacted communities of color [21]. Studies also suggest that primary CS risk factors are limited or no prenatal care, methamphetamine

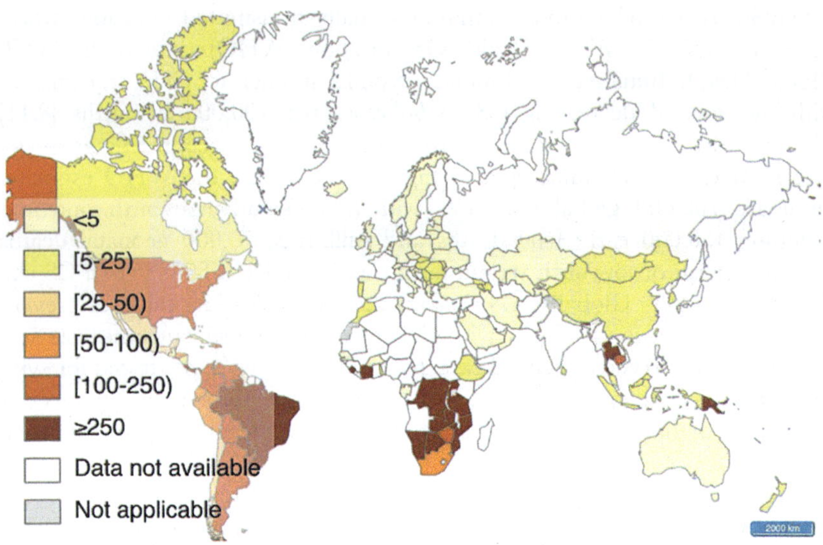

Fig. 1. Global CS rates by country per 100,000 live births. Countries in dark brown have highest CS rates. Note: Map lines delineate study areas and do not necessarily depict accepted national boundaries. (*Data from* WHO, last updated July 2025 [64].)

or other intravenous (IV) drug use, sexually transmitted infections during pregnancy, high-risk sexual activity, recent incarceration, housing insecurity, unemployment, history of adverse childhood events, and mental health concerns [22–26].

NATIONAL, STATE, AND LOCAL CONGENITAL SYPHILIS INTERVENTIONS

Given the alarming increase in US syphilis infections in pregnant women and CS cases, efforts have been made at national, state, and local levels to stem this rising tide of CS cases. Previously, the US Department of Health and Human Services established a National Syphilis and Congenital Syphilis Syndemic Federal Task Force to implement strategies such as increasing availability of treatment, hosting workshops for high-risk communities, and increasing funding for prevention and treatment initiatives in early 2024 [27].

In addition, over the past several years, various statewide public health agencies have created new guidelines for providers to expand syphilis detection for pregnant women and women who may become pregnant. For instance, in California in December 2020, new provider guidelines were released and updated in 2024, and a 2022 State Senate bill was also passed [28,29]. In California, early recommendations were made to increase the frequency of syphilis screening in pregnancy. Most recent recommendations were to screen for syphilis 3 times during pregnancy including in the first trimester, again in the third

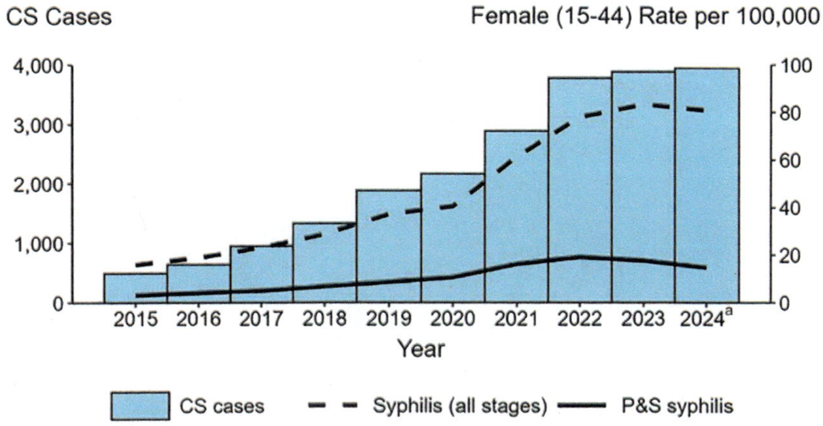

Fig. 2. US congenital syphilis cases by year of birth and rates of primary and secondary syphilis cases in women (15–44 years) from 2015 to 2024. [a]2024 data are provisional as of August 14, 2025. CS, congenital syphilis; P&S syphilis, primary and secondary syphilis. (*Data from* CDC [19].)

trimester (ideally at 28–32 weeks) and also at delivery regardless of risk factors. Similarly, in April 2024, the American College of Obstetrics and Gynecology also changed their recommendations to screen for syphilis 3 times in pregnancy [30]. Providers have received reminders that women with stillbirths should be tested for syphilis. Other recommendations adopted by state public health departments such as California include increasing syphilis testing through annual testing of all sexually active young people (15–44 years of age) and enhancing screening of pregnant women for syphilis at nontraditional sites of care such as emergency departments, urgent care clinics, jails, mental health facilities, drug treatment centers, and homeless outreach services [28,29,31].

CONGENITAL SYPHILIS CLINICAL CONSIDERATIONS AND MANIFESTATIONS

Congenital syphilis definition, transmission

CS refers to in utero (ie, transplacental) syphilis infection of the developing fetus from the bacteria *T pallidum.* Nearly all CS cases result from transplacental passage of *T pallidum* to the fetus in the setting of a disseminated maternal infection. Occasionally exposure to maternal genital lesions at the time of delivery (ie, *intrapartum*) can cause neonatal infection [32]. *T pallidum* is not transmitted via human milk, but transmission to the infant during breastfeeding may occur if an infected lesion is present on the mother's breast [1,33].

The risk of vertical transmission from mother to infant varies by maternal syphilis stage and pregnancy trimester [34]. The risk of vertical transmission is estimated to be 60% to 90% with untreated primary or secondary syphilis but decreases to 40% in early latent and less than 10% in late latent infection

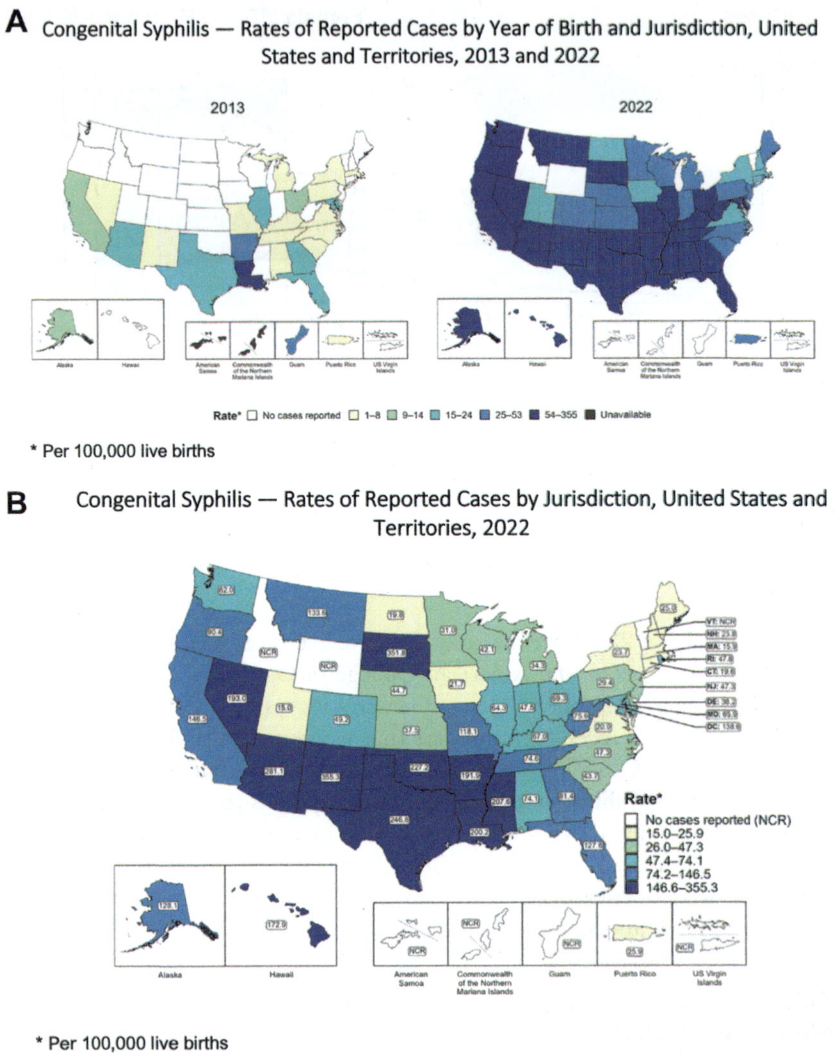

Fig. 3. Changing US CS rates over time and CS rates by US states. (*A*) US and territories map showing rates of reported CS cases per year of birth and jurisdiction in 2013 to 2022. CS cases per 100,000 live births. States in dark blue have the highest CS and increasing number of states over time with high CS rates. (*B*) US and territories with CS rates of reported cases by Jurisdiction in 2022, [a]Please note color scale in maps in (*A*) and (*B*) are different. Note: Map lines delineate study areas and do not necessarily depict accepted national boundaries. (*Data sourced from* the Centers for Disease Control [18].)

[1,3,33,35,36]. In particular, for a woman with untreated syphilis infection, there is a 70% chance of fetal syphilis infection in the 4 years following the initial infection if she remains untreated [37]. Maternal infection can be asymptomatic or associated with nonspecific symptoms such as rash, fever, or genital ulcers [38]. For recently acquired syphilis in pregnancy, the risk of syphilis transmission to the fetus increases with gestational age [1,33]. Recent Australian data suggest the risk of fetal transmission increases when infection is acquired after 18 weeks' gestation; there is a 26% risk if CS is treated by 24 weeks and rises as high as 60% if CS is untreated by the third trimester [39]. CS can cause spontaneous abortion, often after the first trimester, as well as late-term stillbirth in up to 40% of cases [37,40]. Stillbirth is thought to be secondary to reduced blood flow to the fetus in a syphilitic placenta [37]. Studies have demonstrated that maternal coinfection with human immunodeficiency virus (HIV) also increases the risk of syphilis vertical transmission [41,42].

Fetal ultrasound findings

CS fetal ultrasound findings are often varied and nonspecific. A 2022 review examining postnatal and antenatal anomalies in 432 known CS cases over the past 50 years attempted to quantify the incidence of these findings. Hepatomegaly was the most common organ anomaly in 83% of cases, followed by splenomegaly in 16%. Ascites was seen in 19% of cases and bowel hyperechogenicity or dilation in 2.4% of cases. Nonspecific fetal growth restriction was a frequent finding in 14% of cases. Hydrops was seen in 12% of cases with isolated subcutaneous edema in 7%, pericardial effusion in 2%, and pleural effusion in 1% [43]. The study cited that the finding of anemia with elevated middle cerebral artery peak systolic velocity noted in 38% (in the context of ascites or atypical hydrops) should raise clinical suspicion for CS [43]. The study also observed placentomegaly in 34% of cases, polyhydramnios in 11%, and oligohydramnios in 9% [43]. It is well documented that placentas of CS fetuses are enlarged (ie, placentomegaly) secondary to local inflammatory responses [22,44]. In 75% of cases, the CS fetal placenta is heavier (>90th percentile). Thus, all mothers with placental weight at the 90th percentile or higher should be tested for CS [44]. Placenta histologic examination often demonstrates necrotizing funisitis (ie, "barber's pole" appearance), enlarged hypercellular villi, proliferative vascular changes, and acute or chronic villitis [45].

Clinical manifestations

As with other congenital infections, CS infants may present with a range of clinical findings. The extent of infection-related injury to the developing fetus depends on the gestational age when maternal infection occurs and the duration of exposure prior to maternal treatment [3]. Untreated infection early in pregnancy may lead to fetal demise in the first trimester, stillbirth, or neonatal death [3] (Fig. 4). However, fortunately, the majority of live-born CS infants will appear normal at birth without clinical or laboratory evidence of infection. In a series of 173 infants born to mothers with untreated syphilis, only 6 (3.5%) had clinical findings at birth [42]. However, a troubling feature of CS is that if CS infants remain untreated, they may develop disease months to many years later. There are 2 primary clinical syndromes of CS: *early and late CS* [1,2,34].

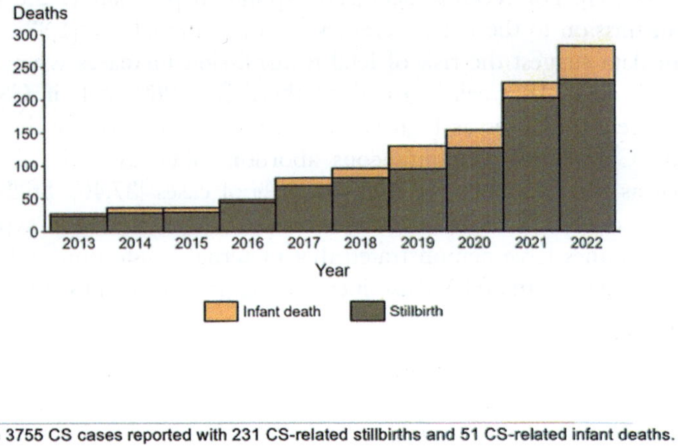

Fig. 4. CS-related stillbirths and infant deaths in the US from 2013 to 2022. (*Data sourced from* the Centers for Disease Control [18].)

Early CS refers to clinical manifestations occurring in the first 2 years of life (Fig. 5A–D, Table 1). Severely affected CS infants have been depicted throughout history as premature, ill-appearing infants with "old" facies, "withered" or "wrinkled," rash-marked skin, and distended abdomens [3,46]. Among the most commonly seen CS features is hepatomegaly and may be accompanied by transaminitis, elevated alkaline phosphatase, and direct hyperbilirubinemia with jaundice [2]. Hepatitis from CS may initially worsen with penicillin G treatment and may take months to resolve [2,34]. Splenomegaly may also occur due to extramedullary hematopoiesis. Thrombocytopenia, which may present as petechiae or purpura, is a frequent finding and may be the only CS manifestation in the first few months of life [34].

Rhinitis or "snuffles" refers to a copious, watery nasal discharge that may turn purulent and serosanguinous and may also be accompanied by laryngitis [2,3]. Nasal discharge and mucocutaneous lesions are infectious with high numbers of spirochetes, thus appropriate contact precautions should be taken, particularly before and during the first 24 hours of treatment [1–3,34]. Mucocutaneous lesions are common findings and may be seen in 40% to 60% of affected CS infants. The rashes are classically red, oval, and maculopapular prior to becoming copper-colored [1–3]. The rashes are usually most prominent on the hands and feet and may be accompanied by desquamation of the palms and soles. The rash may be reminiscent of secondary syphilis seen in adults. Another less common form of CS rash is known as pemphigus syphiliticus, which may begin as red papules and evolve to a fluid-filled bullous eruption with skin crusting, wrinkling, and desquamation [2,3,34]. This condition may even be confused with staph scalded skin syndrome or epidermolysis bullosa. Fissures or mucus patches may be seen, especially in the perioral, perianal, or genital regions [2]. Rare mucocutaneous manifestations include

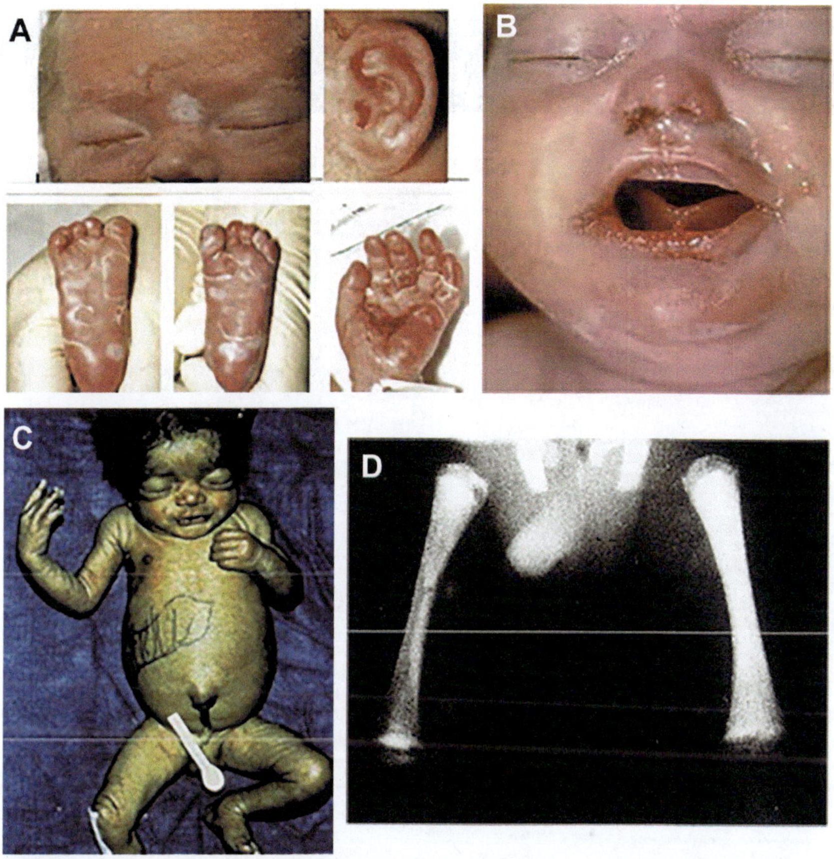

Fig. 5. Examples of early CS clinical manifestations. Left to right clockwise: Early manifestations of congenital syphilis: (*A*) desquamating, maculopapular lesions including erosions and blisters especially of palms and soles; (*B*) "snuffles" or mucopurulent nasal discharge; (*C*) jaundice and hepatosplenomegaly; (*D*) xray with bone metaphysitis including R-sided decreased density of shaft ends and destruction of proximal tibia. (Photos courtesy of the CDC [Dr Ronald Ballard] [65].)

condylomata lata, which are hypertrophic wart-like papular lesions typically in perioral or perianal regions [1,2,34,47] (see Fig. 5, Table 1).

CS may affect the bones in 60% to 80% of infants with other CS clinical findings and usually occurs from periostitis or cortical demineralization [2,3,34]. Bony involvement may occur in 20% of well-appearing, otherwise asymptomatic CS infants [34]. Long bones (especially the humerus and femur), ribs, and cranium are the mostly common places that CS osteochondritis or periostitis may occur. Bone involvement is typically symmetric and frequently affects the lower extremities [34]. Classic radiologic findings include a "celery stalk" appearance due to alternating dense and radiolucent bands; Wimberger's sign, which is localized bony destruction of the medial proximal tibial

Table 1
Infant congenital syphilis clinical findings: Early and late congenital syphilis [2,3,34,48,50,66–68]

EARLY CS FINDINGS Manifest under 2 years of age, usually in first 8 weeks of life	
Skeletal[a] • May see bony involvement in 20% well-appearing infants • **Osteochondritis** • **Periostitis** (primarily long bones) • Pseudoparalysis, painful limbs (can be mistaken for nonaccidental trauma)	**Mucocutaneous lesions** • Maculopapular small **dark, red copper lesions** especially hands/feet • **Desquamation palms, soles** • **Pemphigus syphiliticus** (bullous eruption that may peel, crust) • **Condyloma lata** (plaques perioral/perianal) • Mucous patches • Perioral/perianal fissures • Patchy alopecia

Central nervous system
• Clinical signs neurosyphilis are rare in infants
  ○ Bulging fontanelle, seizures, leptomeningitis, cranial nerve palsies, hydrocephalus, cerebral infarction
  ○ Pituitary gland dysfunction, diabetes insipidus
• CSF abnormalities (CSF elevated cell count, protein)
Ophthalmologic
• Chorioretinitis
Salt and pepper fundus
• Iritis
• Cataract
• Glaucoma
ENT/Pulmonary
• **"Snuffles"** (rhinitis with copious nasal secretions)
• Pneumonitis (Pneumonia alba, fibrosing pneumonitis with diffuse infiltrates)
GI/Renal/Cardiac
• **Hepatomegaly**[a]
• **Hyperbilirubinemia/ Jaundice**
• **Splenomegaly**
• GI tract fibrosis, inflammation
  ○ Ileitis, necrotizing enterocolitis, rectal bleeding, malabsorption
• Pancreatitis
• Nephrotic syndrome
• Myocarditis
	Hematologic
	• **Cytopenias** (anemia may be hemolytic, leukopenia, **thrombocytopenia**[a])
	• Rare reports of pancytopenia mistaken for congenital hemophagocytic lymphohistiocytosis (HLH)
	Lymphadenopathy (LAD)
	• Generalized LAD (uncommon, nodes firm and nontender)
	• Epitrochlear nodes (may be seen, characteristic)
	Other
	• Low birth weight <2500g/SGA, intrauterine growth restriction
	• Failure to thrive
	• Preterm birth
	• Hydrops (nonimmune), diffuse edema
	• **Stillbirth**
	• Placenta (villitis, vasculitis, **large placenta**)
	Rare severe presentations
	• Hypoxic ischemic encephalopathy (HIE)
	• Disseminated intravascular coagulopathy
	• Persistent pulmonary hypertension (PPHN)

LATE CS FINDINGS Manifest when older than 2 years of age, usually in adolescence or early adult years	

Skeletal
• **Frontal bossing**
• **Saddle nose**
• **Short maxilla, high palate arch**
• **Higoumenakis sign** (periostitis of clavicle)
• **Mandible protuberance**
• Clutton joints-symmetric painless swelling of knees
• Anterior bowing of shins (Saber shins)
• Rhagades (perioral fissures)
Teeth
• Hutchinson teeth (peg-shape, notched central incisors)
• Mulberry molars (extra molar cusps)
Other
• Gummas of skin or mucous membranes
	Ophthalmologic
	• Interstitial keratitis, corneal scarring
	  ○ May see 5-20 yrs later
	• Optic nerve atrophy
	• Healed chorioretinitis, uveitis, secondary glaucoma
	Central nervous system
	• Developmental delay
	• Hydrocephalus
	• Seizures
	• Cranial nerve palsies
	• Paralysis
	• Hearing loss from cranial 8th nerve impairment
	  ○ May see 10-40 yrs later

[a]Most common.

metaphysis leading to a "moth eaten" appearance; or Wegner sign with "sawtooth metaphysis" with serrated metaphyseal findings. Some of the bone lesions can be painful, and may lead to subepiphyseal fractures or epiphyseal dislocations that can be mistaken for nonaccidental trauma, or "pseudoparalysis" of Parrot. Bone lesions often heal within 6 months even without antibiotic therapy [2,3,34] (see Fig. 5, Table 1).

Central nervous system involvement (neurosyphilis) may also occur in 41% to 50% of CS infants who have clinical, laboratory, or radiographic CS signs [2,34]. However, actual clinical signs of neurosyphilis (bulging fontanelle, seizures, leptomeningitis, cranial nerve palsies, hydrocephalus, and cerebral infarction) are considered rare in infants. In addition, neurosyphilis may surreptitiously complicate CS even in infants without other CS signs and symptoms [3]. Other less common findings include anemia that may be hemolytic, ocular involvement (chorioretinitis, cataracts, glaucoma, and uveitis), pneumonitis including pneumonia alba with complete bilateral opacification of lung fields, nephrotic syndrome, myocarditis, pancreatitis, and gastrointestinal tract fibrosis with inflammation [2,34].

CS also remains an important cause of stillbirth and infant death. Of the 3755 CS US cases in 2022, 231 CS-related stillbirths and 51 CS-related infant deaths were reported (see Fig. 4). One recent small case series from a US neonatal intensive care unit academic center also reported several severe CS infant presentations with hypoxic ischemic encephalopathy, persistent pulmonary hypertension, and disseminated intravascular coagulation that providers should keep in mind [48]. In addition, providers should note that infants with CS may present beyond the neonatal period. One study reported 67 symptomatic CS infants with a median age of over 2 months who presented most commonly with rash, "snuffles," or hepatomegaly [49]. There are also rare reports of infants presenting with pancytopenia, hepatosplenomegaly, and lymphadenopathy initially mistaken for hemophagocytic lymphohistiocytosis [50].

Features of *late CS* may result from persistent inflammation or "scars" of early CS [3]. These findings may occur after 2 years of life, although more often in adolescence or early adult years, regardless of whether there were prior CS signs or symptoms [2,3]. Classic dental findings due to vasculitic injury of developing tooth buds include Hutchinson's teeth, which may show peg-shaped or widely spaced, barrel-shaped or notched central incisors; Mulberry molars, where the first lower molars may have many small cusps instead of the normal 4 [1,3]. Deafness due to osteochondritis of the otic capsule may affect the eighth cranial nerve, but may not occur until 10 to 40 years later. Ocular changes (uveitis, interstitial keratitis, and optic nerve atrophy) may also not occur for 5 to 20 years later, and interstitial keratitis, a form of corneal inflammation, can lead to blindness. Late CS manifestations such as Hutchinson's triad refers to interstitial keratitis, cranial nerve 8 deafness, and Hutchinson's teeth. Other late CS findings include tibial bowing (Saber shins) from tibial periostitis; skull periostitis (frontal bossing), rhagades (perioral fissures), short maxilla and high arch palates from syphilitic rhinitis, saddle nose deformity with perforation of the palate and nasal septum from inflammation of the nasal mucosa extending to cartilage and bone, Higoumenakis sign (periostitis of the clavicle), and Clutton joints (painless joint swelling) [1,2,34]. Other neurologic manifestations of late congenital neurosyphilis may be similar to those seen in acquired syphilis and include intellectual disability, hydrocephalus, seizure disorders, general paresis, and cranial nerve abnormalities [2,3,34] (Fig. 6A, B, see Table 1).

Congenital syphilis diagnosis and testing methodologies

There are 2 main types of syphilis serologic tests: *nontreponemal and treponemal tests* [51–53]. The main nontreponemal tests used include rapid plasma reagin (RPR) and Venereal Disease Research Laboratory (VDRL). Nontreponemal tests, first developed in 1906, are quantitative tests that detect reactivity to antigens (cardiolipin, lecithin or phosphorylcholine, and cholesterol) in *T pallidum* membranes [51–54]. They may be falsely positive with other types of

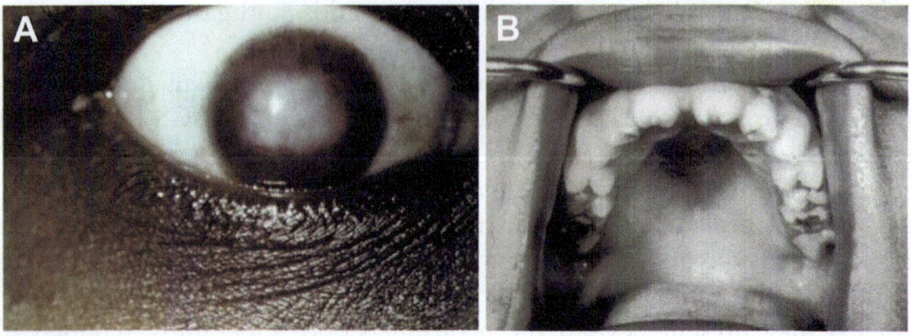

Fig. 6. Examples of late CS clinical manifestations. Left to right: Late manifestations of congenital syphilis: (*A*) interstitial keratitis from inflammation of corneal connective tissue; (*B*) Hutchinson teeth, a congenital abnormalities leading to narrow and notched permanent incisor teeth and notched, screwdriver shaped central incisors. (Photos courtesy of CDC [65].)

treponemal infections, pregnancy, autoimmune diseases, and other infections. Nontreponemal tests are the primary tests used in the evaluation and management of CS infants and titers typically decline with treatment. The same test form (eg, RPR) should be used for both mother and infant to allow for titer comparisons.

Treponemal tests are qualitative serum assays that detect antibodies to various *T pallidum* antigens [52]. In contrast to nontreponemal assays, treponemal assays typically remain positive even after appropriate treatment and are not used to evaluate treatment responses. Treponemal tests resembling ones used today were first developed in 1960s [54]. The main treponemal tests now used are *T pallidum* particle agglutination test (TP-PA) and fluorescent treponemal antibody-absorption (FTA-ABS). Other treponemal tests that are more automated with a faster turnaround time include treponemal enzyme immunoassay (EIA) and treponemal chemiluminescence immunoassay (CIA); these assays are well-suited for syphilis maternal screening, especially in high-volume clinical laboratories [52].

Many institutions have traditionally used nontreponemal tests in pregnancy to evaluate women for syphilis infection, and positive testing is confirmed with a treponemal test (ie, *traditional algorithm*) [1] (Fig. 7). However, given the increase in syphilis cases, some institutions have switched to the *reverse algorithm,* where treponemal tests are done first and then confirmed with a nontreponemal test since treponemal tests can become reactive before nontreponemal tests [1] (see Fig. 7). Similar to nontreponemal tests, false positives with treponemal testing can occur with other treponemal infections, Lyme disease, and autoimmune diseases. Nevertheless, pregnant patients with positive treponemal and nontreponemal tests should be treated for syphilis in a timely manner that is appropriate for their syphilis stage (Table 2).

It is important to remember that maternal nontreponemal and treponemal immunoglobulin G antibodies are transferred transplacentally to the fetus and may be present for up to 18 months, which confounds serologic CS

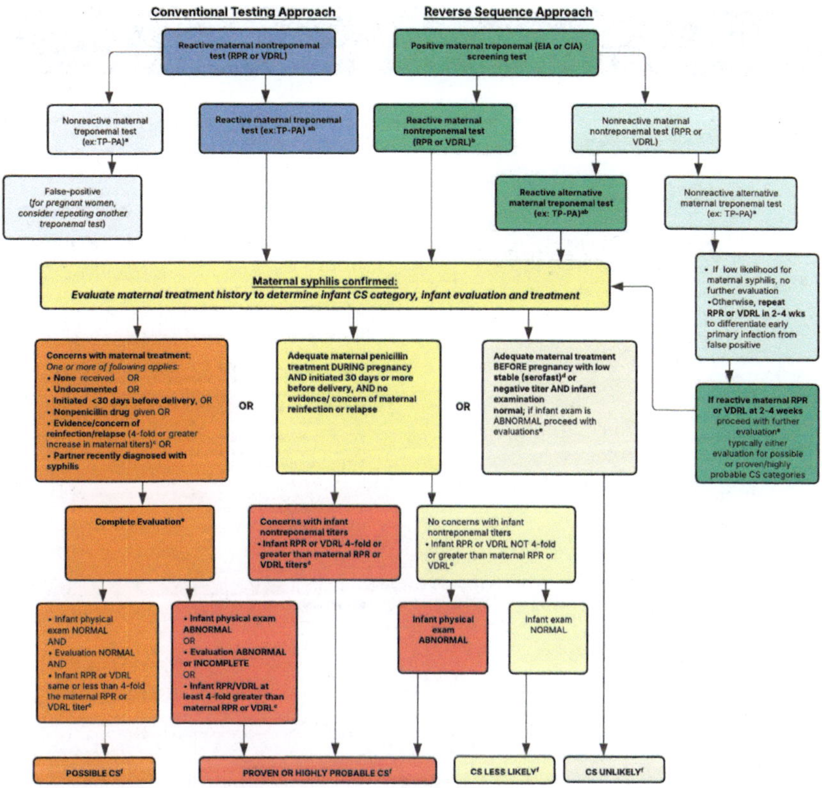

Fig. 7. Approach to evaluating infants born to mothers with reactive syphilis serologic tests. RPR, rapid plasma reagin; VDRL, Venereal Disease Research Laboratory. [a]Treponema pallidum particle agglutination (TP-PA) (which is the preferred treponemal test) or fluorescent treponemal antibody absorption (FTA-ABS). [b]Mothers with confirmed syphilis testing should also be tested for HIV. Infants of HIV-infected mothers do not require different evaluation or treatment for syphilis. [c]A fourfold change in titer is the same as a change of 2 dilutions. Example: titer of 1:64 is fourfold greater than a titer of 1:16, and a titer of 1:4 is fourfold lower than a titer of 1:16. Same type of nontreponemal test should be used to compare titers (either RPR or VDRL). [d]Stable VDRL titers 1:2 or less or RPR 1:4 or less beyond 1 year after successful treatment are considered low serofast. [e]Complete evaluation includes: complete blood cell (CBC) and platelet count; cerebrospinal fluid (CSF) examination for cell count, protein, and quantitative VDRL, long bone radiographs as well as other tests as clinically indicated (eg, chest radiographs, eye examination, liver function tests, neuroimaging, and auditory brainstem response). For neonates, pathologic examination of the placenta or umbilical cord with specific fluorescent antitreponemal antibody staining, if possible. HIV testing of infants should also be done, especially those where congenital syphilis is proven or highly probable. [f]Refer to Table 2 for further CS infant evaluation and treatment recommendations. (Used with permission of American Academy of Pediatrics, from Red Book: 2024–2027 Report of the Committee on Infectious Diseases, 33rd Edition, 2024; permission conveyed through Copyright Clearance Center, Inc.)

Table 2
Approach to maternal prenatal syphilis screening and management [1,61]

Approach to Maternal Prenatal Syphilis Screening: Screen, Stage, Treat, Monitor to Prevent Congenital Syphilis		
Screen	Screen all patients 3 times in pregnancy • At pregnancy confirmation (1st prenatal encounter, ideally 1st trimester) • Early 3rd trimester (~28 wks gestation) • At delivery *Diagnosis of maternal syphilis in pregnancy requires positive non-treponemal test (RPR or VDRL) and positive confirmatory treponemal test (TP-PA, FTA-ABS or EIA/CIA)*	
Stage	**Syphilis Stage**	**Symptoms**
	Primary	**+Chancre** (classically painless indurated ulcers but may be painful with localized lymphadenopathy)
	Secondary • 1-2 months later	**+Rash** (polymorphic, maculopapular, often includes palms and soles) and/other signs • **Condyloma lata** (hypertrophic papular lesions of perineum), **patchy alopecia, mucous patches** • May also see fever, sore throat, muscle aches, hepatitis, generalized lymphadenopathy, arthralgia, headache, malaise
	Early-Latent	No symptoms and **infection occurred within 1 year** • Within prior 12 mo had either a) seroconversion or sustained 4-fold titer rise (RPR or VDRL) • Unequivocal symptoms of primary and secondary syphilis • Sexual partner with primary, secondary or early latent syphilis
	Late-Latent or Unknown Duration	No symptoms and infection **not meet criteria for early latent**
	Neurosyphilis/Ocular/Otic[a]	+CNS signs or symptoms +CSF findings on lumbar puncture
Treat	**Stage**	**Treatment**
	Primary, Secondary, Early Latent	**Benzathine penicillin G** 2.4 million units IM x1
	Late-Latent or Unknown Duration	**Benzathine penicillin G** 2.4 million units IM (intramuscular) q7 days x 3 doses *(6-8 day interval acceptable but if late or missed doses, restart whole 3-dose course)*
	Neurosyphilis/Ocular/Otic	**Aqueous penicillin G** 3-4 million units IV q4 hours for 10 to 14 days
Monitor	• If treated at or prior to 24 weeks gestation, wait at least 8 weeks to repeat maternal syphilis titers unless concerns for primary/secondary stage symptoms/signs present or suspect treatment failure • Nontreponemal titers (RPR or VDRL) should be repeated at delivery *Post-treatment serologic response in pregnancy varies widely. Many pregnant patients do not have 4-fold decline in titers by delivery If see sustained (>2 week) 4-fold increase in titers after completed treatment, should be evaluated for reinfection and neurosyphilis*	

[a]Neurosyphilis, ocular, otic syphilis may occur at any syphilis stage. Requires neurologic exam including ophthalmic and otic exam, CSF evaluation is typically recommended if there are signs/symptoms of CNS involvement (cranial nerve palsies etc). If only ocular or otic manifestations without other neurologic abnormalities, CSF evaluation may not be necessary.

Abbreviations: IM, intramuscular; IV, intravenous; mo, month; q4 hours, every 4 hours; q7 days, every 7 days.

Data from CADPH (California Department of Public Health) and California Prevention Training Center (CAPTC) "Prenatal Syphilis Screening, Staging, and Management for Congenital Syphilis Prevention Pocket Card, Revision 5/2025".

diagnosis. As a result, treponemal tests are not helpful in the evaluation and management of CS [1,52].

CS definitive diagnosis is based on the detection of *T pallidum* from body fluid or tissues either by dark field microscopy (not typically available at most institutions), polymerase chain reaction (PCR), fluorescent antibody or silver staining [1,55]. However, for most infants, the diagnosis of CS is inferred from serology through comparison of maternal and infant titers. Infant CS infection is confirmed by an infant quantitative nontreponemal titer (eg,

RPR) that is 4 fold higher than maternal titer [1]. However, this is an uncommon finding, and its absence does not rule out congenital infection as most CS infants have nontreponemal serologic titers that are the same or 1 to 2 dilutions less than the maternal titer [2,34].

The diagnosis of congenital neurosyphilis is also challenging as most of these infants do not have clinical neurologic abnormalities [2,34]. Central nervous system (CNS) involvement is often inferred from cerebral spinal fluid (CSF) abnormalities noted with a reactive CSF VDRL and/or CSF pleocytosis, or an elevated CSF protein for infant age, which may be most commonly seen as suggested by a recent study [2,34,56]. Animal studies have previously found that CNS invasion may occur in over 40% to 50% of infants with clinical, laboratory, or imaging findings suggestive of CS and in over 60% of infants with abnormal physical examination consistent with CS [2,34]. This is one of the reasons it is important for CS infants to be treated conservatively with regimens that have CNS penetration (ie, aqueous penicillin G IV).

Congenital syphilis management

All infants born to mothers with positive syphilis serology (any positive nontreponemal titer and positive treponemal testing) require careful evaluation, testing, and follow-up to prevent missed or untreated CS cases, since clinical manifestations of disease may develop years later. These infants require a thorough examination at birth to evaluate for early signs of CS and nontreponemal testing (either RPR or VDRL), which should be the same type of assay used for maternal testing to enable comparison of titers. Additional evaluation of the infant beyond this depends on the infant CS category (Table 3, see Fig. 7).

A complete CS evaluation includes CSF analysis including VDRL, cell count, protein, long bone radiographs, and CBC with differential. Other tests as clinically indicated may be done such as hepatic function tests, chest x-ray (CXR), neuroimaging, ophthalmologic examination, and hearing evaluation (auditory brain stem response) [1,55]. *T pallidum* (syphilis) PCR testing can be performed if there is significant nasal discharge or exudative skin lesions. For women diagnosed with syphilis during pregnancy, it is recommended that placental and umbilical cord pathology be requested including silver staining and/or *T pallidum* PCR [55]. These infants, especially those with proven or highly probable CS, should be tested for HIV via either DNA or RNA PCR [1,55]. Mothers should be tested for other sexually transmitted infections, if not previously done, including chlamydia, gonorrhea, HIV, hepatitis B, and hepatitis C.

It is important to remember that penicillin is considered the only effective treatment to prevent vertical transmission of *T pallidum* and treat fetal infection and CS [1]. The Centers for Disease Control and Prevention (CDC) still considers data for other antimicrobials agents including ampicillin to be "insufficient" [55]. Thus, even for infants initially treated with ampicillin for possible sepsis, it is still recommended to complete the recommended full course of penicillin for CS treatment [1,55]. Those with penicillin allergy should be desensitized and still treated with penicillin G [1,55]. In addition, aqueous

Table 3
Infant congenital syphilis category evaluation and treatment

Category	Criteria	Evaluation	Treatment
CS proven or highly probable	• **Abnormal infant PE** cw CS OR • Serum quantitative nontreponemal titer **4-fold or higher** than birthing parent's at delivery (ex: maternal 1:2; neonatal titer ≥1:8) OR • + darkfield test or PCR of lesions/body fluid (CDC also acknowledges PCR or silver stain of placenta)	• **CSF (VDRL, cell count, protein)** • **CBC with diff** • **Long bone radiographs** **Other tests as indicated** • CXR • Transaminases • Neuroimaging • Ophthal eval • Auditory brain stem response • **HIV testing**	**Aqueous PCN G (preferred) IV x 10 days** • 50 000U/kg, IV, q12 hours (1 wk or younger), then q8 h for infants older than 1 wk OR Procaine PCN G daily IM x 10 days • 50 000 U/kg/day
CS possible	• Normal infant exam AND • Infant nontreponemal titer <4-fold birthing parent titer at delivery (ex: maternal 1:8, neonatal titer ≤1:16) **Plus one of below:** • Birthing parent not tx, inadequate tx, or no documentation of tx OR • Tx with non-PCN regimen OR • **Tx received but <u>initiated <30 days before delivery</u>**	• **CSF (VDRL, cell count, protein)** • **CBC with diff** • **Long bone radiographs**	**Aqueous PCN G IV (preferred) x10 days** OR Procaine PCN G IM daily x 10 days OR Benzathine PCN G IM x1 • (50 000 U/ kg, IM x1 dose) **only if all components of eval obtained, normal and **followup is certain**)*
CS less likely	• Normal infant exam AND • Infant nontreponemal titer < 4-fold birthing parent titer at delivery AND • Birthing parent **tx appropriately during pregnancy** (for syphilis stage), **tx initiated ≥ 30 days before delivery** AND • No reinfection or relapse	None	**Benzathine PCN G IM x1 (preferred)** • Other less preferred option: • If birthing parent's nontreponemal titers decreased at least 4-fold after tx for early syphilis or remain stable low titer (VDRL ≤ 1:2 or RPR ≤1:4) can follow serology q2-3 mo without treatment until nonreactive
CS unlikely	• Normal infant exam AND • Infant nontreponemal titer < 4-fold birthing parent titer at delivery AND • Birthing parent tx adequately **before pregnancy** AND • Birthing parent nontreponemal titer low and stable (serofast) before, during pregnancy and at delivery (ex: VDRL ≤ 1:2, RPR ≤ 1:4)	None	**None** • **Some experts consider giving benzathine PCN G IMx1** if uncertain followup and reactive test • **Follow nontreponemal titers if positive** • If infant with negative nontreponemal test at birth and birth parent with seroreactive at delivery, **recheck 3 mo** to ensure not incubating CS

Abbreviations: +, positive; CS, Congenital syphilis; cw, consistent with; CXR, chest xray; IM, intramuscular; IV, intravenous; kg, kilogram; ophthal eval, ophthalmology evaluation; PCN, penicillin; PE, physical exam; q12 hours, every 12 hours; q2-3mo, every 2-3 months; q8 hours, every 8 hours; tx, treatment; U, units; wk, week.

Data from AAP Red Book 2024: Chapter Syphilis, Table 3.72. Evaluation and Treatment of Infants Up To 1 Month of Age With Possible, Probable, or Confirmed Congenital Syphilis [1].

penicillin G IV is the only form of treatment with adequate CNS penetration, which is important for infants with congenital neurosyphilis or at risk for this condition. Rare CS treatment complications include the Jarisch-Herxheimer reaction, which is an acute inflammatory response from rapid killing of spirochetes, which can lead to fever, tachypnea, hypotension, and accentuation of cutaneous lesions within the first 24 hours of penicillin treatment.

Determining infant congenital syphilis category

Key factors to consider in determining infant CS category and thus evaluation and management include the following 4 factors: (1) *maternal diagnosis and treatment timing in pregnancy*; (2) *infant examination findings*; (3) *comparison of infant/maternal nontreponemal titers*; (4) *results of additional infant workup* if warranted (see Table 3, see Fig. 7). Within this first category, there are several features of maternal syphilis treatment that need to be fulfilled for the mother to be considered appropriately treated for syphilis. Maternal treatment during pregnancy should always be appropriate for syphilis stage (see Table 2). Treatment should have been completed with penicillin G and initiated early enough (≥30 days prior to delivery) to minimize the risk of syphilis transmission to the fetus [1,55]. Treatment should be documented, and there should be an appropriate response to maternal treatment. A maternal nontreponemal titer with a 4 fold or more increase in titer after treatment would be concerning for either relapse or reinfection. In addition, it is important to ensure maternal sexual partners have been treated for syphilis to prevent risks of reinfection after treatment during pregnancy [1].

Primary CS categories include the following: (1) *CS proven or highly probable* (examination consistent with CS or infant nontreponemal titer 4 fold or higher than maternal titer or positive darkfield test or PCR of lesions or body fluid); (2) *CS possible* (normal examination and infant nontreponemal titers not diagnostic and at least one element of concern regarding maternal treatment (eg, treatment not done, inadequate treatment, nonpenicillin regimen used, treatment without documentation, or treatment initiated <30 days before delivery; (3) *CS less likely* (normal examination and infant nontreponemal titers not diagnostic and maternal treatment appropriate during pregnancy for syphilis stage and started at least 30 days or more before delivery and no concerns for reinfection or relapse); and (4) *CS unlikely* (normal examination and infant nontreponemal titers not diagnostic, maternal treatment completed adequately before pregnancy and mother maintained low, stable nontreponemal titer before, during pregnancy, and at delivery) [1,55] (see Table 3, see Fig. 7).

Evaluation and management based on infant congenital syphilis category

Infants in CS proven or highly probable (group 1) should have the full evaluation including CBC with differential, CSF studies (VDRL, cell count, and protein), long bone radiographs, and other tests as clinically indicated (transaminases or preferably hepatic function tests, CXR, neuroimaging, ophthalmologic evaluation, hearing evaluation [auditory brain stem response], and HIV testing) [1,55]. These infants should be treated most conservatively with aqueous penicillin G IV for 10 days with dosing adjusted for infant age after 1 week (q8 hours instead of q12 hours). If 1 day of therapy is missed, the entire course needs to be restarted (see Table 3, see Fig. 7).

For those with CS possible (group 2), similar workup should be done with CBC with differential, CSF studies, and long bone radiographs [1,55]. Most providers would still treat these infants with aqueous penicillin G IV for 10 days, although procaine penicillin intramuscular (IM) × 10 days or benzathine penicillin (PCN) G IM × 1 dose is a possibility if all components of evaluation are done, all results are normal, and infant follow-up is certain. *For CS less likely infants (group 3)*, no additional workup is initially needed [1,55]. However, most providers would still give 1 dose of benzathine penicillin G IM. *For CS unlikely infants (group 4)*, no further evaluation of the infant is initially needed, and treatment is not necessarily required [1,55]. However, some experts would still consider giving one dose of benzathine PCN G IM, especially if follow-up is uncertain and if the infant had a reactive nontreponemal test at birth. *All CS infants in these 4 categories require repeat serology after discharge, regardless of whether the infant serology is positive at birth* [1] (see Table 3, see Fig. 7).

While CS is a treatable infection, infant prognosis largely depends on the extent of damage incurred prior to treatment [34]. Fortunately, most CS infants treated early in infancy, particularly those treated prenatally or within the first 3 months of life, do well [1,2,34]. All CS infants require careful follow-up at well-child visits. Most importantly, nontreponemal testing should be done every 2 to 3 months until nonreactive, and serology should be nonreactive by 6 months of age [1,55]. If infant nontreponemal testing is initially negative at birth, these infants should be retested at 3 months to ensure it remains negative. Infants with increasing or persistently stable titers 6 to 12 months after treatment should be re-evaluated with repeat CSF evaluation and typically retreated as appropriate [1,55]. Serial CSF studies after treatment during outpatient follow-up for infants suspected of congenital neurosyphilis are no longer required as long as they do not have persistently positive nontreponemal serologic tests at 6 to 12 months of age [1,55].

Providers should report all CS cases to their local public health departments, ideally before discharge from the hospital. Pediatric infectious diseases (ID) consultation is often involved in these cases after birth, if available at one's health care institution. Providers should consider having CS infants followed by pediatric ID specialists if available locally. Infants with confirmed or highly probable CS should also have audiology, ophthalmology, and developmental (regional center) follow-up as appropriate [57,58].

Other helpful congenital syphilis provider resources

Decisions regarding infant CS category and thus evaluation and management may be challenging for providers given complex algorithms in standard reference guidelines such as the American Academy of Pediatrics (AAP) Red Book, CDC sexually transmitted disease (STD) treatment guidelines, and individual state guidelines [1,55]. In response to this, the AAP Red Book created a new CS website interactive algorithm, available since August 2024 [1,59]. The AAP has also made additional CS provider clinical and patient tool kits to aid in the care of patients with CS [60].

Many local public health departments consider CS a high priority and have STD consult lines, which can advise providers and review their local STD database to identify prior maternal syphilis laboratory results and treatment received. Many will provide clinical consultations to assist with syphilis diagnosis, staging, and treatment as well as information regarding accessing penicillin treatment of pregnant women and partners at no additional cost. Other national resources are now mentioned in the AAP Red Book 2024 chapter [1]. For CS and other STDs, expert consultation within 1 to 5 business days can be provided from the *National Network of STD Clinical Prevention Training Centers (NNPTC) STD Clinical Consultation Network*, which is supported by the CDC Division of STD Prevention, at www.stdccn.org. Other helpful training CS resources include sites from NNPTC and the University of Washington STD Prevention Training Center: www.nnptc.org; https://www.std.uw.edu. The California Department of Public Health (CDPH) has a helpful clinical pocket card summarizing appropriate treatment of syphilis in pregnancy by syphilis stage [61] (see Table 2).

FUTURE CONSIDERATIONS

Syphilis prevention initiatives are critical to curtail the rising global CS epidemic. The creation of successful syphilis vaccines has eluded scientists for decades as infection does not induce immunity. Studies focused on pathogen persistence and immune evasion are critical for the development of immune-based strategies to prevent disease [62]. It is speculated that *T pallidum* outer membrane proteins are the most likely syphilis vaccine candidates for the future despite animal studies demonstrating only partial protection [63]. Benzathine penicillin shortages across the world have triggered a quest for studying other antibiotics for syphilis treatment, including agents such as amoxicillin, doxycycline, ceftriaxone, cefixime, and dalbavancin [63]. In the absence of effective vaccines, treatment for prevention is the best alternative approach to curtail rising syphilis rates. Clinical trials are ongoing to evaluate syphilis prep (preexposure prophylaxis) strategies in pregnancy to reduce CS rates in high-risk settings (NCT07189208).

CLINICS CARE POINTS

- CS, caused by the bacteria *T pallidum*, remains an important cause of preventable fetal and infant morbidity and mortality in the United States and globally.
- CS can be prevented by timely screening and treatment of pregnant women and their partners for syphilis.
- CS has become a US public health crisis as rates have dramatically increased (7–10 fold) in the past decade, reflecting growing community sociodemographic disparities.
- In response, many states and professional societies have recommended increasing the frequency of syphilis testing in pregnancy. Recommended testing is now 3 times in pregnancy (first trimester, third trimester, and delivery).
- Careful evaluation and nontreponemal titers are important in diagnosis, evaluation, and management of infants at risk or with CS.
- Evaluation and management of the CS infant depends on infant CS category: (1) CS proven or highly probable; (2) CS possible; (3) CS less likely; or (4) CS unlikely (see Fig. 7, Table 3).

- Infants with CS or possible CS require full evaluation, including physical examination; nontreponemal titer to compare to maternal titer (often RPR); CBC with differential; CSF studies (including VDRL); and long bone radiographs and other tests as clinically indicated (see Table 3). Infants with CS or high risk for CS require conservative treatment with 10 days of aqueous penicillin G IV (see Table 3).
- All infants at risk for CS or with CS require close follow-up including serial nontreponemal titers to ensure these have normalized by 6 months of age. If nontreponemal infant titers are negative at birth, repeat testing at 3 months of age is still needed to ensure the infant does not have asymptomatic CS.
- Local public health departments, AAP Red Book, and the NNPTC STD Clinical Consultation Network can provide support to providers that may not have pediatric ID services readily available for consultation of potential CS cases.
- Most infants do well if diagnosed and treated early for CS.

Funding

This study was supported by the National Institute of Allergy and Infectious Diseases, United States (AI187414 to K. Nielsen-Saines).

Disclosure

N. Pithia, K. Nielsen-Saines, and K. Adachi have no other disclosures.

References

[1] Committee on Infectious Diseases AAP. Red book: 2024–2027 Report of the Committee on Infectious Diseases. Itasca (IL): American Academy of Pediatrics; 2024.
[2] Syphilis JW. Feigin and Cherry's Textbook of Pediatric Infectious Diseases. Amsterdam, Netherlands: Elsevier; 2025. p. 1333–50, chap 145.
[3] Kollman TR, Dobson SRM. Syphilis. In: Wilson CB, Nizet V, Maldonado Y, et al, editors. Remington and Klein's Infectious Diseases of the Fetus and Newborn. 8th edition; 2015. 2015. p. 512–43.
[4] Hemarajata P. Revisiting the great imitator: the origin and history of Syphilis. American Society for microbiology. Available at: https://asm.org/articles/2019/june/revisiting-the-great-imitator,-part-i-the-origin-a.
[5] CDC. About The Untreated Syphilis Study at Tuskegee. 10-27-2025, 2025. Available at: https://www.cdc.gov/tuskegee/about/index.html
[6] Chae DHCK. Hunter EA Health justice remains elusive 50 years after Tuskegee Syphilis Study. 10-27-2025. 2025. Available at: https://sph.tulane.edu/health-justice-remains-elusive-50-years-after-tuskegee-syphilis-study.
[7] Gainty C. What newly digitized records reveal about the Tuskegee Syphilis Study. Smithsonian magazine. Available at: https://www.smithsonianmag.com/history/what-newly-digitized-records-reveal-about-the-tuskegee-syphilis-study-180983568.
[8] David A, Posfay-Barbe KM, Aguiar Nogueira C, et al. Congenital syphilis in Switzerland: a marker of inequality? A mini-review. Front Public Health 2023;11:1265725; https://doi.org/10.3389/fpubh.2023.1265725.
[9] Moore A, Freyne B, Nourse C. The global crisis of congenital syphilis: vulnerable and disenfranchised women most at risk. Res Rep Neonatol 2023;13(null):65–79.
[10] Glasier A, Gulmezoglu AM, Schmid GP, et al. Sexual and reproductive health: a matter of life and death. Lancet 2006;368(9547):1595–607.
[11] Gilmour LS, Walls T. Congenital syphilis: a review of global epidemiology. Clin Microbiol Rev 2023;36(2); https://doi.org/10.1128/cmr.00126-22.

[12] Borg SA, Tenneti N, Lee A, et al. The reemergence of syphilis among females of reproductive age and congenital syphilis in Victoria, Australia, 2010 to 2020: a Public Health Priority. Sex Transm Dis 2023;50(8):479–84.
[13] Organization WH. Mother-to-Child transmission of syphilis. 2025. Available at: https://www.who.int/teams/global-hiv-hepatitis-and-stis-programmes/stis/prevention/mother-to-child-transmission-of-syphilis. Accessed August 22, 2025.
[14] Moseley P, Bamford A, Eisen S, et al. Resurgence of congenital syphilis: new strategies against an old foe. Lancet Infect Dis 2024;24(1):e24–35.
[15] Pascoal LB, Carellos EVM, Tarabai BHM, et al. Maternal and perinatal risk factors associated with congenital syphilis. Trop Med Int Health 2023;28(6):442–53.
[16] Paixao ES, Ferreira AJ, Dos Santos IO, et al. Mortality in children under 5 years of age with congenital syphilis in Brazil: a nationwide cohort study. PLoS Med 2023;20(4):e1004209; https://doi.org/10.1371/journal.pmed.1004209.
[17] McDonald R, O'Callaghan K, Torrone E, et al. Vital signs: missed opportunities for preventing congenital Syphilis — united States, 2022. MMWR Morbidity and Mortality Weekly Report 2023;72(46):1269–74.
[18] CDC. CDC STI Statistics. Available at: https://www.cdc.gov/sti-statistics/?CDC_AAref_Val=https://www.cdc.gov/std/statistics/2019/data.zip https://www.cdc.gov/std/statistics/2022/data.zip.
[19] CDC. Slides from 2024 STI Surveillance (Provisional). Available at: https://www.cdc.gov/sti-statistics/annual/index.html.
[20] Liang Y, Menzies NA, Ronn MM. Trends in Syphilis Prevalence by Race and Ethnicity among people who are pregnant in the United States, 2016 to 2023. Sex Transm Dis 2025;52(9):535–41.
[21] U.S. syphilis cases in newborns continue to increase: a 10-Times increase over a decade. 2023. Available at: https://www.cdc.gov/media/releases/2023/s1107-newborn-syphilis.html.
[22] Villarreal DD, Lewis KA, Cielo M, et al. Patterns of congenital syphilis in a large public hospital: maternal risk factors and infant outcomes. Sex Transm Dis 2025;52(7):395–401.
[23] Menza TW, Zlot A, Gonzalez-Pena Y, et al. Multilevel Drivers of Congenital Syphilis, Oregon, 2013 to 2021. Sex Transm Dis 2025;52(1):1–8.
[24] Rahman MM, Hoover A, Johnson C, et al. Preventing congenital syphilis-opportunities identified by congenital syphilis case review boards. Sex Transm Dis 2019;46(2):139–42.
[25] Smullin C, Wagman J, Mehta S, et al. A Narrative Review of the Epidemiology of Congenital Syphilis in the United States from 1980 to 2019. Sex Transm Dis 2021;48(2):71–8.
[26] Johnson KA, Snyder RE, Tang EC, et al. Geospatial social determinants of health correlate with disparities in Syphilis and congenital Syphilis cases in California. Pathogens 2022;11(5):547.
[27] CDC. CDC: Call to Action: Let's Work Together to Stem the Tide of Rising Syphilis in the United States. 2017.
[28] CDPH. Expanded syphilis screening recommendations for the Prevention of Congenital Syphilis: guidelines for California medical providers 2020. 2020. Available at: https://www.cdph.ca.gov/Programs/CID/DCDC/CDPHDocumentLibrary/Expanded-Syphilis-Screening-Recommendations.pdf.
[29] CDPH. Healthcare providers California department of public health (CDPH) updates syphilis screening recommendations. 2024. Available at: https://www.cdph.ca.gov/Programs/OPA/Pages/CAHAN/CDPH-Updates-Syphilis-Screening-Recommendations.aspx.
[30] ACOG. Screening for Syphilis in Pregnancy: practice Advisory April 2024. Available at: https://www.acog.org/clinical/clinical-guidance/practice-advisory/articles/2024/04/screening-for-syphilis-in-pregnancy.
[31] LACDPH. Syphilis in women action toolkit. Available at: http://publichealth.lacounty.gov/dhsp/SyphilisInWomen-ActionKit.htm. Accessed October 27, 2025.

[32] Stafford IA, Workowski KA, Bachmann LH. Syphilis complicating pregnancy and congenital Syphilis. N Engl J Med 2024;390(3):242–53.
[33] Kimberlin DWBE, Lynfield R, Sawyer MH. Red book: 2021-2024 report of the committee on infectious diseases. American Academy of Pediatrics; 2021.
[34] Cooper JM, Sánchez PJ. Congenital syphilis. Semin Perinatol 2018;42(3):176–84.
[35] Braccio S, Sharland M, Ladhani SN. Prevention and treatment of mother-to-child transmission of syphilis. Curr Opin Infect Dis 2016;29(3):268–74.
[36] Fang J, Partridge E, Bautista GM, Sankaran D. Congenital syphilis epidemiology, prevention, and management in the United States: a 2022 update. Cureus 2022;14(12):e33009.
[37] De Santis M, De Luca C, Mappa I, et al. Syphilis infection during pregnancy: fetal risks and clinical management. Infect Dis Obstet Gynecol 2012;2012:1–5.
[38] Fanella S, Bitnun A, Barton M, et al. Diagnosis and management of congenital syphilis: avoiding missed opportunities. Paediatr Child Health 2024;29(7):472–9.
[39] Centre MSH. Syphilis in pregnancy treatment guidelines. Alfred health. Available at: www.mshc.org.au/health-professionals/treatment-guidelines/syphilis-in-pregnancy-treatment-guidelines. Accessed August 26, 2025.
[40] Yang L, Cambou MC, Segura ER, et al. Patterns of pregnancy loss among women living with and without HIV in Brazil, 2008-2018. AJOG Glob Rep 2022;2(4):100121; https://doi.org/10.1016/j.xagr.2022.100121.
[41] Adachi K, Xu J, Yeganeh N, et al. Combined evaluation of sexually transmitted infections in HIV-infected pregnant women and infant HIV transmission. PLoS One 2018;13(1):e0189851; https://doi.org/10.1371/journal.pone.0189851.
[42] Yeganeh N, Watts HD, Camarca M, et al. Syphilis in HIV-infected mothers and infants: results from the NICHD/HPTN 040 study. Pediatr Infect Dis J 2015;34(3):e52–7.
[43] David M, Hcini N, Mandelbrot L, et al. Fetal and neonatal abnormalities due to congenital syphilis: a literature review. Prenat Diagn 2022;42(5):643–55.
[44] Pillay S, Horn AR, Tooke L. Placental weights of neonates born with symptomatic congenital syphilis. Front Pediatr 2023;11:1215387.
[45] Genest DR, Choi-Hong SR, Tate JE, et al. Diagnosis of congenital syphilis from placental examination: comparison of histopathology, Steiner stain, and polymerase chain reaction for Treponema pallidum DNA. Hum Pathol 1996;27(4):366–72.
[46] Tsigkouli I. The Centenary Series - STIs through the ages: 'the Sins of the Fathers are visited upon the Children': the history of congenital syphilis. Sex Transm Infect 2025;101(5):283–6.
[47] Aires Figueiredo L, Botelho Brito T, Labrusco M, et al. A rare but pathognomonic sign of congenital syphilis. J Pediatr 2023;262:113622; https://doi.org/10.1016/j.jpeds.2023.113622.
[48] Aleem S, Walker LS, Hornik CD, et al. Severe congenital syphilis in the neonatal intensive care unit: a retrospective case series. Pediatr Infect Dis J 2022;41(4):335–9.
[49] Kimball A, Bowen VB, Miele K, et al. Congenital syphilis diagnosed beyond the neonatal period in the United States: 2014-2018. Pediatrics 2021;148(3); https://doi.org/10.1542/peds.2020-049080.
[50] Krueger C, Nourse C, Penner J, et al. #41: curious congenital conundrums – in the eye of the beholder. Febrile: a cultured podcast. Available at: https://player.captivate.fm/episode/b786c3a8-0297-479f-b0e0-f8c43bc1d628.
[51] Papp JR, Park IU, Fakile Y, et al. CDC laboratory recommendations for syphilis testing, United States, 2024. MMWR Recomm Rep (Morb Mortal Wkly Rep) 2024;73(1):1–32.
[52] Satyaputra F, Hendry S, Braddick M, et al. The laboratory diagnosis of syphilis. J Clin Microbiol 2021;59(10):e0010021; https://doi.org/10.1128/JCM.00100-21.
[53] Cao W, Thorpe PG, O'Callaghan K, et al. Advantages and limitations of current diagnostic laboratory approaches in syphilis and congenital syphilis. Expert Rev Anti Infect Ther 2023;21(12):1339–54.

[54] Hemarajata P. A brief history of laboratory diagnostics for syphilis. American Society for Microbiology. Available at: https://asm.org/articles/2020/january/a-brief-history-of-laboratory-diagnostics-for-syph. Accessed September 14, 2025.
[55] Workowski KA, Bachmann LH, Chan PA, et al. Sexually transmitted infections treatment guidelines, 2021. MMWR Recomm Rep 2021;70(4):1–187.
[56] McCleery EJ, Plotzker RE, Partridge E. The utility of cerebrospinal fluid analysis in guiding management of infants exposed to Syphilis in utero. Pediatr Infect Dis J 2025;44(8):813–7.
[57] Amjad Hafeeez A, Cavalcanti Bezerra K, Jimoh Z, et al. Scoping review of hearing loss attributed to congenital syphilis. PLoS One 2024;19(4):e0302452; https://doi.org/10.1371/journal.pone.0302452.
[58] Oliveira TDS, Dutra MRP, Nunes-Araujo A, et al. The prevalence of risk for hearing impairment in newborns with congenital syphilis in a newborn hearing screening program (NHS). Front Public Health 2023;11:1214762; https://doi.org/10.3389/fpubh.2023.1214762.
[59] AAP. Red book interactive algorithms: congenital syphilis. Available at: https://publications.aap.org/redbook/module/29684/section/dd33dfb6-1ba5-4ca0-9b80-810a70439398?target=module-content.
[60] AAP. Congenital syphilis toolkit. Available at: https://www.aap.org/en/patient-care/congenital-syphilis/congenital-syphilis-toolkit/.
[61] Prenatal syphilis screening, staging, and management for Congenital syphilis Prevention. 2025. Available at: https://www.cdph.ca.gov/Programs/CID/DCDC/CDPHDocumentLibrary/Prenatal-Syphilis-Prevention-Treatment-Considerations_Pocket-Card.pdf.
[62] Kojima N, Konda KA, Klausner JD. Notes on syphilis vaccine development. Front Immunol 2022;13:952284; https://doi.org/10.3389/fimmu.2022.952284.
[63] Hawley KL, Montezuma-Rusca JM, Delgado KN, et al. Structural modeling of the Treponema pallidum outer membrane protein repertoire: a road map for deconvolution of syphilis pathogenesis and development of a syphilis vaccine. J Bacteriol 2021;203(15):e0008221; https://doi.org/10.1128/JB.00082-21.
[64] WHO. Congenital syphilis reported rate per 100 000 live births, reported. Available at: https://www.who.int/data/gho/data/indicators/indicator-details/GHO/congenital-syphilis-rate-per-100-000-live-births.
[65] CDC. CDC archives. Available at: https://archive.cdc.gov/www_cdc_gov/ncbddd/birthdefects/surveillancemanual/quick-reference-handbook/congenital-syphilis.html.
[66] Dorrough S, Vicetti Miguel CP. Approach to prevention, diagnosis, and treatment of congenital Syphilis. Pediatr Clin North Am 2025;72(4):685–99.
[67] Easterlin MC, Ramanathan R, De Beritto T. Maternal-to-Fetal transmission of Syphilis and Congenital Syphilis. NeoReviews 2021;22(9):e585–99.
[68] Medoro AK, Sanchez PJ. Syphilis in neonates and infants. Clin Perinatol 2021;48(2):293–309.

Advances in Pediatrics 73 (2026) 25–40
ADVANCES IN PEDIATRICS

Opioids and Adolescents

How to Prevent and Treat Addictions Early

Gloria Sanchez, MD, FASAM[a,*],
Shona Lowe, MD, MPH, FASAM[b],
Theresa Nevarez, MD, MBA[c], Karen Olmos, MD, MPH[c]

[a]David Geffen School of Medicine at UCLA, Medications Addiction Treatment Harbor UCLA Medical Center, Torrance, CA, USA; [b]Los Angeles General Primary Care West, Los Angeles, CA, USA; [c]David Geffen School of Medicine at UCLA, Harbor UCLA Family Medicine, Torrance, CA, USA

Keywords

• Adolescent • Opioid use • Early identification • Prevention • And treatment

Key points

- Substance use has become increasingly fatal due to the use of non-prescribed drugs that may contain fentanyl.
- Early identification with universal screening and treatment that includes medications can be very effective for at-risk opioid use and use disorders.
- Prevention and harm reduction including naloxone distribution can help decrease the morbidity and mortality of illicit opioid use.
- Treatment that emphasizes motivational interviewing and family-based treatment can be highly effective with adolescents who use illicit substances.
- Using FDA-approved medications like buprenorphine can help adolescents decrease mortality and improve outcomes for opioid use disorder.

INTRODUCTION

Addiction is a treatable, chronic condition of pediatric onset. Early identification of opioid misuse, trauma-informed care, and low-barrier use of medications for opioid use disorder (MOUD) saves lives and helps at-risk adolescents. Most adults who have a substance use disorder begin use during

*Corresponding author. Harbor UCLA Medical Center, Department of Family Medicine, Box 433, 1000 West Carson Street, Torrance, CA 90502. *E-mail address:* gsanchez@dhs.lacounty.gov

https://doi.org/10.1016/j.yapd.2026.01.001

Abbreviations

COWS	Clinical Opiate Withdrawal Scale
IMF	illicitly manufactured fentanyl
MOUD	medications opioid use disorder
OTP	opioid treatment program
S2BI	Screener to Brief Intervention
SBIRT	screening, brief intervention, and/or referral to treatment

adolescence, so early intervention is critical during this period of development [1]. Stigma, as well as health care and societal disparities, are barriers for adolescents receiving evidence-based care for substance use; this care can help people using opioids to successfully achieve and maintain sobriety [2–4].

Since 1975, the Monitoring the Future: A Continuing Study of the Lifestyles and Values of Youth Report has demonstrated an overall decrease in the use of illicit substances [5]. Despite this downward trend, overdose deaths due to opioids have significantly increased for adolescents and young adults [6,7].

Opioid overdose deaths are the 3rd leading cause of death in adolescents and sadly, adolescents struggling with opioid misuse and/or opioid use disorders can be negatively impacted by providers and treatment centers not offering MOUD, or by parents and patients themselves declining these critical medications.[8–10].

According to the CDC's State Unintentional Drug Reporting System between 2019 and 2021, the median monthly overdose deaths of persons aged 10 to 19 years increased by 182% for illicitly manufactured fentanyl (IMF) and 109% for overdose deaths [11]. The distribution of IMF, availability of counterfeit pills meant to resemble prescription medications which might contain IMF, and the ever-increasing ability to purchase pills via social media are all contributing to the increase in overdose deaths [11].

Since 2011, the American Academy of Pediatrics has recommended substance use disorder screening and in 2023 reaffirmed the need to provide medications for addiction treatment and behavioral therapies [12]. Despite rising overdose deaths, national calls for action, and many years of data demonstrating that early initiation of MOUD decreases morbidity and mortality and can dramatically improve recovery from OUD, less than 5% of adolescents receive these life-saving medications [2,10,13,14].

Given the rising number of overdoses and unintentional deaths due to illicit substances including stimulants and counterfeit pills, and the increasing prevalence of IMF in these substances, this article aims to help clinicians who care for adolescents better screen and treat with evidenced-based modalities including behavioral interventions, MOUD, and harm reduction strategies with adolescents and their families [6,15,16].

Health care disparities and stigma in the era of fentanyl

There are many barriers to receiving evidence-based opioid use disorder treatment that include: provider lack of knowledge and comfort prescribing

MOUD, lack of MOUD access, healthcare and patient stigma towards substance use disorder care, identification of use versus use disorder, adolescent ability to engage in discussions about use and treatment options, physicians' ability to have trauma-informed care discussions about substance use and treatment options, confidentiality, and insurance status [2,10,14]. Additionally, studies have identified that similarly to adult populations, adolescents and their families perceive being on MOUD as stigmatizing [3,16–18].

Another important limitation of MOUD could be the perception that it's a "replacing one drug with another" or a "crutch" for sobriety. Adolescents, like adults, expressed concern for withdrawal symptoms, side effects, and the unknown duration of MOUD treatment. Fortunately, many adolescents feel MOUD can assist with being fully functional in their lives and avoid lethal overdose [19].

Certain subsets of adolescent populations are at higher risk for substance use and Substance Use Disorder (SUD). Marginalization, higher rates of adverse child experiences, and stigma are risk factors for this disparity in use [20–22].

Black, Native American, and Latinx represent another tragic health care disparity given that the overdose rates for these historically marginalized populations have dramatically increased and are nearly 2 fold greater than White Americans [4,23].

Gender and sexual minority adolescents

Lesbian, gay, bisexual, transgender, queer/questioning, and other gender and sexual minority (LGBTQ+) adolescents experience varying levels of stigma, with a number of studies identifying the experience of minority stress: "excess stress to which individuals from stigmatized social categories are exposed as a result of their social, often a minority, position [24]" as a predictor of substance use [20].

Studies have found higher rates of alcohol, tobacco, and marijuana use among LGBTQ + youth, but data regarding opioid use in particular and use among transgender and gender nonconforming adolescents are more sparse [22,25]. In 2023, the National Survey on Drug Use and Health added questions regarding sexual orientation for respondents 12 to 17 years of age for the first time but did not ask specifically about gender identity [25]. The most recent Youth Risk Behavior Surveillance Survey, completed in 2023, asks high school students about misuse of prescription opioids within the last 30 days and at any point in time; LGBTQ + high school students have higher rates of misuse compared to their cisgendered heterosexual counterparts for both use during last 30 days (7% vs 3%, respectively) and for use at any point in time (18% vs 8%, respectively) [26].

Justice-involved adolescents

Adolescents who have been engaged in the legal system have significantly higher rates of opioid use than non-justice-involved youth; one study identified that 20% of adolescents with prescription opioid misuse had a history of justice involvement [27].

Efforts are underway to identify not only best practices for the screening and treatment of substance use in juvenile justice settings [28] but also to identify interventions for the prevention of opioid use initiation and OUD among justice-involved youth [29].

Adolescents in foster care

Individuals who have been in foster care at some point during their youth have higher rates of substance use, both during adolescence and as adults. In one study, 34% of youth with a lifetime history of foster care reported using drugs other than alcohol within the last year, nearly double the rate among youth without a history of foster care (18.1%) [30]. In a study of Medicaid recipient youth receiving care in a large academic center in the Midwest, youth aged 10 to 20 years who had ever been in foster care initiated substance use at an earlier age and had 1.5 times higher rates of lifetime substance use compared to demographically matched youth who had never been in foster care [30].

Screening and diagnosis

The American Academy of Pediatrics recommends universal substance use screening, brief intervention, and referral to treatment (SBIRT) as part of routine pediatric care [12]. Despite these recommendations and the validity of SBIRT, one study demonstrated that only 11% of pediatricians surveyed were able to complete parts of this screener due to time restraints and concern for lack of treatment options for positive screens [31].

Fortunately, two brief electronic screeners, Screener to Brief Intervention (S2BI) and Brief Screener for Tobacco, Alcohol, and other Drugs have demonstrated feasibility in multiple settings including primary care, adolescent clinics, and substance use disorder clinics [32] The S2BI tool can be administered by the clinician or completed by the patient (Fig. 1).

The American Academy of Pediatrics recommends multiple tobacco and substance use screeners for use with patients between the ages 11 and 21 years [34]. Using both S2BI and CRAFFT [35] can provide the best assessment of use and risk of using tobacco, alcohol, and other drugs because when given in combination, they assess overall use and frequency [36,37].

Screening can assist with the early identification of substance use and provide an opportunity for intervention. However, an adolescent experimenting with substances does not always equate to an adolescent with a substance use disorder. Given the risk of overdose death, it is imperative to begin immediate harm reduction and offer MOUD to any adolescent who uses opioids for recreation. In the era of fentanyl, it is critical that the health care system provides immediate and low-barrier MOUD and harm reduction including naloxone [13,38,39].

The Diagnostic and Statistical Manual of Mental Disorders V (DSM V) defines opioid use disorder via 11 criteria. It is important to use clinically relevant, feasible, translatable language when working with adolescents and their families. According to National Institute Drug Abuse Clinical Addiction Research

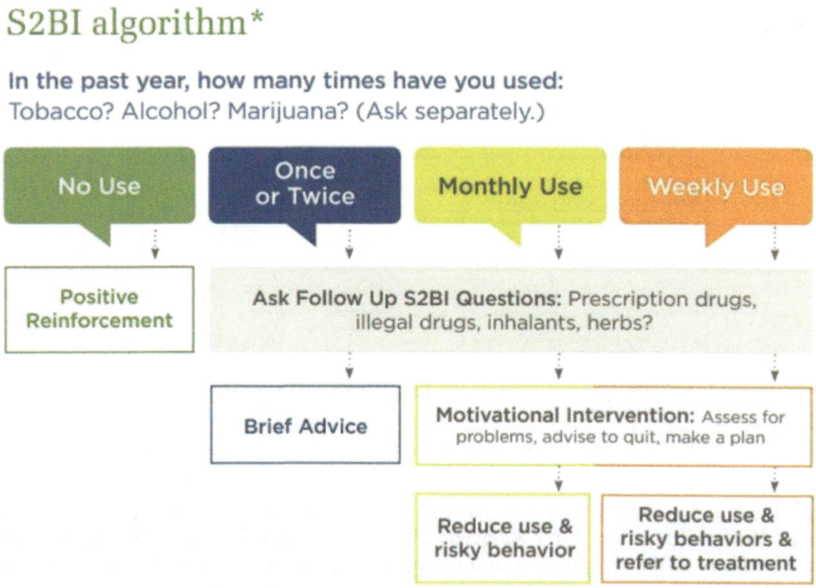

Fig. 1. The Screener to brief intervention algorithm [33]. (*From* Levy S. MD, MPH, Chief, Division Addiction Medicine, Boston Children's Hospital, Professor of Pediatrics, Harvard University. Creative Commons Attribution-Non Commercial 40 International License. Boston Children's Hospital, 2014.)

and Education Program at Boston University Chobanian and Avedisian School of Medicine, a helpful strategy is using language that summarizes the DSM V criteria in three general categories: loss of control, compulsive use, and consequences related to opioid use (Fig. 2). Using these categories may be more tangible for adolescents and their families to understand.

TREATMENT

Family-based interventions and behavioral interventions

There are multiple nonpharmacologic treatments that are critical to supporting adolescents who use opioids or other substances and their families (Fig. 3).

Opioid use disorder treatments are limited by many factors including cost, regional availability, provider knowledge, and patient and family preference. Vulnerable populations that are underfunded or rely on Medicaid may not have access to all of these critical therapeutic options that save lives [41]. In addition, cultural and language non-concordance can significantly limit adolescents' and their families' ability to engage in a therapeutic relationship within a system that primarily serves patients that speak English [42].

Community reinforcement approach (CRAFT + A-CRA) may be better for an entire family since it can increase patient treatment entry and completion, decrease patient drug use, and support family mental health and improve family depression scores.

Criteria Type	Description
Impaired Control	1. Opioids are often taken in larger amounts or over a longer period of time than intended.
	2. There is a persistent desire or unsuccessful efforts to cut down or control opioid use.
	3. A great deal of time is spent in activities necessary to obtain the opioid, use the opioid, or recover from its effects.
	4. Craving, or a strong desire to use opioids.
Social Impairment	5. Recurrent opioid use resulting in failure to fulfill major role obligations at work, school or home.
	6. Continued opioid use despite having persistent or recurrent social or interpersonal problems caused or exacerbated by the effects of opioids.
	7. Important social, occupational or recreational activities are given up or reduced because of opioid use.
Risky Use	8. Recurrent opioid use in situations in which it is physically hazardous.
	9. Continued use despite knowledge of having a persistent or recurrent physical or psychological problem that is likely to have been caused or exacerbated by opioids.
Pharmacologic Properties	10. Tolerance, as defined by either of the following: (a) a need for markedly increased amounts of opioids to achieve intoxication or desired effect (b) markedly diminished effect with continued use of the same amount of an opioid. *Note: This criterion not considered to be met for those individuals taking opioids solely under appropriate medical supervision.
	11. Withdrawal, as manifested by either of the following: (a) the characteristic opioid withdrawal syndrome (b) the same (or a closely related) substance are taken to relieve or avoid withdrawal symptoms. *Note: This criterion not considered to be met for those individuals taking opioids solely under appropriate medical supervision.
Severity	Mild: 2-3 symptoms. Moderate: 4-5 symptoms. Severe: 6 or more symptoms

1. Loss of Control
2. Compulsive use
3. Consequences

Adapted from The Immersion Training in Addiction Medicine Program

Fig. 2. Opioid use disorder via 11 criteria [40]. (*Adapted from* National Institute Drug Abuse, The Immersion Training in Addiction Medicine Program, Clinical Addiction Research and Education (CARE) Program at Boston University Chobanian and Avedisian School of Medicine 2022.)

Multisystemic therapy is a comprehensive family and community-based approach that has not only demonstrated decreased substance use but also criminal activity.

Motivational interviewing is an evidenced-based counseling method that aims to resolve ambivalence, strengthen motivation and commitment to change, and ultimately self-efficacy [43]. Adolescents have responded well to this patient-centered approach, and health care systems should require training of all health care staff to use this effective method of engaging youth in care [44].

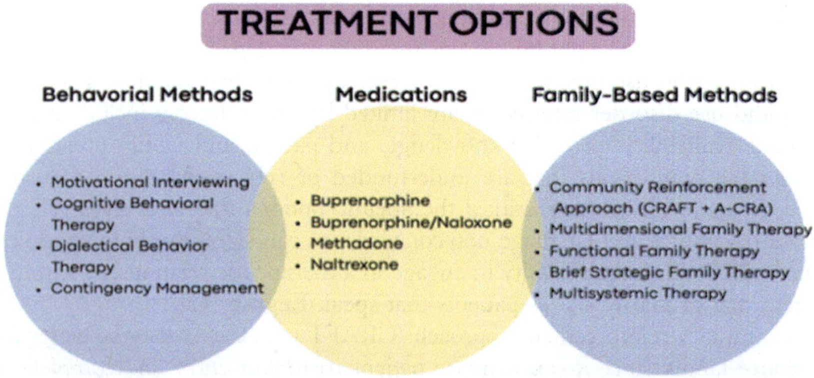

Fig. 3. Nonpharmacologic treatments.

Ultimately, it is the responsibility of both the provider and health care system to identify and expedite opioid use treatment options that emphasize affordability, family strength-oriented therapies, low-barrier MOUD, cultural humility, and using methods that incorporate innovative options like digital and mindfulness-based therapies [1,41,45].

Trauma-informed care: shifting from "What's wrong with you?" to "what happened to you?"

Taking care of vulnerable populations like adolescents who use opioids requires a trauma-informed approach. Substance Abuse and Mental Health Services Administration's concept of trauma and guidance for a trauma-informed approach emphasizes the 6 principles of trauma-informed care [46]:

Safety
Trustworthiness and transparency
Peer Support
Collaboration and mutuality
Empowerment, voice, and choice
Cultural, historical context, and gender.

Helping adolescents feel safe and empowering their voices and choices can help engage and sustain youth in treatment and recovery. Trauma-informed care approaches not only improve patient outcomes but also help decrease provider burnout [47].

Identify and treat co-occurring mental health disorders

According to multiple studies, adolescents who use substances can have upwards of 60% to 75% co-occurring mental health disorders [48,49]. Adolescents who have not used substances and experience major depressive disorder are 16% more likely to try an illicit substance use after diagnosis [48]. Universal substance use and mental health screening can help adolescents with either condition receive early pharmacologic and behavioral health treatment [49].

Pharmacologic treatments

The Food and Drug Administration (FDA) has approved 3 classes of medications for treatment of OUD: full opioid agonist (methadone), partial opioid agonist (buprenorphine), and opioid antagonist (naltrexone). There is state-to-state variability in laws regarding the age of consent for adolescent patients, so it is recommended to check specific state requirements with the National Center for Youth Law [50].

Buprenorphine sublingual formulation is FDA-approved for individuals 16 years and older and data show this medication is safe and effective for adolescents [13,51,52]. Buprenorphine is also available in an extended-release injection, which is currently FDA-approved for individuals 18 years and older. Methadone and naltrexone are also FDA-approved medications for opioid use disorder for individuals 18 years and older.

Buprenorphine is a high-affinity, partial *mu*-opioid receptor agonist, and *k*-opioid antagonist. It has a favorable safety profile due to the "ceiling effect," meaning that higher doses will not cause respiratory depression, in contrast to full opioid agonists. Given the high affinity of buprenorphine, it may displace full opioid agonists and precipitate withdrawal.

Studies have shown that longer durations of buprenorphine treatment are more effective at preventing return to use, reduce mortality, and is a cost-effective treatment option [14,53]. Research among adults with OUD has shown that buprenorphine doses of 16 mg and higher can improve abstinence from illicit opioids.

Physicians who treat adolescents have a role in prescribing these life-saving medications to expand patient access to MOUD. If a patient is endorsing at-risk use of any opioids or has had a prior unintentional opioid overdose after using another substance with opioids or IMF, it is recommended to offer buprenorphine with low barriers to initiation. No baseline labs are required prior to starting buprenorphine, nor are specific labs required to monitor after initiation.

Naltrexone is a long-acting opioid antagonist. It is available in an oral formulation, which is taken daily at a usual dose of 50 mg and in a long-acting formulation that is administered as a 380 mg intragluteal injection every 4 weeks. As administration of naltrexone can precipitate withdrawal in patients with recent opioid use, patients must be abstinent from short-acting opioids for at least 7 days or up to 14 days for long-acting opioids prior to initiation of naltrexone.

Methadone is a full opioid agonist that is administered daily and taken orally. There is limited access for youth due to federal regulations, including that methadone must be administered through a licensed opioid treatment program (OTP) so dosing is not discussed in this chapter [54].

Starting MOUD needs to be individualized to the adolescent (Table 1). Multiple hotlines and resources exist for providers if they need assistance with MOUD initiation. National Clinical Consultation Center [55] and Bridge to Treatment [56] can assist providers in providing low-barrier and timely MOUD. For patients, families, or providers trying to identify MOUD providers or OTP programs, the Substance Abuse Mental Health Services Administration web site can be a resource [57].

We highly encourage providers to use the multiple national hotlines or resources available to initiate immediate MOUD for adolescents and/or parents

Table 1
MOUD pharmacotherapy

Indication	Medication	Adolescent-Specific Considerations
Opioid use	Buprenorphine Buprenorphine/Naloxone Methodone	• FDA approved for age $\geq$16 y.o • IM formulation insufficiently studied in youth • Many states require parental consent for <18 y.o • Very limited access for youth
	Naltrexone	• FDA-approved for age >18 y.o

who agree to this life saving treatment. There have been multiple national calls to provide MOUD at all levels of health care, yet only 1 in 3 substance use programs that treat youth offer MOUD [58]. Sadly, these efforts have not led to an increase in MOUD initiation despite the increasing overdose rates [9,39].

When initiating buprenorphine for MOUD treatment, using the Clinical Opiate Withdrawal Scale (COWS) and opioid withdrawal adjunct therapy can be helpful (Fig. 4). Typically, when a COWS score is 8 or higher, buprenorphine can be initiated in either a "micro" buprenorphine 2 mg dose or "macro" buprenorphine 8 mg dose given with repeated doses the first day until withdrawal symptoms are controlled. The total dose used the first day can be divided into split doses for subsequent days and increased if needed to manage cravings. Opioid withdrawal can present with flu-like symptoms and anxiety, hence the need to provide standing or as-needed acetaminophen, antiemetics, antidiarrheal, and anxiety medications like gabapentin or even benzodiazepines for the first few days of buprenorphine initiation. MOUD treatment is safe for adolescents, decreases mortality, and increases retention in substance use treatment [13,52,59].

Harm reduction: "anticipatory guidelines" for adolescents

Adolescence is a time of risk-taking, and data strongly support health care providers should use harm reduction and a collaborative approach with youth who experiment or have at-risk use of substances (Fig. 5) [38].

Despite providers recognizing the high risk and prevalence of illicit fentanyl, they often lack confidence and ability to distribute harm reduction supplies like naloxone, safer injection supplies, and fentanyl test kits [60]. For example, there is a high risk of fentanyl contamination in sitmulants and counterfeit prescirption pills such as benzodiazepines, so any patient or caregiver should be

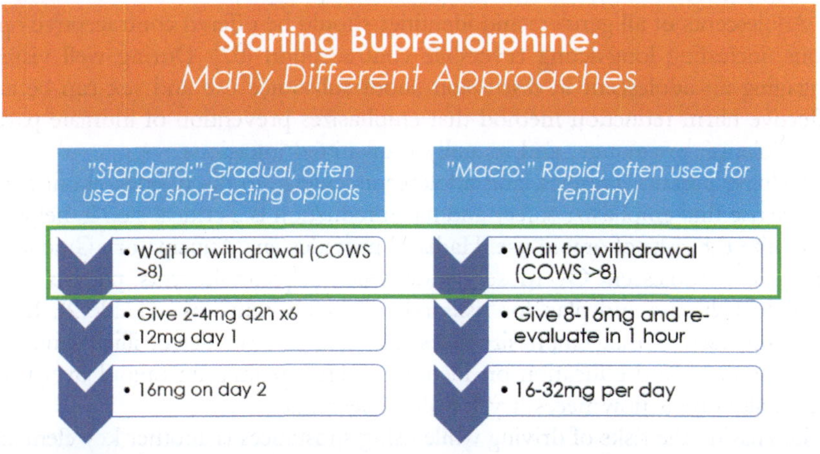

Fig. 4. Different approaches when initiating buprenorphine for medications opioid use disorder treatment.

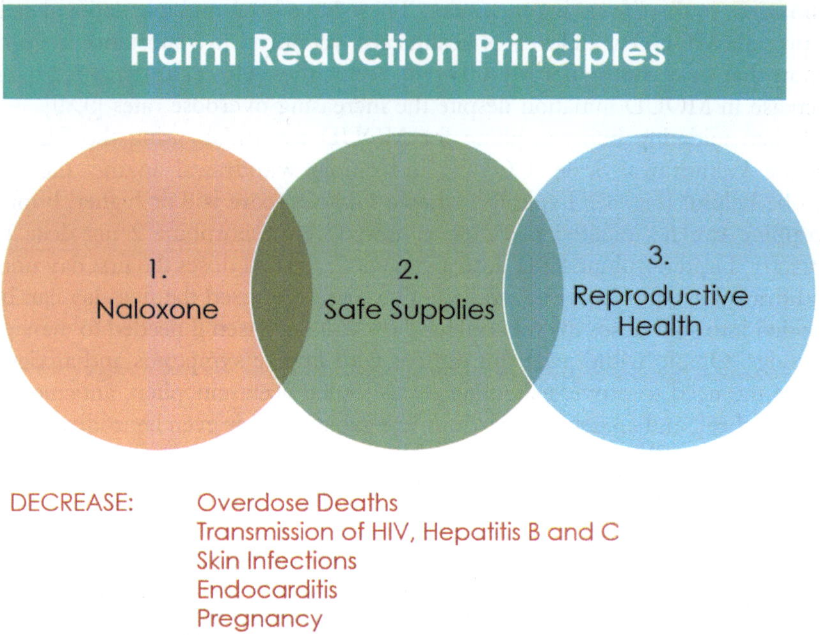

Fig. 5. Harm reduction principles.

educated about opioid overdoses and provided naloxone. For youth identified as using intravenous routes for any substance, educating and offering safer injection supplies can decrease morbidity and mortality. Syringe service programs (SSPs) are supported by the CDC and have demonstrated upwards of 50% reduction in transmission of HIV and Hep C [61].

Adolescents of all genders and identities should be offered contraceptive options, including long-acting reversible contraception [62]. During well visits, engaging an adolescent in discussion about substance use and sex can be an effective harm reduction method that emphasizes prevention of intimate partner violence, pregnancy, and sexually transmitted infections.

Helping parents, families, and adolescents engage in discussions about substance use that emphasize safety and harm reduction is a critical step in helping minimize the risks of opioid use. Hadland provides an "Anticipatory Guidance to Prevent Adolescent Overdose" guide which helps adolescents, parents, and providers discuss and plan for risks related to substance use (Table 2). Initiating discussions that emphasize risks, learning how to detect illicit fentanyl in substances, and education on identifying and treating an opioid overdose with naloxone is now necessary for all adolescents.

Discussing the risks of driving while using substances is another key element for harm reduction. Discussing an "Exit Plan" with an adolescent that emphasizes how they would avoid driving and/or riding with someone under the influence can decrease morbidity and mortality. For example, practicing with an

Table 2
How to talk to teens and families about overdose risk [63]

Concept	Sample Statements to an Adolescent and/or Family Member
Initiate conversation	"It's important that we talk about safety. As you might know, the number of teen drug overdoses has been increasing. I now talk all my teen patients and their families about how to prevent and respond to an overdose."
Provide education about fentanyl	"What do you know about fentanyl?"
	"Fentanyl is potent opioid that is causing a record number of teen overdose. Most of the prescription pills that people sell—including on social media—are fake and contain fentanyl, and can cause someone to overdose. If a medication isn't prescribed by a doctor and provided by a pharmacy, it's likely to be fake."
Review signs of overdose	"Do you know what an overdose looks like? Have you seen one?"
	"Someone who is having an overdose looks sleepy, or might even be unconscious. Their breathing is slow, or they might have stopped breathing altogether. They often look pale, and might be blue around their lips or fingertips."
Review how to respond to an overdose	"How would you respond if you thought someone was having an overdose?"
	"If you suspect someone has overdosed, immediately call 911. Then, if you have naloxone nasal spray, use it. If the person is not breathing and you know how give rescue breaths, do so."
Discuss naloxone and how to find it	"What do you know about naloxone? Do you have any?"
	"I recommended everyone carry naloxone with tem and have it in their home. Naloxone can save someone's life. And it's safe to use even if someone isn't having an overdose. I can prescribe it to you today. You can also but it over the counter—though it's more expensive this way—and its often available at school or in the community."
Confidentially assess previous fentanyl use/exposure	Discussed confidentially with adolescent only:
	"In our practice, we ask every teen about their use of drugs and alcohol. Thanks for completing the screening questionnnaire. To your knowledge, have uou ever used fentanyl?"
	"Do you have any friends who use pills that might not have been prescribed by a doctor or filled by areal pharmacy? Have you ever used a pill that someone gave or sold you? Have you ever been approached in real life or on social media to buy one?"

adolescent how to find alternative transportation or stay at their current location can prepare the adolescent if they were to find themselves in such a situation.

According to a national survey, a large majority of clinicians recognize the risk of "non-pharmaceutical fentanyl" and the need to assess and prepare for the risk of an overdose, however they lack comfort and knowledge on how to provide harm reduction supplies like naloxone nasal spray and fentanyl test strips. Clinicians serving only pediatric patients had limited familiarity and comfort applying harm reduction strategies. There remains a critical need to help fund educational efforts for adolescents, parents, and clinicians on prevention and timely treatment of opioid use and overdose [60].

Consent and confidentiality

Laws regulating minor consent for substance use disorder care and medications and privacy vary across the country. Unfortunately, this is a real and lethal barrier to adolescents receiving evidenced-based care for opioid misuse and/or opioid use disorder. In addition, many state laws do not reflect pediatric professional standards of care. The lack of consistency among laws is a barrier to implementing equitable, evidence-based care and protecting adolescent privacy [64].

For information on state and federal laws regarding minor consent and confidentiality, providers can access the National Center for Youth Law [50]. Engaging youth in discussions that maintain confidentiality can be challenging and begins with knowing local and federal laws pertaining to the treatment of minors. Ultimately, conversations with both adolescents and families that emphasize prevention, identification, harm reduction, and treatment for substance use have a new urgency in the era of fentanyl.

SUMMARY

Adolescent overdose deaths are preventable if we implement universal emergency public health and educational efforts that help eliminate health care and societal barriers [4,38,58]. Clinicians are urged to provide immediate harm reduction resources like naloxone nasal spray and low barrier MOUD to any youth who endorses opioid use [14]. It is imperative that substance use programs that serve youth also provide low-barrier and continuous MOUD [13,14,58,63].

Providers can help decrease the lethal treatment gap for adolescents who use opioids in the era of fentanyl.

CLINICS CARE POINTS

- Universal screening for substance use with tools such as CRAFFT should be implemented at all clinics that serve pediatric patients.
- For patients identified at risk for opioid overdose, provide naloxone and education around identifying and treating an overdose for both the patient and caregiver.

- Immediate treatment with medications such as buprenorphine is the standard of care for treating opioid use disorder and can be started by any licensed provider that has a DEA registration.
- While medications can be started without the patient engaging in other forms of treatment, often the combination with behavioral treatments can be effective in sustaining recovery and engaging family support.

Acknowledgments

We thank Dr Brian Hurley and Dr Clay Thibodeaux for their support in this publication.

Disclosure

The authors have nothing to disclose.

References

[1] Fadus MC, Squeglia LM, Valadez EA, et al. Adolescent substance use disorder treatment: an update on evidence-based strategies. Curr Psychiatry Rep 2019;21(10):96.

[2] Hadland SE, Burr WH, Zoucha K, et al. Treating adolescent opioid use disorder in primary care. JAMA Pediatr 2024;178(4):414–6.

[3] Bagley SM, Hadland SE, Carney BL, et al. Addressing stigma in medication treatment of adolescents with opioid use disorder. J Addict Med 2017;11(6):415–6.

[4] Friedman JR, Tiako MJN, Hansen H. Understanding and addressing widening racial inequalities in drug overdose. Am J Psychiatr 2024;181(5):381–90.

[5] Miech R, Johnston L, Patrick M, et al. Monitoring the future study annual report: national survey results on drug use, 1975-2024:Overiview and detailed results for seconday school students. 2025. Available at: https://monitoringthefuture.org/wp-content/uploads/2024/12/mtf2025.pdf. Accessed September 13, 2025.

[6] Panchal N, Zitter S. Teens, drugs, and overdose: contrasting pre-pandemic and current trends. Kasier family foundation. Available at: https://www.kff.org/mental-health/teens-drugs-and-overdose-contrasting-pre-pandemic-and-current-trends/. Accessed September 15, 2025.

[7] Warren LK, Adams J, Bobashev G. Trends in opioid misuse among individuals aged 12 to 21 years in the US. JAMA Netw Open 2023;6(6):e2316276.

[8] Goldstick JE, Cunningham RM, Carter PM. Current causes of death in children and adolescents in the United States. N Engl J Med 2022;386(20):1955–6.

[9] Ball A, Winstead T, Singh S, et al. Adolescent and young adult access to opioid use disorder care. Pediatrics 2025;156(1); https://doi.org/10.1542/peds.2024-070224.

[10] Pilarinos A, Bromberg DJ, Karamouzian M. Access to medications for opioid use disorder and associated factors among adolescents and young adults: a systematic review. JAMA Pediatr 2022;176(3):304–11.

[11] Tanz LJ, Dinwiddie AT, Mattson CL, et al. Drug overdose deaths among persons aged 10-19 years - united States, July 2019-December 2021. MMWR Morb Mortal Wkly Rep 2022;71(50):1576–82.

[12] Levy SJL, Williams JF, USE COS, et al. Substance use screening, brief intervention, and referral to treatment. Pediatrics 2016;138(1); https://doi.org/10.1542/peds.2016-1211.

[13] Hadland SE, Bagley SM, Rodean J, et al. Receipt of timely addiction treatment and Association of Early Medication treatment with retention in care among youths with opioid use disorder. JAMA Pediatr 2018;172(11):1029–37.

[14] Robinson CA, Wilson JD. Management of opioid misuse and opioid use disorders among youth. Pediatrics 2020;145(Suppl 2):S153–64.
[15] Yule AM, Lyons RM, Wilens TE. Opioid use disorders in adolescents-updates in assessment and management. Curr Pediatr Rep 2018;6(2):99–106.
[16] Saloner B, McGinty EE, Beletsky L, et al. A public health strategy for the opioid crisis. Public Health Reports® 2018;133(1_suppl):24S–34S.
[17] Burke KN, Krawczyk N, Li Y, et al. Barriers and facilitators to use of buprenorphine in state-licensed specialty substance use treatment programs: a survey of program leadership. J Subst Use Addict Treat 2024;162:209351.
[18] Fishman M, Wenzel K, Gauthier P, et al. Engagement, initiation, and retention in medication treatment for opioid use disorder among young adults: a narrative review of challenges and opportunities. J Subst Use Addict Treat 2024;166:209352.
[19] Bagley SM, Schoenberger SF, dellaBitta V, et al. Ambivalence and stigma beliefs about medication treatment among young adults with opioid use disorder: a qualitative exploration of young adults' perspectives. J Adolesc Health 2023;72(1):105–10.
[20] Kidd JD, Jackman KB, Wolff M, et al. Risk and protective factors for substance use among sexual and gender minority youth: a scoping review. Curr Addict Rep 2018;5(2):158–73.
[21] Swedo EA, Sumner SA, de Fijter S, et al. Adolescent opioid misuse attributable to adverse childhood experiences. J Pediatr 2020;224:102–9.e3.
[22] Mammadli T, Mack LM, Deng Y, et al. Substance use among transgender and gender non-conforming youth and young adults living in the US: a systematic review. Soc Sci Med 2025;383:118330.
[23] Wu LT, Woody GE, Yang C, et al. Racial/ethnic variations in substance-related disorders among adolescents in the United States. Arch Gen Psychiatry 2011;68(11):1176–85.
[24] Meyer IH. Prejudice, social stress, and mental health in lesbian, gay, and bisexual populations: conceptual issues and research evidence. Psychol Bull 2003;129(5):674–97.
[25] Grigsby TJ, Hoopsick R, Barker D, et al. Substance use and sexual orientation among adolescents: differences by age group and sex in the 2023 National Survey of Drug Use and Health. Am J Addict 2025;1–8; https://doi.org/10.1111/ajad.70087.
[26] Centers for Disease Control and Prevention. Youth Risk Behavior Survey Data Summary & Trends Report: 2013–2023. U.S. Department of Health and Human Services; 2024.
[27] Sung HE, Richter L, Vaughan R, et al. Nonmedical use of prescription opioids among teenagers in the United States: trends and correlates. J Adolesc Health 2005;37(1):44–51.
[28] Goldman PN, Hull I, Wilson JD. "No excuses anymore": substance use screening and treatment for justice-involved youth. J Addict Med 2023;17(4):454–62.
[29] Ahrens K, Blackburn N, Aalsma M, et al. Prevention of opioid use and disorder among youth involved in the legal System: innovation and implementation of four studies funded by the NIDA HEAL initiative. Prev Sci 2023;24(Suppl 1):99–110.
[30] Radenhausen M, Unkrich J, Beal SJ, et al. Young people in foster care and substance use. Semin Pediatr Neurol 2024;50:101136.
[31] Hammond CJ, Parhami I, Young AS, et al. Provider and practice characteristics and perceived barriers associated with different levels of adolescent SBIRT implementation among a national sample of US pediatricians. Clin Pediatr 2021;60(9–10):418–26.
[32] Levy S, Brogna M, Minegishi M, et al. Assessment of screening tools to identify substance use disorders among adolescents. JAMA Netw Open 2023;6(5):e2314422.
[33] Levy S, Division Addiction Medicine, Boston Childrens Hospital, Professor of Pediatrics, Harvard Univeristy. Creative commons attribution-non commercial 40 international license. Boston (MA): Boston Children's Hospital; 2014.
[34] Bright futures toolkit: links to commonly used screening instruments and tools. Available at: https://publications.aap.org/toolkits/resources/15625/Bright-Futures-Toolkit-Links-to-Commonly-Used?autologincheck=redirected. Accessed September 14, 2025.
[35] Knight JRMD. Reproduced with permission from the Center for Adolescent behavioral health research (CABHRe), Boston Children's Hospital. 2020. Available at: www.crafft.org.

[36] Ebersole AM, Gallup J, Rockwell A, et al. Implementing Evidence-Based, electronic, substance-use screening in a primary care clinic. J Adolesc Health 2023;73(1): 127–32.
[37] Shenoi RP, Linakis JG, Bromberg JR, et al. Predictive validity of the CRAFFT for substance use disorder. Pediatrics 2019;144(2); https://doi.org/10.1542/peds.2018-3415.
[38] Winer JM, Yule AM, Hadland SE, et al. Addressing adolescent substance use with a public health prevention framework: the case for harm reduction. Ann Med 2022;54(1): 2123–36.
[39] Friedman J, Hadland SE. The overdose crisis among U.S. adolescents. N Engl J Med 2024;390(2):97–100.
[40] National Institute Drug Abuse. The immersion training in addiction medicine program, clinical addiction research and education (CARE). Boston (MA): Program at Boston University Chobanian and Avedisian School of Medicine; 2022.
[41] Welsh JW, Krishnan SD, Terranella A. Prevention and management of opioid use disorder and overdose in adolescents and young adults. Curr Psychiatry Rep 2025;663–4; https://doi.org/10.1007/s11920-025-01638-0.
[42] Burrow-Sánchez JJ, Minami T, Hops H. Cultural accommodation of group substance abuse treatment for Latino adolescents: results of an RCT. Cultur Divers Ethnic Minor Psychol 2015;21(4):571–83.
[43] Emery RL, Wimmer M. Motivational interviewing, . StatPearls [Internet]. Treasure Island (FL): StatPearls Publishing; 2025. p. 1.
[44] Knight DK, Joe GW, Becan JE, et al. Effectiveness of an intervention for improving intrinsic motivation among adolescent males in a secure substance use treatment setting. Crim Justice Behav 2019;46(1):101–14.
[45] Horigian VE, Anderson AR, Szapocznik J. Family-based treatments for adolescent substance use. Child Adolesc Psychiatr Clin N Am 2016;25(4):603–28.
[46] Strategies TICIRCbCfHC. What is trauma informed care?. Available at: https://www.traumainformedcare.chcs.org. Accessed October 9, 2025.
[47] Şimşek Z, Uğur B. Trauma-informed healthcare systems: an evaluation of trauma-informed care training for hospital-based healthcare professionals in the aftermath of the 2023 earthquakes in Türkiye. Health Policy Plan 2025;40(2):234–43.
[48] Youth.gov. Co-occurring disorders. Available at: https://youth.gov/youth-topics/substance-use/co-occurring-disorders. Accessed October 9, 2025.
[49] Welsh JW, Knight JR, Hou SS, et al. Association between substance use diagnoses and psychiatric disorders in an adolescent and young adult clinic-based population. J Adolesc Health 2017;60(6):648–52.
[50] NCfY Law. Minor consent and confidentiality: a compendium of state and federal laws. Available at: https://www.teenhealthlaw.org/state-federal-compendium. Accessed October 12, 2025.
[51] Polsky D, Glick HA, Yang J, et al. Cost-effectiveness of extended buprenorphine-naloxone treatment for opioid-dependent youth: data from a randomized trial. Addiction 2010;105(9):1616–24.
[52] Borodovsky JT, Levy S, Fishman M, et al. Buprenorphine treatment for adolescents and young adults with opioid use disorders: a narrative review. J Addict Med 2018;12(3): 170–83.
[53] Marsch LA, Moore SK, Borodovsky JT, et al. A randomized controlled trial of buprenorphine taper duration among opioid-dependent adolescents and young adults. Addiction 2016;111(8):1406–15.
[54] Mattick RP, Breen C, Kimber J, et al. Buprenorphine maintenance versus placebo or methadone maintenance for opioid dependence. Cochrane Database Syst Rev 2014;2014(2): CD002207.
[55] National clinical consultation center. Available at: https://nccc.ucsf.edu/clinical-resources/substance-use-resources/.

[56] Bridge to treatment clinical resources. Available at: https://bridgetotreatment.org/tools/resources/.
[57] Substance abuse and mental health services administration. Available at: https://www.samhsa.gov/find-help. Accessed October 5, 2025.
[58] Cano M, Hernandez N, Mendoza NS, et al. Fewer than 1 in 3 adolescents with past-year opioid use disorder received substance use treatment, 2022-23. Health Aff (Millwood) 2025;44(9):1060–9.
[59] Woody GE, Poole SA, Subramaniam G, et al. Extended vs short-term buprenorphine-naloxone for treatment of opioid-addicted youth: a randomized trial. JAMA 2008;300(17):2003–11.
[60] Whitney E, Weyer G, Perri M, et al. Understanding clinician knowledge, attitudes, and practices relating to nonpharmaceutical fentanyl and harm reduction. Subst Use Addctn J 2025;46(1):120–6.
[61] CDC. Strengthening syringe service programs. Available at: https://www.cdc.gov/hepatitis-syringe-services/php/about/.
[62] Ott MA, Hoopes AJ, Sucato GS, et al. Contraception for adolescents: policy statement. Pediatrics 2025;156(1); https://doi.org/10.1542/peds.2025-072217.
[63] Hadland SE, Schmill DM, Bagley SM. Anticipatory guidance to prevent adolescent overdoses. Pediatrics 2024;153(5); https://doi.org/10.1542/peds.2023-065217.
[64] Sharko M, Jameson R, Ancker JS, et al. State-by-State variability in adolescent privacy laws. Pediatrics 2022;149(6); https://doi.org/10.1542/peds.2021-053458.

Advances in Pediatrics 73 (2026) 41–63

ADVANCES IN PEDIATRICS

Updates in Adolescent Contraception

Claudia M. Douglas, MD, MS[a,b,*],
Janis L. Sethness, MD, MPH[a,b]

[a]Seattle Children's Hospital and Research Institute, Seattle, WA, USA; [b]Department of Pediatrics, University of Washington, Seattle, WA, USA

Keywords

• Adolescent contraception • Reproductive equity
• Long-acting reversible contraception • Shared decision-making
• Contraceptive access

Key points

- Despite declining adolescent sexual activity and birth rates, the United States continues to have persistent racial, ethnic, and geographic disparities.
- Although LARC methods offer the highest effectiveness, counseling should be nondirective and align with adolescents' preferences and reproductive goals.
- Emerging safety data have prompted updates to DMPA guidance, although absolute risks remain low for most adolescents.
- New contraceptive formulations and delivery systems increase the importance of individualized, adolescent-centered counseling and shared decision-making.

ADOLESCENT CONTRACEPTION

The landscape of adolescent contraception in the United States continues to shift. New contraceptive technologies, rapidly changing legal and political environments, and evolving societal norms all contribute to this change. Now more than ever, health professionals play a key role in protecting and expanding adolescents' access to comprehensive sexual and reproductive health (SRH) services. We must recognize that adolescents' experiences within the health care

*Corresponding author. M/S CSB 200, PO Box 5371, Seattle, WA 98145-5005. *E-mail address:* claudia.douglas@seattlechildrens.org

https://doi.org/10.1016/j.yapd.2026.05.001

Abbreviations

AAP	American Academy of Pediatrics
ACOG	American College of Obstetricians and Gynecologists
BMD	bone mineral density
CHC	combined hormonal contraceptive
CDC	Centers for Disease Control and Prevention
DMPA	depot medroxyprogesterone acetate
IUD	intrauterine device
LARC	long-acting reversible contraception
MEC	Medical Eligibility Criteria
SPR	Selected Practice Recommendations
SRH	sexual and reproductive health
STI	sexually transmitted infection
VTE	venous thromboembolism
YRBS	Youth Risk Behavior Survey

system today will shape their trust and engagement with SRH care in the future.

While there is a wide range of contraceptive options, many adolescents still face barriers to affordable, confidential, and effective contraception [1,2]. These inequities disproportionately impact adolescents from marginalized communities [1,2]. This reality makes innovative and adolescent-centered approaches to contraceptive care increasingly urgent [3].

In this context, the American Academy of Pediatrics (AAP) has updated its 2014 policy statement on adolescent contraception, providing evidence-based, equity-informed guidance for clinical care [1]. The American College of Obstetricians and Gynecologists (ACOG) has also issued updated recommendations emphasizing shared decision-making, reproductive autonomy, and the removal of structural barriers to contraceptive access [2]. Together, these guidelines highlight the importance of adolescent-centered visits, confidentiality protections, and a commitment to adolescent SRH equity.

In addition, the Centers for Disease Control and Prevention (CDC) US Medical Eligibility Criteria (US MEC) and Selected Practice Recommendations (US SPR) provide essential, evidence-based guidance for contraceptive use and management in adolescents. The US MEC outlines medical eligibility criteria for contraceptive use across a variety of health conditions, while the US SPR provides guidance on how to use various contraceptive methods safely and effectively, including initiation, management of side effects, and special populations. Given the scope and complexity of these updates, a recently published adolescent-focused review serves as a practical resource for health professionals to apply the latest US MEC and US SPR recommendations in adolescent SRH care [4].

This article reviews trends in adolescent contraception and teen birth rates, examines the evolving landscape of the adolescent SRH visit, and highlights novel contraceptive methods and clinically meaningful updates to contraceptive guidelines.

TRENDS IN SEXUAL ACTIVITY AND TEEN PREGNANCY

Recent trends in adolescent sexual activity and pregnancy rates provide important context for understanding current contraceptive needs and guiding clinical care. According to the 2023 Youth Risk Behavior Survey (YRBS), adolescent sexual activity has declined over the past decade, with 32% of high school students reporting sexual intercourse in 2023 compared to 47% in 2013 [5]. Rates vary by developmental stage, with 16% of 9th graders and 48% of 12th graders reporting intercourse in 2021 (grade-level data not available in the 2023 survey), highlighting the need for developmentally appropriate, individualized counseling [6]. However, interpreting these trends requires caution as YRBS response rates dropped from 71% in 2011 to 35% in 2023 [7]. Despite these methodological limitations, early data suggest that declines in adolescent sexual activity are genuine and likely multifactorial [7,8]. Increased smartphone and social media utilization since the early 2010s has reduced opportunities for in-person social interactions that have traditionally facilitated romantic relationships [9]. Broader generational delays in dating initiation and other adult milestones have also been observed. These patterns have been further amplified by the social isolation many adolescents experienced during the COVID-19 pandemic [8].

Adolescent birth rates in the United States have continued to decline, with a rate of 13.1 births per 1000 females aged 15 to 19 in 2023, a 4% drop from 2022, a 68% decrease since 2007, and a 79% decrease since 1991 [10]. Declines have occurred across age groups, with rates falling 8% annually among younger adolescents (15–17) and 6% annually among older adolescents (18–19) between 2007 and 2023 [11]. Despite this progress, the United States still has one of the highest adolescent birth rates among industrialized nations [11]. In 2021, the US adolescent birth rate of 13.9 per 1000 females aged 15 to 19 was higher than that of the United Kingdom (8.2), France (5.1), Canada (4.9), and Sweden (2.5), reflecting systemic disparities in sex education, access to contraception, and social safety nets [12]. Notably, most adolescent pregnancies are unintended, carrying significant health and socioeconomic consequences for adolescent parents and their children [1,12].

Racial, ethnic, and geographic disparities in adolescent pregnancies continue to persist despite overall declines. Between 2016 and 2023, birth rates fell across all racial and ethnic groups, declining 35% among Hispanic adolescents and 34%, 41%, and 54% respectively among non-Hispanic Black, White, and Asian adolescents [12]. However, in 2023, birth rates for Hispanic adolescents and non-Hispanic American Indian or Alaska Native, Native Hawaiian or Other Pacific Islander, and Black adolescents were each more than double those of non-Hispanic White adolescents and over 10 times those of non-Hispanic Asian adolescents [12]. Geographic disparities in adolescent birth rates also exist, with the highest rates of adolescent birth rates concentrated in rural areas and Southern states, where structural disparities in access to contraception and SRH services are well-documented [3,12].

Ultimately, declines in adolescent pregnancy rates reflect multiple intersecting factors, including increased use of highly effective contraceptive methods, particularly long-acting reversible contraception (LARC) and multimethod approaches, as well as broader societal and economic shifts, such as expanded educational and economic opportunities. Understanding the interplay between trends in adolescent sexual behavior, declining pregnancy rates, and evolving patterns of contraceptive use, including where disparities and gaps in access persist, is essential for informing care that is clinically responsive to the full spectrum of adolescent contraceptive needs [1,12].

OVERVIEW OF CONTRACEPTIVE METHODS

A wide range of contraceptive methods is available for adolescents, differing in effectiveness, duration of action, hormonal exposure, and level of user involvement [13,14] (Table 1). Contraceptive counseling for adolescents should present the full spectrum of options in a nondirective manner that prioritizes patient preferences, reproductive goals, and individual health considerations [1,14,15]. Methods are commonly categorized as LARC, short-acting hormonal methods, on-demand methods, emergency contraception, and barrier methods [13,14].

Contraceptive effectiveness is commonly reported using typical-use failure rates, which reflect how methods perform under real-world conditions, including inconsistent or incorrect use [13,14]. These rates differ from perfect-use failure rates, which reflect effectiveness when a method is used consistently and correctly [13,14]. Because adolescents may face challenges with adherence to user-dependent methods, typical-use effectiveness is particularly relevant when counseling adolescents about contraceptive options [1,13,14].

Long-acting reversible contraception

LARC methods include intrauterine devices (IUDs) and the etonogestrel implant. These are the most effective forms of reversible contraception available to adolescents. Fewer than 1% of users become pregnant during the first year of use [13,16]. In addition to their high effectiveness, LARC methods have high continuation rates. In a large prospective cohort study of adolescents aged 14 to 19 years, the 12-month continuation rate for LARC methods was 81%, compared with 44% for non-LARC methods [17]. Contraceptive failure rates are also substantially lower with LARC methods; pregnancy rates among individuals using combined oral contraceptive pills, patches, or vaginal rings were 20 times higher than those using LARC methods, with this difference particularly pronounced among individuals younger than 21 years [16].

Available LARC methods include one progestin subdermal implant and several IUDs, including both copper and levonorgestrel-releasing IUDs. The implant suppresses ovulation through continuous release of progestin, whereas IUDs primarily prevent fertilization through local effects on sperm motility and viability. In addition to pregnancy prevention, some LARCs provide important noncontraceptive benefits, particularly for the management of heavy menstrual

Table 1
Contraceptive methods reference guide 2026

Highly Effective

Method	Perfect Use	Typical Use	Hormone	Description
Hormonal implant	>99%	>99%	Progestin	• Thin rod inserted under the skin of the upper arm • Lasts up to 5 years • If used only for menstrual suppression, may not be effective after 3 years • May cause irregular bleeding or spotting for some
Hormonal IUD	>99%	>99%	Progestin	• T-shaped device in the uterus releasing low-dose progesterone • Lasts 3–8 years depending on type • Can reduce or eliminate periods • Some types can be used as emergency contraception up to 5 days after unprotected sex

Method	Perfect Use	Typical Use	Hormone	Description
Copper IUD (non-hormonal)	>99%	>99%	N/A	• Hormone-free copper device that prevents fertilization • Lasts up to 10–12 years • The most effective emergency contraception if inserted within 5 days. • May cause heavy periods and cramping • Miudella® IUD was FDA approved in 2025, lasts up to 3 years; ongoing studies are evaluating extended use
Sterilization (tubal ligation, vasectomy)	~99%	~95-99%	N/A	• Permanent surgical procedure, reversal is difficult • Tubal ligation closes the fallopian tubes • Vasectomy cuts the vas deferens • Newer studies have shown higher failure rates for tubal sterilization; 2.9% and 5.2% at 1 and 5 years respectively [73]

Very Effective

Method	Perfect Use	Typical Use	Hormone	Description
Combined hormone pill	99%	93%	Estrogen & Progestin	• Daily oral pill that prevents ovulation, many formulations available • Used to manage conditions such as painful and heavy periods, acne, etc.
Progestin-only pill (mini pill)	99%	93%	Progestin	• Daily pill with no estrogen • Requires strict daily timing • May be used to make monthly bleeding less painful and regular
Injection (Depo-Provera)	99%	96%	Progestin	• Injection given ~3 months (13 weeks), can be given in medical setting or can be given by individual • May cause weight gain (~5lbs), mood changes, and decreased bone mineral density (improves after stopping) • Fertility may take ~10 months to return after stopping injection
Hormonal patch	99%	93%	Estrogen & Progestin	• Skin patch changed weekly for 3 weeks, followed by a patch-free week • Used to manage conditions such as painful and heavy periods, acne, etc. • May cause skin irritation
Vaginal ring	99%	93%	Estrogen & Progestin	• Flexible ring inserted vaginally • Monthly ring (NuvaRing®) or yearly ring (Annovera®) • Used to manage conditions such as painful and heavy periods, acne, etc. • Can increase vaginal discharge

Effective with Correct Use

Method	Perfect Use	Typical Use	Description
Vaginal pH modulator	96%	~86–89%	• Phexxi® is a non-hormonal gel that maintains an acidic vaginal pH that neutralizes sperm • Requires application within 1 hour before sex • Requires prescription
External condom	98%	87%	• Latex or polyurethane sheath worn over the penis • Protects against most STIs • Widely available, no prescription needed
Internal condom	95%	79%	• Nitrile pouch inserted into the vagina before sex • Protects against most STIs
Diaphragm	~92–96%	~83–88%	• Silicone or latex dome inserted before sex to cover the cervix, used with spermicide (frequent spermicide use can increase risk of HIV) • Must be fitted by health care professional • Reusable, must be left in for 6 hours after sex, but no more than 24 hours
Spermicide alone	~82%	~79%	• Chemical barrier of gel, foam, jelly, cream, or suppository that inactivates sperm • Inserted in vagina close to cervix before sex, remains in place 6-8 hours after sex • Frequent use of spermicides can increase risk of HIV
Fertility awareness methods (FAM)	~95–99%	~76–88%	• Tracks cycles, basal body temperatures, and cervical mucus to identify fertile days • Effectiveness varies widely • Can be difficult if periods are irregular • App-based tools can help improve accuracy
Withdrawal (pull-out method)	~96%	~80%	• Withdrawing the penis before ejaculation • Requires reliable execution every time. • Can disrupt sexual pleasure

Emergency Contraception

Method	Timing	Effectiveness	Description
Progestin Only	Within 3 days	~81–90%	• Commonly known as Plan B One-Step®, AfterPill, ® Morning After®, My Way®, and others • Available over the counter (state and local laws may vary); 1 tablet, 1.5mg levonorgestrel or 2 tablets, .75mg each levonorgestrel • Should be taken as soon as possible after unprotected sex, most effective on days 1-3 • Stops or delays ovulation to prevent pregnancy • Effectiveness may decrease for individuals over 165lbs
Ulipristal acetate	Within 5 days	~94-98%	• Brand name is Ella®, selective progesterone receptor modulator prevents ovulation • Requires a prescription • More effective than levonorgestrel on days 3-5 and in people with higher body weight (efficacy may decrease above 195lbs)
Copper IUD	Within 5 days	>99%	• Most effective emergency contraception method • Must be inserted by a health care professional • Effective up to 5 days, although some studies have shown 10 days without failure • No weight limitation concerns
Combined hormone pill	Within 5 days	56-86%	• Estrogen and progestin birth control pills taken in higher than usual amounts, most effective on days 1-3 • Requires 2 doses, 12 hours apart • Commonly known as Yuzpe method • Exact dosing depends on brand of pill • May be associated with more nausea and vomiting than other methods

Note: Effectiveness rates are based on ACOG and CDC guidance, current as of 2026.

bleeding and dysmenorrhea [13,14]. Levonorgestrel-releasing IUDs are available in several doses and durations of action and often lead to lighter menstrual bleeding or amenorrhea with continued use. Copper IUDs provide highly effective hormone-free contraception and may be used for extended durations. The etonogestrel implant, Nexplanon, provides continuous progestin release and is approved for 5 years of use [13].

Although LARC methods offer highly effective and convenient contraception, both initiation and removal require clinical procedures. For some adolescents, these procedures may be anxiety-provoking or potentially retraumatizing, particularly for those with histories of sexual violence or medical trauma [14,18]. Current guidance from the ACOG and the CDC recommends offering pain-management options during IUD insertion and removal, including local or topical anesthetics, oral or intravenous medications, or anxiolytics when appropriate [14,18]. Importantly, eligibility for IUD placement is not restricted by age, parity, or confirmed negative sexually transmitted infection (STI) test results, and same-day initiation of contraception is recommended when pregnancy can reasonably be excluded [13,14].

Improving procedural experience

Concerns about procedural discomfort remain an important barrier to IUD uptake among adolescents. The updated US SPR provides expanded guidance on evidence-based strategies to improve the IUD placement experience [14]. Recommended approaches include local anesthetic techniques such as paracervical lidocaine blocks or topical cervical anesthetics [14]. Routine use of misoprostol prior to IUD insertion is not recommended due to limited evidence of benefit and potential side effects [14,18]. The guidance also emphasizes the importance of anticipatory counseling and trauma-informed care [14,18]. Adolescents with anxiety, prior negative health care experiences, or a history of trauma may benefit from individualized counseling and supportive strategies designed to reduce procedural distress [14,18].

Managing long-acting reversible contraception side effects

Irregular bleeding is the most common reason adolescents discontinue the etonogestrel implant [14,19]. The updated US SPR outlines several management strategies for bothersome bleeding, including short courses of nonsteroidal anti-inflammatory medications, combined hormonal contraceptives (CHCs), or antifibrinolytic agents [14]. While these treatments may improve bleeding patterns temporarily, health professionals should also emphasize that implant removal should be available at any time if the patient desires discontinuation [1,14]. Providing anticipatory counseling about expected bleeding patterns and offering timely management strategies may improve satisfaction and continuation of the method [14,19,20].

Short-acting hormonal methods

Short-acting hormonal contraceptives include CHC methods and progestin-only methods. CHCs contain both estrogen and progestin and are available as daily oral pills, vaginal rings, and transdermal patches [21]. Short-acting progestin-only methods include progestin-only pills and an injectable contraceptive [21]. Although highly effective when used consistently and correctly, short-acting hormonal methods require regular adherence and therefore have higher typical-use failure rates than LARC methods [21]. Pregnancy rates among adolescents using pills, patches, or rings are approximately twice as high in individuals younger than 21 years compared with older users [16]. Additionally, many adolescents discontinue short-acting hormonal contraceptives within 6 months of initiation, most commonly due to perceived side effects [22].

Oral contraceptive pills remain the most commonly used reversible contraceptive method among adolescents in the United States [23]. Typical-use pregnancy rates range from 4% to 7% per year [13,21]. CHCs are associated with a small increase in venous thromboembolism (VTE) risk from approximately 2 to 10 events per 10,000 women-years in nonusers to 7 to 10 events per 10,000 women-years among users, although serious complications remain rare in adolescents without underlying risk factors [13,21]. Progestin-only and nonhormonal methods are generally preferred for individuals with medical conditions in which estrogen use is contraindicated [13,21].

Hormonal contraceptives also offer important noncontraceptive benefits for adolescents. These potentially include regulation of menstrual cycles, reduction of dysmenorrhea, treatment of acne, and management of conditions influenced by hormonal fluctuations, such as endometriosis and premenstrual dysphoric disorder [1,23,24]. These methods may also be used for menstrual suppression through extended-cycle or continuous dosing, which reduces or eliminates scheduled withdrawal bleeding [23,24]. Continuous use of combined oral contraceptive pills or vaginal rings can safely suppress menstruation and may be particularly beneficial for adolescents with heavy menstrual bleeding, dysmenorrhea, or menstrual-related symptoms [24]. Amenorrhea rates vary by method and duration of use, but with continuous combined hormonal contraception, rates may approach 49% to 88% after 1 year of use [24]. Extended or continuous use of the transdermal patch can also reduce bleeding frequency; however, because the patch delivers higher systemic estrogen exposure than most oral contraceptive pills and potentially incurs a higher VTE risk, some experts recommend extended-cycle use with periodic hormone-free intervals rather than fully continuous dosing [23,24]. Counseling adolescents about expected bleeding changes with extended or continuous use can improve satisfaction and continuation [24].

Depot medroxyprogesterone acetate efficacy and administration

Depot medroxyprogesterone acetate (DMPA) is an injectable progestin-only contraceptive that provides effective contraception for approximately 3 months per injection and may be appealing to adolescents who prefer a method that does not require daily adherence. The intramuscular formulation is administered every 11 to 13 weeks in a clinic setting, while a lower-dose subcutaneous formulation can be self-administered in appropriately trained patients, potentially improving convenience and autonomy [14]. DMPA suppresses ovulation and has a typical-use failure rate of approximately 4% per year [13,23]. Many users experience decreased menstrual bleeding or amenorrhea with continued use, although irregular bleeding is common during the first months of therapy [14,24].

Depot medroxyprogesterone acetate side effects and safety considerations

Two potential concerns relevant to adolescent counseling are changes in bone mineral density (BMD) and weight gain. DMPA use has been associated with modest reductions in BMD due to suppression of ovarian estrogen production [1,13]. Since adolescence is a critical period for bone mass accrual, these effects have been closely studied; however, available evidence indicates that BMD loss with DMPA is generally reversible after discontinuation [25]. Current guidance from ACOG and the AAP states that concerns about bone density alone should not preclude DMPA use or continuation beyond 2 years when the method aligns with a patient's preferences [25]. Counseling should include strategies to support bone health, including adequate calcium and vitamin D intake and regular weight-bearing exercise [25].

Weight gain is another commonly cited side effect. Average weight gain during the first year of use ranges from approximately 3 to 5 kg, though individual responses vary, and early weight gain may predict continued increases over time [23,26].

Recent updates to the US MEC reflect emerging evidence suggesting a modest increase in VTE risk with DMPA use compared with nonuse, resulting in revised eligibility classifications for individuals with conditions associated with elevated baseline thrombotic risk [13]. For adolescents, it is important to contextualize these changes within the broader framework of absolute risk. The overall risk of VTE among healthy adolescents remains low, and the risk associated with DMPA is still lower than that associated with estrogen-containing contraceptive methods [13,23]. Accordingly, DMPA continues to be considered an acceptable contraceptive option for most adolescents without significant underlying thrombotic risk [13].

Beyond BMD concerns, weight gain, and thrombotic risk, an emerging concern is the potential association between DMPA and intracranial meningioma. A 2024 study from France found an increased risk with long-term progestogen exposure, including DMPA [27]. A subsequent US cohort study reported a 2.43-fold higher relative risk among DMPA users compared with nonusers [28]. However, this risk was limited to individuals with more than 4 years of use or initiation after age 31 and was not observed with other contraceptive methods, including IUDs, implants, or combined oral contraceptives [28]. The absolute risk for DMPA remains low, with a number needed to harm greater than 1000 [28]. For adolescents who initiate DMPA at younger ages and use it for shorter durations, the clinical implications are likely limited; however, these data should be incorporated into shared decision-making regarding method selection and duration of use.

Depot medroxyprogesterone acetate self-administration

The US SPR continues to support self-administration of subcutaneous DMPA as a safe and effective option for individuals who prefer this approach [14]. Self-administration may improve contraceptive continuation by reducing the need for in-person clinic visits and allowing greater flexibility in dosing schedules [14]. For adolescents facing barriers such as transportation challenges, school schedules, or confidentiality concerns, this approach can expand access to a longer-acting contraceptive method [3,14].

Emergency contraception

While ongoing contraceptive methods have traditionally formed the cornerstone of pregnancy prevention, emergency contraception provides an important safety net following unprotected intercourse, contraceptive failure, or sexual assault and contributes meaningfully to reductions in unintended adolescent pregnancy [1,29]. Available options include oral emergency contraception pills and IUDs.

The copper IUD is the most effective form of emergency contraception when inserted within 5 days of unprotected intercourse [14]. Evidence suggests that the 52 mg levonorgestrel-releasing IUD may offer similar effectiveness when used for this indication, although it is not formally U.S. Food and Drug Administration (FDA)-approved for emergency contraception [14,29]. Both methods provide ongoing highly effective contraception after placement [14,29].

Among oral options, ulipristal acetate (ella) is the most effective emergency contraception pill when used within 120 hours of intercourse [14,29]. However, because ulipristal acetate acts as a progesterone receptor modulator, initiation of other hormonal contraceptive methods should be delayed for at least 5 days after its use to avoid reducing the effectiveness of emergency contraception [14]. Oral levonorgestrel 1.5 mg is widely available over the counter and is most effective when taken within 72 hours, although some effectiveness persists up to 5 days [14,29]. Levonorgestrel emergency contraception may have reduced effectiveness among individuals with a body mass index greater than 30 kg/m^2 [13,29].

Providing anticipatory counseling about emergency contraception, including advance prescriptions when appropriate, can improve timely access and reduce unintended pregnancy risk among adolescents [1,29].

Barrier and on-demand contraception

Barrier and on-demand contraceptive methods remain important options for adolescents, particularly for those who prefer user-controlled methods, desire contraception only at the time of sexual activity, or are unable or unwilling to use hormonal or long-acting methods [30–32]. External (male) condoms and internal (female) condoms are the most commonly used barrier methods among adolescents and offer the added benefit of protection against STIs [30]. When used consistently and correctly, condoms are effective for pregnancy prevention and should be recommended for dual protection, even when another contraceptive method is used [30,31]. Other barrier and on-demand options include diaphragms, cervical caps, contraceptive sponges, and spermicides [13,33]. More recently, prescription, nonhormonal vaginal pH modulators have emerged as additional on-demand options that are used prior to intercourse [34]. These methods may be particularly appealing to adolescents seeking nonhormonal, user-controlled contraception.

While barrier and on-demand methods offer flexibility and autonomy, they generally have higher typical-use failure rates compared with long-acting and hormonal methods, largely due to reliance on correct and consistent use [33]. Counseling should therefore include discussion of effectiveness, ease of use, and strategies to improve adherence, such as advance provision and education on proper use [1,31,32]. Importantly, many barrier methods are available over the counter, which may reduce access barriers for adolescents and support confidential care [30,31]. Clinicians should present these methods within a shared decision-making framework, emphasizing that barrier and on-demand options can be appropriate choices depending on patient preferences, sexual patterns, and goals, and encouraging dual protection to support both pregnancy and STI prevention [1,32].

EMERGING AND UPDATED CONTRACEPTIVE OPTIONS

In recent years, the range of available contraceptive methods has expanded with the introduction of new formulations, delivery systems, and updated dosing options [34–37] (Fig. 1). These innovations offer adolescents greater flexibility in choosing methods that align with their preferences regarding hormonal exposure, dosing frequency, privacy, and user control.

The introduction of a prefilled, self-injectable formulation of DMPA represents one of the more meaningful recent shifts in contraceptive delivery, extending the reach of an established method to adolescents who might otherwise face barriers to clinic-based administration [3,14].

Recent developments in oral contraceptive formulations have also expanded options for adolescents. The FDA approval of an over-the-counter progestin-only oral contraceptive pill containing norgestrel represents a significant milestone in contraceptive access [35]. Because this medication can be obtained without a prescription, it may reduce structural barriers to care for adolescents who face challenges related to transportation, confidentiality, or access to health professionals [35,36].

Additional oral contraceptive options include a drospirenone-only pill, Slynd, which provides a longer window for missed pills compared with traditional progestin-only pills, potentially improving adherence for adolescents managing daily dosing [34]. Nextstellis is a combined oral contraceptive that contains estetrol, a naturally occurring estrogen [34]. This newer formulation may offer an alternative hormonal profile compared with traditional ethinyl estradiol–containing pills [34].

Nondaily CHC methods have also expanded. A newer transdermal patch, Twirla, delivers a lower estrogen dose than earlier patch formulations, while

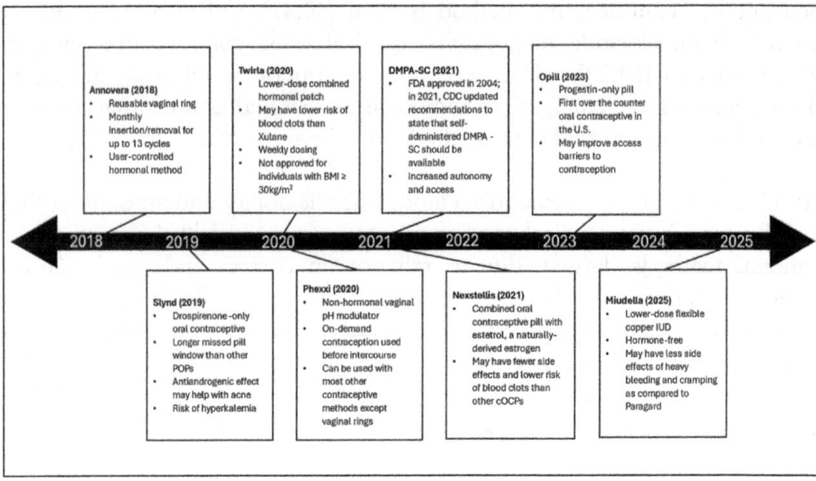

Fig. 1. Timeline of recent contraceptive innovations relevant to adolescents. COCPs, combined oral contraceptive pills; POPs, progestin-only pills.

Annovera, a reusable combined hormonal vaginal ring, provides up to 1 year of contraception through monthly cycles of insertion and removal [34]. These options allow adolescents to use combined hormonal contraception without the need for daily pill-taking while maintaining user control over method initiation and discontinuation [34].

Innovations in nonhormonal contraception have also emerged. Miudella, a newer copper IUD with a smaller and more flexible frame, has been introduced as an additional hormone-free long-acting option [37]. In addition, Phexxi, a vaginal pH modulator, provides an on-demand contraceptive method that works by maintaining an acidic vaginal environment that impairs sperm motility [34]. Although Phexxi is less effective than long-acting options with a typical use failure rate of approximately 14%, it may appeal to adolescents seeking hormone-free or episodic contraception [34,38,39].

Taken together, the growing diversity of contraceptive options underscores the importance of individualized counseling that considers adolescents' preferences regarding effectiveness, convenience, hormonal exposure, and degree of user involvement.

TRENDS IN CONTRACEPTIVE USE

Over the past decade, adolescent contraceptive use in the United States has increasingly shifted toward more effective and longer-acting methods, alongside rising use of emergency contraception and continued reliance on user-dependent methods such as condoms. In 2021, 52% of sexually active high school students reported condom use at last intercourse, compared with 33% who reported use of an effective hormonal method (oral contraceptive pills, IUDs, implants, injections, patches, or rings) [40].

Use of LARCs among adolescents has increased significantly, from 3% at last intercourse in 2006 to 2010 to 15% in 2015 to 2019 among adolescents (15–19) [41]. Overall, 19.2% of adolescents reported ever using a LARC method [42]. Among LARC users, implant use (10%) exceeds IUD use (5%), a pattern that has been consistent across national surveys [41]. Increasing uptake of LARC methods among adolescents reflects their appeal as methods that do not require daily adherence or ongoing user action, factors that are particularly important for adolescents who may face challenges with consistent and correct use of user-dependent contraceptive methods [1,3,41]. However, method selection among LARC users varies by age, with younger adolescents more likely to use implants and older adolescents more likely to use IUDs, likely reflecting differences in comfort with pelvic examinations, parental preferences, and anticipated discomfort with the IUD procedure [41,42].

Despite increased use of highly effective contraceptives like the IUD and implant, a concerning decline in condom use has emerged. Condom use among sexually active adolescents decreased from 59% in 2013 to 52% in 2023 [5,43]. This decline is likely multifactorial; as adolescents increasingly adopt more effective contraception methods for pregnancy prevention, condom use as a primary contraceptive strategy may be used less consistently [1,41,43]. This is particularly concerning given that young people ages 15 to 24 account for nearly half (48%) of all reported cases of chlamydia, gonorrhea, and syphilis [44]. Together, these trends highlight the importance of integrating dual protection counseling into all contraceptive care to address both pregnancy prevention and STI risks. Increasing utilization of emergency contraception use from 8.1% in 2002 to 22.3% in 2015 to 2019 further highlights the need for comprehensive counseling that includes consistent method use, anticipatory guidance on backup options, and STI prevention [42].

While the decline in condom use is concerning, it is equally important to recognize that barrier methods and other nonpharmacologic strategies remain a widely used and clinically relevant source of contraception among adolescents. External condoms, internal condoms, fertility-awareness methods, spermicides, pH modulators, and the withdrawal method are inexpensive, widely accessible, and have few medical contraindications [13,45]. These methods are typically used at the time of intercourse and therefore offer individuals control over contraceptive use without ongoing medication or procedures [43]. Adolescents should be supported in choosing any contraceptive method without stigma or judgment, and counseling should be tailored to support informed decision-making based on individual preferences and needs. Health professionals should be familiar with the full range of contraceptive options and facilitate access to these methods for adolescents [14,15].

REPRODUCTIVE JUSTICE AND EQUITY

Discussion of adolescent contraception must be grounded in a reproductive justice framework. SisterSong Women of Color Reproductive Justice Collective defines reproductive justice as "the human right to maintain personal bodily autonomy, have children, not have children, and parent the children we have in safe and sustainable communities." [46] This framework extends beyond just legal access and choice to center the structural, economic, and social conditions that shape adolescents' ability to exercise reproductive autonomy, particularly for those from marginalized communities [46,47]. It is important to remember that experiences of discrimination, stigma, and historical reproductive coercion continue to influence trust and engagement in SRH care [14,48].

Geographic access is another often-underrecognized dimension of reproductive equity. More than 19 million individuals in the United States live in contraceptive deserts, counties without any health centers that can offer a full range of contraceptive options [47,49]. For adolescents in these areas, traditional clinic-based care is often infeasible, making innovative, low-barrier delivery models essential to achieving meaningful reproductive equity [47,50].

CENTERING ALL ADOLESCENTS IN CONTRACEPTIVE CARE

Centering all adolescents in contraceptive care begins with recognizing that every young person deserves care that is affirming and reflective of their individual needs, regardless of ability, identity, or background [1,14,15]. Contraceptive care must prioritize autonomy, informed choice, and protection from coercion, particularly for populations that have been historically marginalized. The 2024 US SPR emphasizes that all individuals should be supported in selecting the contraceptive method that best aligns with their preferences and reproductive goals [14].

Despite this, many adolescents remain underserved. Adolescents with physical disabilities, developmental disabilities, and chronic health conditions frequently have more complex contraceptive needs yet often face substantial barriers to contraceptive care. For example, adolescents with developmental disabilities are more likely to experience menstrual disorders yet are less likely to access care or use hormonal contraceptives [51]. Similarly, adolescents with disabilities are also less likely to receive comprehensive sexual health education and counseling, despite experiencing higher rates of STIs, unintended pregnancies, and sexual violence [51,52]. It is important to note that these disparities reflect structural barriers, including inaccessible health care facilities, limited provider knowledge and biases, and challenges related to consent or guardianship, rather than the disability itself [51,52].

Adolescents who are sexual and gender minorities represent another group whose contraceptive needs are frequently overlooked. Transmasculine and gender-nonbinary adolescents assigned female at birth who receive testosterone therapy may still be at risk for pregnancy and should be counseled accordingly [53,54]. It is important for health professionals to recognize that contraceptives may be used for a variety of reasons, including menstrual suppression or as part of an individual's gender-affirming care [53,54]. Yet, only 7.4% of adolescents who are sexual and gender minorities report receiving sex education that includes positive representations of sexual orientation and gender identity topics, leaving many without essential SRH knowledge [55].

Delivering equitable contraceptive care requires health professionals to recognize how structural barriers shape access and decision-making across diverse adolescent populations. Counseling must be responsive to each adolescent's lived experience and oriented toward reducing barriers to contraceptive care while supporting informed, autonomous decision making [1,14,15].

ADOLESCENT SEXUAL AND REPRODUCTIVE HEALTH VISITS

Both the AAP and ACOG have issued updated guidance that provides a comprehensive framework for delivering high-quality, adolescent-centered SRH care across a range of clinical settings [1,2,56].

ACOG recommends that the initial reproductive health visit occur between ages 13 and 15, with the primary goals of providing preventive care, education, and anticipatory guidance, while also addressing problem-focused concerns [56]. This first visit does not require a pelvic examination; rather, it provides an opportunity to establish trust, address misconceptions about reproductive health care, and lay the foundation for ongoing dialog. Contraceptive counseling should begin prior to sexual debut, with attention to access even among adolescents who are not yet sexually active [56]. ACOG also recommends obtaining a comprehensive sexual history using the CDC's 5 Ps framework (Partners, Practices, Protection from STIs, Past history of STIs, and Pregnancy Intention) [56–58]. ACOG's Committee Opinion on the Initial Reproductive Health Visit also incorporates gender-inclusive language, expands counseling to include sexual orientation and gender identity, and emphasizes trauma-informed care, recognizing the complex developmental, social, and relational contexts adolescents are navigating [56,57].

In 2025, the AAP also released an updated policy statement on adolescent contraception, replacing its 2014 guidelines [1]. The updated recommendations emphasize a patient-centered, equity-informed approach, with contraceptive counseling prioritizing adolescents' reproductive goals and guided by shared decision-making rather than efficacy alone [1]. The AAP also highlights the importance of integrating STI screening, human papillomavirus vaccination, and counseling on healthy relationships and consent into comprehensive SRH care [1].

CONFIDENTIALITY AND CONSENT

One-on-one time between adolescents and health professionals remains a core component of SRH care, according to guidance from both AAP and ACOG [1,56]. The AAP recommends initiating private conversations regardless of caregiver presence and exploring reproductive goals, knowledge, and preferences without assumptions [1]. ACOG similarly affirms that all adolescents should have access to confidential care, as concerns about privacy may lead adolescents to delay or forgo SRH services [59].

Both organizations also recognize that parental and caregiver involvement, when possible and safe, can play an important role in adolescent SRH care [1,59]. The AAP recommends that clinical practices establish clear confidentiality policies and discuss them regularly with adolescents and caregivers [1,60]. Parents and caregivers should be included in broader conversations about adolescent health, while preserving the adolescent's right to confidential care [1,60]. When supported with accurate information and a nonjudgmental approach, families can serve as important partners in promoting healthy sexual development [1]. Resources to support these conversations are available through the AAP's Bright Futures guidelines and parent portal [1,61].

Confidentiality within modern health systems remains an ongoing challenge. Insurance billing processes, electronic health records, and patient portals may inadvertently disclose sensitive information, highlighting the need for safeguards at all levels of care, from individual clinical encounters to practice and institutional-level policies [1,60].

Minor consent laws vary by state, so adolescents, families, and caregivers must understand how these laws impact their ability to receive contraceptive and SRH services [1]. As of 2024, 25 states and the District of Columbia allow minors to consent to contraceptive services, although this landscape is rapidly changing [62]. In recent years, a growing number of states have moved to restrict minor consent protections and expand parental notification requirements, changes that disproportionately affect adolescents who may be likely to forgo SRH care entirely if confidentiality cannot be assured [1,60,62]. Federal protections, including Title X and HIPAA, offer additional safeguards, and the AAP advises using clinical judgment to protect confidentiality when appropriate and to document it [1,60]. Clear communication and understanding of these laws is critical in supporting adolescents' access to confidential and timely SRH care.

CREATING AN ADOLESCENT-FRIENDLY OFFICE ENVIRONMENT AND EXPANDING ACCESS TO CARE

The clinical environment plays an important role in adolescents' sense of safety and willingness to engage in SRH care. ACOG recommends creating adolescent-friendly spaces with age-appropriate materials, inclusive intake forms, and accessible educational resources, providing information to both adolescents and caregivers at the conclusion of the visit [56]. Clinical spaces should implement clear policies affirming adolescents' right to confidential care and ensure that all staff are trained to protect privacy across all aspects of care delivery, including medical records, test results, billing, and patient portals [1,60]. Identifying pharmacies that support confidential prescribing, offering flexible hours, walk-in appointments, same-day access, and telehealth options further reduces scheduling barriers and increases the likelihood that adolescents will seek and continue care [1].

Creating a nonstigmatizing clinical culture is also important. The AAP recommends that SRH counseling be offered universally to all adolescents, not just those perceived as *high risk*, to minimize bias and ensure equitable care [1]. Health professionals should also recognize the roles that stigma, discrimination, and structural racism have played, and continue to play, in shaping adolescents' willingness to engage with care, and embed nondiscriminatory policies and trauma-informed practices throughout all aspects of care delivery, including care delivered beyond the traditional office setting [1,14,48].

Historically, adolescents have obtained contraception through traditional clinical settings, including pediatric primary care, adolescent medicine clinics, family planning clinics, and obstetrics and gynecology practices. Increasingly, however, a growing range of novel and nontraditional settings are expanding access to SRH and contraceptive care, including school-based health centers, mobile health clinics, and outreach programs through youth-serving organizations [1,3] (Fig. 2). School-based health centers represent a particularly important access point, reducing barriers related to transportation, scheduling, and cost by bringing services directly into the school environment [1,63]. Community-based delivery models can further extend reach to adolescents

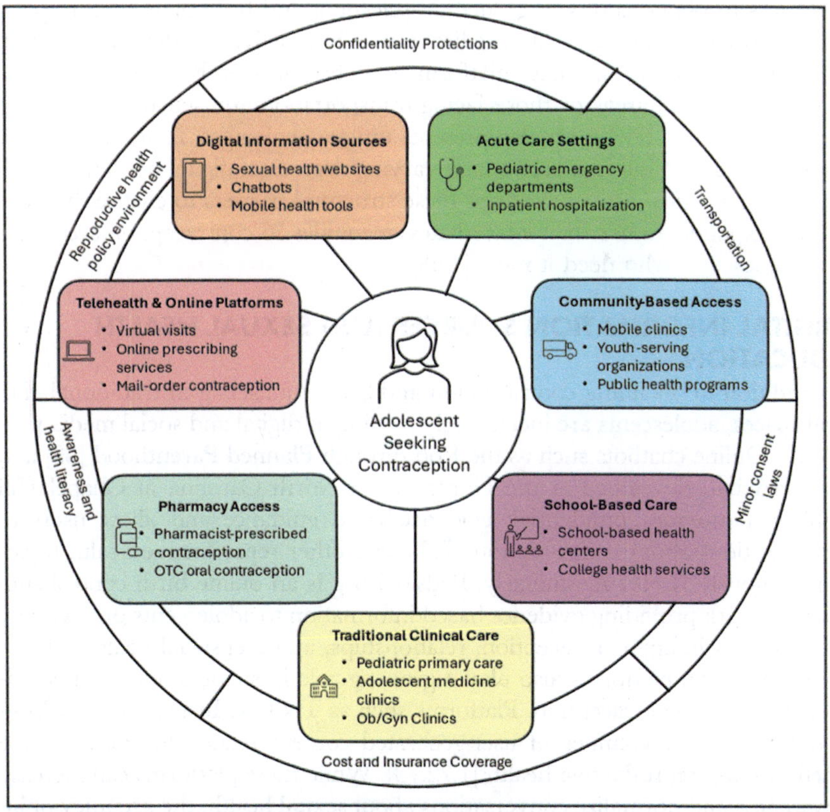
Confidentiality Protections
Digital Information Sources
Sexual health websites
Chatbots
Mobile health tools
Acute Care Settings
Pediatric emergency departments
Inpatient hospitalization
Reproductive health policy environment
Transportation
Telehealth & Online Platforms
Virtual visits
Online prescribing services
Mail-order contraception
Community-Based Access
Mobile clinics
Youth-serving organizations
Public health programs
Adolescent Seeking Contraception
Awareness and health literacy
Minor consent laws
Pharmacy Access
Pharmacist-prescribed contraception
OTC oral contraception
School-Based Care
School-based health centers
College health services
Traditional Clinical Care
Pediatric primary care
Adolescent medicine clinics
Ob/Gyn Clinics
Cost and Insurance Coverage

Fig. 2. Pathways to contraceptive access for adolescents.

who face structural barriers to traditional clinic-based care, making these settings not merely convenient alternatives, but essential components of an equitable contraceptive care infrastructure [1].

Publicly funded safety net programs, particularly the Title X Family Planning Program, remain essential for adolescents who are uninsured, underinsured, or seeking confidential care outside of their primary health care setting [1,64]. The *quick start* or same-day initiation approach, which allows contraception to be initiated at the time of a clinical encounter, can reduce delays associated with follow-up appointments and is particularly valuable for adolescents who face barriers to returning for additional visits [14,65]. Additionally, integration of reproductive health services into acute care settings, including pediatric emergency departments and inpatient units, has shown promise in reaching adolescents who have limited contact with outpatient providers and who might otherwise lack access to contraceptive counseling and initiation [3,66,67].

Expanding access beyond physical settings, telehealth has emerged as an increasingly important modality for adolescent contraceptive care, allowing adolescents to obtain counseling, method selection, and hormonal contraceptive prescriptions remotely, with medications often delivered directly through mail-order pharmacies. These platforms may be particularly beneficial for adolescents in rural areas or those facing transportation and scheduling barriers [1,68]. However, telehealth also presents unique challenges, including privacy concerns, limited internet access, and varying degrees of digital literacy. Health professionals must actively address these structural barriers to ensure that telehealth expands, rather than exacerbates, inequities in contraceptive access for the adolescents who need it most [1,68].

DIGITAL INFORMATION SOURCES AND SEXUAL HEALTH EDUCATION

In addition to obtaining contraception and SRH counseling in traditional clinical spaces, adolescents are increasingly turning to digital and social media platforms. Online chatbots such as the Roo through Planned Parenthood [69] and SARHAchat, developed at the University of North Carolina at Chapel Hill [70], can provide confidential, evidence-based guidance and allow users to ask questions about contraception, STIs, and other reproductive health topics anonymously [1,69,70]. Similarly, Bedsider.org is an online birth control support network providing evidence-based information to adolescents on a variety of topics, including contraception, relationships, and menstrual health [71].

Social media platforms also play a growing role in shaping adolescents' understanding of contraception. Platforms such as TikTok, Instagram, and YouTube host large volumes of user-generated content related to contraceptive methods and reproductive health [1,72,73]. While these platforms can increase awareness and normalize conversations about sexual health, the accuracy of information varies widely. Studies have found that misinformation regarding contraceptive safety, side effects, and effectiveness is common on social media, and adolescents may have difficulty distinguishing evidence-based information from anecdotal or misleading claims [1,72,73]. In an increasingly digital world, health professionals should be prepared to address misinformation and guide adolescents to reliable, evidence-based contraceptive resources.

SUMMARY

Adolescent contraceptive care is rapidly evolving, shaped by expanding options, updated clinical guidance, and a growing emphasis on reproductive autonomy. High-quality care requires individualized, developmentally appropriate counseling that centers adolescent preferences, alongside efforts to expand access through flexible models such as telehealth, school-based care, and over-the-counter options. Addressing structural barriers and adopting innovative approaches to care delivery are essential to improving access and ensuring contraceptive care that is responsive to adolescents' needs.

CLINICS CARE POINTS

- Confidential, developmentally appropriate counseling ensures that adolescents' autonomy is prioritized and that shared decision-making is supported.
- The updated US Medical Eligibility Criteria and US Selected Practice Recommendations expand method eligibility and allow same-day initiation of contraceptives when clinically appropriate.
- Telehealth, school-based care, and over-the-counter options can help adolescents overcome structural barriers to contraceptive access.
- Routine integration of sexually transmitted infection screening, human papillomavirus vaccination, and counseling on healthy relationships and consent is essential to comprehensive adolescent contraceptive care.
- Anticipatory counseling on side effects, adherence, and method continuation can improve satisfaction and reduce early discontinuation.

DECLARATION OF AI AND AI-ASSISTED TECHNOLOGIES IN THE WRITING PROCESS

During the preparation of this work the authors used GenAI. After using this tool/service, the authors reviewed and edited the content as needed and take full responsibility for the content of the publication.

Disclosure

The authors have nothing to disclose.

References

[1] Ott MA, Hoopes AJ, Sucato GS, et al, Committee on Adolescence. Contraception for adolescents: policy statement. Pediatrics 2025;156(1):e2025072217.

[2] American College of Obstetricians and Gynecologists. Access to contraception. ACOG Committee statement No. 21. Obstet Gynecol 2025;146(5):e88.

[3] Reilly K, Schmuhl KK, Bonny AE. Removing barriers to contraceptive access for adolescents. J Pediatr Pharmacol Ther 2024;29(3):331–5.
[4] Sethness JL, Simmons KB, Zhang Y, Hoopes AJ. Key takeaways for adolescent-serving clinicians in the 2024 U.S. medical eligibility criteria for contraceptive use and selected practice recommendations for contraceptive use. J Pediatr Adolesc Gynecol 2026; https://doi.org/10.1016/j.jpag.2026.02.012.
[5] Centers for Disease Control and Prevention. Youth risk behavior survey data summary & trends report: 2013–2023. Atlanta (GA): US Department of Health and Human Services; 2024. Available at: https://www.cdc.gov/yrbs/dstr/index.html. Accessed March 20, 2026.
[6] Centers for Disease Control and Prevention. Youth risk behavior survey data summary & trends report: 2011–2021. Atlanta (GA): US Department of Health and Human Services; 2022. Available at: https://www.cdc.gov/yrbs/dstr/index.html. Accessed March 20, 2026.
[7] Santelli JS, Malden DE, Moss RA, et al. Age bias, missing data, and declining response rates in the National Youth Risk Behavior Survey and their influence on estimates of trends in adolescent sexual experience, 2011–2023. Sex Res Soc Policy 2025; https://doi.org/10.1007/s13178-025-01223-3.
[8] Yarger J, Gutmann-Gonzalez A, Han S, et al. Young people's romantic relationships and sexual activity before and during the COVID-19 pandemic. BMC Public Health 2021;21(1):1780.
[9] Twenge JM, Spitzberg BH, Campbell WK. Less in-person social interaction with peers among U.S. adolescents in the 21st century and links to loneliness. J Soc Pers Relat 2019;36(6):1892–913.
[10] Osterman MJK, Hamilton BE, Martin JA, et al. Births: final data for 2023. Natl Vital Stat Rep 2025;74(1):1–55.
[11] Hamilton BE, Martin JA, Osterman MJK. *Births: provisional data for 2023*. Vital statistics rapid release; no. 35. National Center for Health Statistics; 2024; https://doi.org/10.15620/cdc/151797.
[12] Mickler AK, Tollestrup J. *Teen births in the United States: overview and recent trends*. CRS report R45184. Washington, DC: Congressional Research Service; 2024. Available at: https://crsreports.congress.gov/product/pdf/R/R45184. Accessed March 20, 2026.
[13] Nguyen AT, Curtis KM, Tepper NK, et al. U.S. medical eligibility criteria for contraceptive use, 2024. MMWR Recomm Rep (Morb Mortal Wkly Rep) 2024;73(RR-4):1–126.
[14] Curtis KM, Nguyen AT, Tepper NK, et al. U.S. selected practice recommendations for contraceptive use, 2024. MMWR Recomm Rep (Morb Mortal Wkly Rep) 2024;73(RR-3):1–77.
[15] Thornton M, Mann ES, Bullington BW, et al. Exploring adolescent-facing US clinicians' perceptions of their contraceptive counseling and use of shared decision-making: a qualitative study. Perspect Sex Reprod Health 2024;56(4):337–46.
[16] Winner B, Peipert JF, Zhao Q, et al. Effectiveness of long-acting reversible contraception. N Engl J Med 2012;366(21):1998–2007.
[17] Rosenstock JR, Peipert JF, Madden T, et al. Continuation of reversible contraception in teenagers and young women. Obstet Gynecol 2012;120(6):1298–305.
[18] American College of Obstetricians and Gynecologists' Committee on Clinical Consensus–Gynecology. Pain management for in-office uterine and cervical procedures: ACOG Clinical Consensus No. 9. Obstet Gynecol 2025;146(1):161–77; https://doi.org/10.1097/AOG.0000000000005911.
[19] Fei YF, Smith YR, Dendrinos ML, et al. Considerations in adolescent use of the etonogestrel subdermal implant: a cohort study. Front Reprod Health 2021;3:780902; https://doi.org/10.3389/frph.2021.780902.
[20] Milliren CE, DiVasta AD, Edwards AJ, et al. Contraceptive implant-associated bleeding in adolescent/young adult clinical practice: associated factors, management, and rates of discontinuation. J Adolesc Health 2023;72(4):583–90.

[21] Teal S, Edelman A. Contraception selection, effectiveness, and adverse effects: a review. JAMA 2021;326(24):2507–18.
[22] Raine TR, Foster-Rosales A, Upadhyay UD, et al. One-year contraceptive continuation and pregnancy in adolescent girls and women initiating hormonal contraceptives. Obstet Gynecol 2011;117(2 Pt 1):363–71.
[23] Daniels K, Abma JC. Current contraceptive status among females ages 15–49: united States, 2022–2023. NCHS Data Brief No. 539. Hyattsville (MD): National Center for Health Statistics; 2025; https://doi.org/10.15620/cdc/174618.
[24] American College of Obstetricians and Gynecologists' Committee on Clinical Consensus–Gynecology. General approaches to medical management of menstrual suppression: ACOG Clinical Consensus No. 3. Obstet Gynecol 2022;140(3):528–41; https://doi.org/10.1097/AOG.0000000000004900.
[25] American College of Obstetricians and Gynecologists. Depot medroxyprogesterone acetate and bone effects. ACOG Committee Opinion No. 602. Obstet Gynecol 2014;123(6):1398–402; https://doi.org/10.1097/01.AOG.0000450758.95422.c8.
[26] Bonny AE, Secic M, Cromer B. Early weight gain related to later weight gain in adolescents on depot medroxyprogesterone acetate. Obstet Gynecol 2011;117(3):616–22.
[27] Roland N, Neumann A, Hoisnard L, et al. Use of progestogens and the risk of intracranial meningioma: national case-control study. BMJ 2024;384:e078078; https://doi.org/10.1136/bmj-2023-078078.
[28] Xiao T, Kumar P, Lobbous M, et al. Depot medroxyprogesterone acetate and risk of meningioma in the US. JAMA Neurol 2025;82(11):1094–102.
[29] Committee on Adolescence. Emergency contraception. Pediatrics 2019;144(6):e20193149; https://doi.org/10.1542/peds.2019-3149.
[30] Grubb LK, Committee on Adolescence. Committee on Adolescents. Barrier protection use by adolescents during sexual activity. Pediatrics 2020;146(2):e2020007245; https://doi.org/10.1542/peds.2020-007245.
[31] Gerancher KR. Counseling adolescents about contraception. Washington, DC: American College of Obstetricians and Gynecologists; 2017. Available at: https://www.acog.org/-/media/project/acog/acogorg/clinical/files/committee-opinion/articles/2017/08/counseling-adolescents-about-contraception.pdf. Accessed March 24, 2026.
[32] Ott MA, Sucato GS, Leroy-Melamed M, et al, Committee on Adolescence. Contraceptive counseling and methods for adolescents: clinical report. Pediatrics 2025;156(1):e2025072218; https://doi.org/10.1542/peds.2025-072218.
[33] Centers for Disease Control and Prevention. Contraception: birth control methods. Atlanta (GA): US Department of Health and Human Services, CDC; 2024. Available at: https://www.cdc.gov/reproductive-health/contraception/index.html. Accessed March 24, 2026.
[34] Baker CC, Chen MJ. New contraception update — annovera, Phexxi, Slynd, and Twirla. Curr Obstet Gynecol Rep 2022;11(1):21–7.
[35] U.S. Food and Drug Administration. FDA approves first nonprescription daily oral contraceptive. FDA website. 2023. Available at: https://www.fda.gov/news-events/press-announcements/fda-approves-first-nonprescription-daily-oral-contraceptive. Accessed March 24, 2026.
[36] American College of Obstetricians and Gynecologists. First over-the-counter daily contraceptive pill released. ACOG Practice Advisory. ACOG website 2024. Available at: https://www.acog.org/clinical/clinical-guidance/practice-advisory/articles/2024/03/first-over-the-counter-daily-contraceptive-pill-released. Accessed March 24, 2026.
[37] Creinin MD, Gawron LM, Roe AH, et al. Copper 175mm2 IUD Phase 3 Clinical Investigator Group. Three-year efficacy, safety, and tolerability outcomes from a phase 3 study of a low-dose copper intrauterine device. Contraception 2024; https://doi.org/10.1016/j.contraception.2024.110771.
[38] Thomas MA, Chappell BT, Maximos B, et al. A novel vaginal pH regulator: results from the phase 3 AMPOWER contraception clinical trial. Contracept X 2020;2:100031; https://doi.org/10.1016/j.conx.2020.100031.

[39] Schwarz EB, Chiang AY, Lewis CA, et al. Pregnancy after Tubal Sterilization in the United States, 2002 to 2015. NEJM Evid 2024;3(9):EVIDoa2400023; https://doi.org/10.1056/EVIDoa2400023.
[40] Centers for Disease Control and Prevention. High school youth risk behavior Survey: united States, 2021 results. Atlanta (GA): US Department of Health and Human Services; 2023. Available at: https://nccd.cdc.gov/Youthonline/App/Results.aspx. Accessed March 20, 2026.
[41] Lindberg LD, Firestein L, Beavin C. Trends in U.S. adolescent sexual behavior and contraceptive use, 2006–2019. Contracept X 2021;3:100064; https://doi.org/10.1016/j.conx.2021.100064.
[42] Abma JC, Martinez GM. Teenagers in the United States: sexual activity, contraceptive use, and childbearing, 2015–2019. Natl Health Stat Rep 2023;(196):1–23; https://doi.org/10.15620/cdc/124384.
[43] Steiner RJ, Pampati S, Kortsmit KM, et al. Long-acting reversible contraception, condom use, and sexually transmitted infections: a systematic review and meta-analysis. Am J Prev Med 2021;61(5):750–60.
[44] Centers for Disease Control and Prevention. Sexually transmitted infections surveillance, 2023. Atlanta (GA): US Department of Health and Human Services; 2024. Available at: https://www.cdc.gov/sti-statistics/index.html. Accessed March 24, 2026.
[45] Daniels K, Abma JC. Contraceptive methods women have ever used: united States, 2015–2019. Natl Health Stat Rep 2023;(195):1–18.
[46] SisterSong Women of Color Reproductive Justice Collective. Reproductive justice. SisterSong website. Available at: https://www.sistersong.net/reproductive-justice. Accessed March 20, 2026.
[47] Axelson SM, Sealy GA, McDonald-Mosley RE. Reproductive well-being: a framework for expanding contraceptive access. Am J Public Health 2022;112(6):858–61.
[48] Bryson A, Koyama A, Hassan A. Addressing long-acting reversible contraception access, bias, and coërcion: supporting adolescent and young adult reproductive autonomy. Curr Opin Pediatr 2021;33(4):345–53.
[49] Power to Decide. Contraceptive deserts. Power to decide website. Available at: https://powertodecide.org/what-we-do/contraceptive-deserts. Accessed March 20, 2026.
[50] Steward CR, Getahun D, Kuo AA. Expanding adolescent access to hormonal contraception: an update on over-the-counter, pharmacist prescribing, and web-based telehealth approaches. Curr Opin Obstet Gynecol 2019;31(5):363–8.
[51] Ames JL, Cheslack-Postava K, Hillman SL, et al. Reproductive healthcare in adolescents with autism and other developmental disabilities. J Adolesc Health 2024;74(5):897–905.
[52] Grover SR, Whittaker MH. Sexual health education for adolescents and young adults with intellectual and developmental disabilities: recommendations for accessible sexual and reproductive health information. Lancet Child Adolesc Health 2020;4(9):696–708.
[53] Krempasky C, Harris M, Abern L, et al. Contraception across the transmasculine spectrum. Am J Obstet Gynecol 2020;222(2):134–43.
[54] Bonnington A, Dianat S, Kerns J, et al. Society of Family Planning clinical recommendations: contraceptive counseling for transgender and gender diverse people who were female sex assigned at birth. Contraception 2020;102(2):70–82.
[55] Kosciw JG, Clark CM, Menard L. The 2021 national school climate survey: the experiences of LGBTQ+ youth in our nation's schools. New York: GLSEN; 2022. Available at: https://www.glsen.org/research/2021-national-school-climate-survey. Accessed March 24, 2026.
[56] American College of Obstetricians and Gynecologists. The initial reproductive health visit. ACOG Committee Opinion No. 811. Obstet Gynecol 2020;136(4):e70–80; https://doi.org/10.1097/AOG.0000000000004094.

[57] Centers for Disease Control and Prevention. A guide to taking a sexual history. Atlanta (GA): US Department of Health and Human Services; 2015. Available at: https://www.cdc.gov/std/treatment/sexualhistory.pdf. Accessed March 24, 2026.
[58] Workowski KA, Bachmann LH, Chan PA, et al. Sexually transmitted infections treatment guidelines, 2021. MMWR Recomm Rep (Morb Mortal Wkly Rep) 2021;70(RR-4):1–187.
[59] American College of Obstetricians and Gynecologists. Confidentiality in adolescent health care. ACOG Committee opinion no. 803. Obstet Gynecol 2020;135(4):e171–7; https://doi.org/10.1097/AOG.0000000000003770.
[60] Chung RJ, Lee JB, Hackell JM, et al, Committee on Adolescence, Committee on Practice & Ambulatory Medicine. Confidentiality in the care of adolescents: policy statement. Pediatrics 2024;153(5):e2024066326; https://doi.org/10.1542/peds.2024-066326.
[61] Hagan JF, Shaw JS, Duncan PM, editors. Bright Futures: guidelines for health supervision of infants, children, and adolescents. 4th edition. Elk Grove Village (IL): American Academy of Pediatrics; 2017.
[62] Guttmacher Institute. Minors' access to contraceptive services. State Policies in Brief. Guttmacher Institute website. 2024. Available at: https://www.guttmacher.org/state-policy/explore/minors-access-contraceptive-services. Accessed March 24, 2026.
[63] Sullivan EE, Love HL, Fisher RL, et al. Access to contraceptives in school-based health centers: progress and opportunities. Am J Prev Med 2022;62(3):350–9.
[64] Allsbrook JF, Marcella JS. The Title X program: setting standards for contraceptive and health equity. Am J Public Health 2022;112(6):843–5.
[65] Steiner RJ, Liddon N, Swartzendruber AL, et al. Health care provider attitudes and practices related to "quick start" provision of combined hormonal contraception and depot medroxyprogesterone acetate to adolescents. J Adolesc Health 2019;64(2):211–8.
[66] Mollen C, Ketterer T, Min J, et al. Expanding contraceptive access for teens — leveraging the pediatric emergency department. J Adolesc Health 2023;73(1):155–63.
[67] Goldstein RL, Carlson JL, Halpern-Felsher B. Contraception for adolescents and young adults in the inpatient setting: the providers' perspective. Hosp Pediatr 2018;8(4):194–9.
[68] Reilly K, Ebersole A. Confidentiality and privacy considerations for adolescents receiving contraceptive health services via telemedicine: a narrative review. Womens Health (Lond) 2024;20:17455057241233126; https://doi.org/10.1177/17455057241233126.
[69] Planned Parenthood Federation of America. Ask Roo: the sexual health chatbot. Planned Parenthood website. Available at: https://www.plannedparenthood.org/learn/roo-sexual-health-chatbot. Accessed March 24, 2026.
[70] University of North Carolina College of Arts and Sciences. Trust SARHAchat with your reproductive health questions. UNC College of Arts and Sciences website. 2026. Available at: https://college.unc.edu/2026/03/sarhachat/. Accessed March 25, 2026.
[71] Power to Decide. Bedsider: birth control support network. Bedsider website. Available at: https://www.bedsider.org. Accessed March 24, 2026.
[72] Stoddard RE, Pelletier A, Sundquist EN, et al. Popular contraception videos on TikTok: an assessment of content topics. Contraception 2024;129:110300; https://doi.org/10.1016/j.contraception.2023.110300.
[73] Shackleford M, Horvath A, Repetto M, et al. An analysis of oral contraceptive related videos on TikTok. AJOG Glob Rep 2024;4:100364; https://doi.org/10.1016/j.xagr.2024.100364.

[57] Centers for Disease Control and Prevention. A guide to taking a sexual history. Atlanta (GA): US Department of Health and Human Services; 2015. Available at: https://www.cdc.gov/std/treatment/sexualhistory.pdf. Accessed March 24, 2022.
[58] Workowski KA, Bachmann LH, Chan PA, et al. Sexually transmitted infections treatment guidelines, 2021. MMWR Recomm Rep (Morb Mortal Wkly Rep) 2021;70(RR-4):1–187.
[59] American College of Obstetricians and Gynecologists. [illegible]

[60] [illegible] Committee on Adolescence, Committee on Practice and Ambulatory Medicine. Confidentiality in the care of adolescents: policy statement. Pediatrics 2024;153(5):e2024066326. [illegible]

Advances in Pediatrics 73 (2026) 65–81

ADVANCES IN PEDIATRICS

Pain Management in Pediatric Patients with Sickle Cell Disease

Marni Shear, DO, MPH[a,*], Peter Huynh, MD[b], Gloria Sanchez, MD, FASAM[c], Moran Gotesman, MD[a]

[a]Department of Pediatrics, Harbor UCLA Medical Center, The Lundquist Institute of Biomedical Innovation, David Geffen School of Medicine at UCLA, Torrance, CA, USA; [b]Department of Anesthesiology, Harbor UCLA Medical Center, David Geffen School of Medicine at UCLA, Torrance, CA, USA; [c]Department of Family Medicine, Harbor UCLA Medical Center, David Geffen School of Medicine at UCLA, Torrance, CA, USA

Keywords

• Sickle cell disease • Sickle cell pain • Vaso-occlusive episode • Pain management

Key points

- Sickle cell pain presentations are multifactorial, often with both acute and chronic features that require an individualized approach that considers history, previous treatment responses, and psychosocial context.
- Development of individualized pain management plans that incorporate patient preferences, in collaboration with a multidisciplinary care team that includes primary care providers, hematologists, pain specialists, and mental health providers, can improve experiences for patients with sickle cell disease (SCD).
- Awareness of disease-modifying therapies, nonopioid analgesics, newer agents such as buprenorphine, and nonpharmacologic adjuncts to pain management is essential for providers who care for children with SCD.
- Systemic racism and provider bias continue to undermine equitable pain management in SCD, and it is essential for health care providers to recognize their own biases and take active steps to address them.

INTRODUCTION

Sickle cell disease (SCD) affects around 100,000 individuals in the United States, and millions of individuals globally, with sickle cell pain accounting for the most frequent indication for hospitalization among both adult and

*Corresponding author. Department of Pediatrics, Harbor UCLA Medical Center, 1000 W Carson Street, Box 468, Torrance, CA 90509. *E-mail address:* mshear@dhs.lacounty.gov

https://doi.org/10.1016/j.yapd.2025.12.013
0065-3101/26/

Abbreviations

ASH	American Society of Hematology
CNS	central nervous system
CS	central sensitization
FDA	Food and Drug Administration
HbF	fetal hemoglobin
HSCT	hematopoietic stem cell transplant
IV	Intravenous
NHLBI	National Heart, Lung, and Blood Institute
NSAID	nonsteroidal anti-inflammatory drug
OIH	opioid-induced hyperalgesia
OWS	opioid withdrawal syndrome
PCA	patient-controlled analgesia
SCD	sickle cell disease
SNRI	serotonin-norepinephrine reuptake inhibitor
TCA	tricyclic antidepressant
VOE	vaso-occlusive episode

pediatric patients [1,2]. SCD describes a group of inherited blood disorders in which there is a point mutation in the gene that codes for β-globin such that valine is coded instead of glutamic acid at the sixth codon of the beta-hemoglobin chain, resulting in hemoglobin S, an abnormal form of hemoglobin that polymerizes when oxygen levels are low. This polymerization results in elongated structures within the red blood cells that create a sickled or crescent shape. In the setting of repeated episodes of polymerization, erythrocytes sickle irreversibly, predisposing individuals with SCD to vaso-occlusive episodes (VOEs), in which they develop acute episodes of pain that are abrupt in onset and often described as sharp and/or throbbing in nature [1,3–5]. In a 2020 article published in *The Lancet*, Hertz Nazaire, an artist living with SCD, shared his experiences with pain (Fig. 1A, B).

> In these times, I am not really alive anymore, I am not experiencing life, and everything is on hold until the medication wears off and a tidal wave of pain overcomes my body all over again. Then comes the next dose of medication and the cycle repeats [6].

Initial presentations of sickle cell pain begin as early as 6 to 9 months of age, with increasing frequency of pain presentations as children age [7]. Dactylitis, which describes VOE in the hands and feet, is more likely to occur among infants and young children, whereas older children and adolescents are more likely to report pain in their back, chest, and/or extremities.

PATHOPHYSIOLOGY OF PAIN IN SICKLE CELL DISEASE

Acute pain (vaso-occlusive episodes)

The mechanisms of acute sickle cell pain are multifactorial and complex, resulting from tissue hypoxia-reperfusion injury, local inflammation, and activation of nociceptors. VOE occurs when sickled erythrocytes become stuck in small

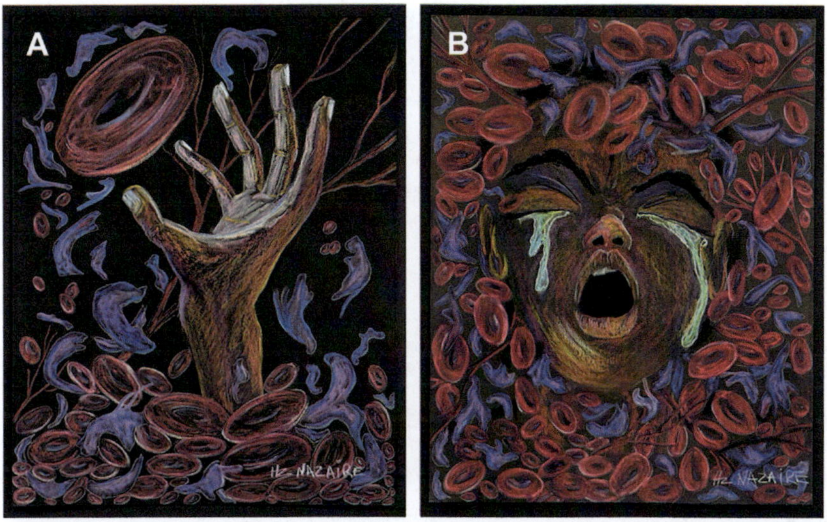

Fig. 1. "Hope" (Panel A) and "Ten Redefined" (Panel B) are two paintings, an artist living with sickle cell disease, who shared his experiences through his art. (Reprinted with permission from Elsevier. The Lancet Haematology. 2020;7(11):e787-e788.)

blood vessels, causing localized tissue ischemia and inflammation (Fig. 2A–D) [4,8]. Interactions between sickled cells and the vascular endothelium result in chronic vascular inflammation, which activates endothelial and blood cells to recruit cells from the innate and adaptive immune system, including macrophages and mast cells, with associated activation of nociceptors [5].

Chronic pain

Chronic pain in SCD is defined as pain that is present on most days for a 6-month period [9]. This is in contrast to the definition of chronic pain in the general population, which is the presence of pain symptoms for at least 3 months [10]. The cause of chronic pain in SCD is varied, often resulting from complications of SCD, such as bone marrow infarction, avascular necrosis, thrombosis, or vertebral collapse [9,11]. Recurrent vaso-occlusive pain, opioid-induced hyperalgesia (OIH), and neuropathic pain can also contribute to central sensitization (CS), in which nociceptors become overly responsive to painful and nonpainful stimuli resulting in hyperalgesia and allodynia, respectively [11]. Symptoms suggestive of neuropathic pain include burning, electric shock sensation, pins and needles, pricking, or shooting sensations [12]. Chronic pain is reported in greater than 50% of older adolescents and young adults with SCD [13].

PAIN PRESENTATIONS IN SICKLE CELL DISEASE

Pain presentations vary significantly across individuals with SCD. Although one individual's VOE may present as a throbbing pain localized deep in a

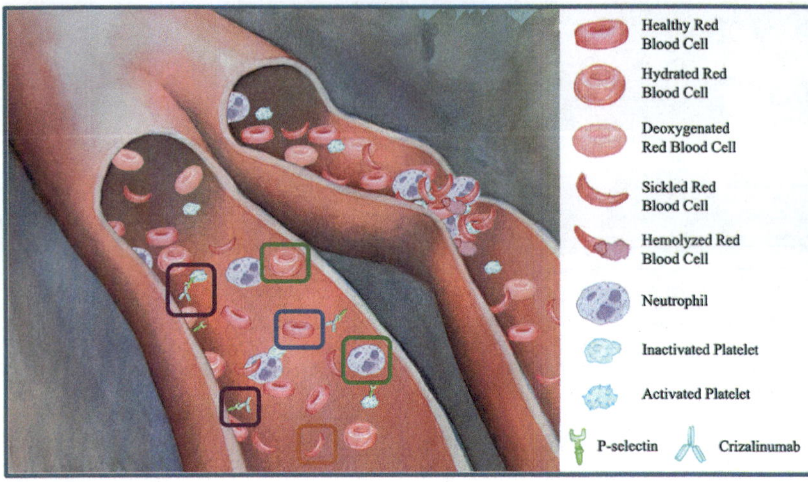

A Hydroxyurea enhances production of fetal hemoglobin, thus reducing hemoglobin polymerization and red blood cell sickling. It also decreases neutrophil and reticulocyte counts and adhesiveness, improves erythrocyte hydration, and increases nitric oxide, which enhances vessel dilation.

B L-Glutamine reduces oxidative damage to red blood cells and increases nicotinamide adenine dinucleotide production, which ultimately increases the redox potential of sickled red blood cells.

C Crizalinumab is humanized monoclonal antibody that blocks P-selectin, a molecule on activated platelets and endothelial cells that promotes platelet aggregation and vaso-occlusion, thereby reducing cellular adhesion.

D Voxelotor stabilizes hemoglobin S to prevent it from polymerizing, thus decreasing sickling and hemolysis and increasing hemoglobin.

Fig. 2. Comparison of a normal blood vessel (*left*) with smooth blood flow and a vessel affected by a sickle cell VOE (*right*), where misshapen red blood cells obstruct circulation, leading to vaso-occlusion and pain. Boxes a through d highlight the proposed mechanisms of four disease modifying therapies: hydroxyurea (A), L-glutamine (B), crizanlizumab (C), and voxelotor (D). The colorful square surrounding each letter indicates the cellular effects of each disease modifying therapy within the figure.

single extremity, another patient may report diffuse and sharp abdominal and back pain with allodynia appreciated on superficial palpation. A significant challenge in managing pain among children with SCD is the risk of missing an alternative diagnosis, as VOE may present concomitantly with other painful manifestations of SCD, such as acute chest syndrome, avascular necrosis, splenic sequestration, hydrops of the gallbladder, or constipation. This can make it difficult to identify the source of pain, and as such, the best way to address the pain of a given individual is to ensure a thorough history has been obtained and that alterative diagnoses have been ruled out.

Triggers of VOE vary significantly across individuals. Inflammatory and environmental triggers have been well described, including injury, infection, hypoxia, dehydration, overexertion, stress, cold weather, or recent menstrual cycle [3]. As such, obtaining a thorough history with a complete physical examination is critical to ruling out alternative causes for pain, which can be easily missed in the setting of SCD. Although sickle cell pain crises that require inpatient hospitalization generally last from 5 to 7 days, there is a large degree of variability between patients, and for some individuals, admissions can last from weeks to months [14].

THE BIOPSYCHOSOCIAL MODEL OF PAIN

The biopsychosocial model is a framework that is helpful to understand the multifaceted and complex nature of pain in SCD (Fig. 3). This model recognizes the complicated relationships between biological, psychological, and social factors on the individual pain experience [15]. Chronic pain in SCD has a known association with anxiety and depression, and it is posited that a negative feedback loop exists such that depression and anxiety result in worsening pain, which can contribute to worsening depression and anxiety [11,16,17]. As

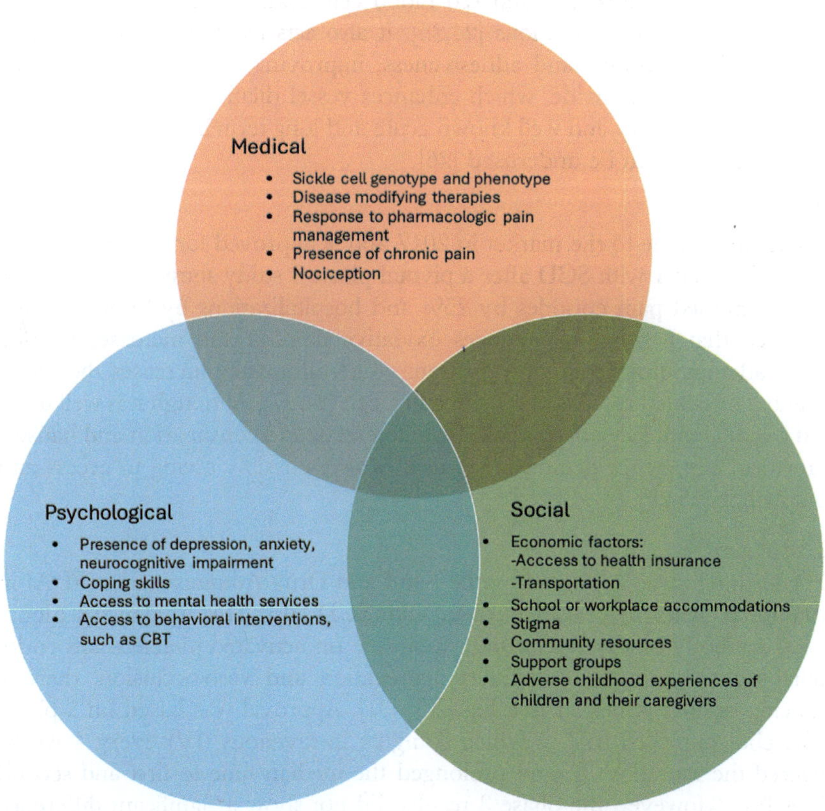

Fig. 3. Biopsychosocial model of pain in SCD. CBT, cognitive behavioral therapy.

such, in considering how best to address sickle cell pain, it is critical to consider how psychological and social factors interplay for a given patient.

DISEASE-MODIFYING THERAPIES

The goal of many disease-modifying medications is to get to the root of the pathophysiology of SCD and ultimately reduce pain [18,19]. Although SCD does not have many treatment options, the landscape is changing, and there are new agents and options on the horizon [20].

Hydroxyurea

Hydroxyurea continues to be the mainstay of treatment options for people with SCD. Currently the National Heart, Lung, and Blood Institute (NHLBI) expert panel report for the management of SCD recommends that hydroxyurea be offered for all children aged 9 months and older with sickle cell anemia (Hemoglobin S-S/Hemoglobin S-Beta Zero thalassemia [HbSS/HbSβ^0]), regardless of clinical severity [19]. The mechanism by which hydroxyurea is thought to work is through enhanced production of fetal hemoglobin (HbF), thus reducing hemoglobin polymerization and red blood cell sickling and reducing known sickle cell–related complications [24,25]. It also acts by decreasing neutrophil and reticulocyte counts and adhesiveness, improving erythrocyte hydration, and increasing nitric oxide, which enhances vessel dilation (see Fig. 2A) [25]. Despite the longevity and well-known acute and long-term benefits of hydroxyurea, it continues to be underused [26].

L-Glutamine

L-Glutamine came to the market in 2017 and is approved for individuals ages 5 years and older with SCD after a pivotal phase 3 study showed that L-glutamine decreased pain episodes by 25% and hospitalizations by 33% [27]. It is proposed that L-glutamine reduces oxidative damage and increases nicotinamide adenine dinucleotide production, which ultimately increases the redox potential of sickled red blood cells (see Fig. 2B) [24,27]. Although it is well tolerated overall, with side effects typically being related to constipation and nausea, real-world experience demonstrates lack of use, possibly owing to access and compliance [28,29].

Crizanlizumab

Crizanlizumab was approved by the Food and Drug Administration (FDA) in 2019 for patients 16 years and older with SCD [30]. This humanized monoclonal antibody blocks P-selectin, a molecule on activated platelets and endothelial cells that promotes platelet aggregation and vaso-occlusion, thereby reducing cellular adhesion (see Fig. 2C) [31]. Approval was based on a phase 2 placebo-controlled trial in which 5 mg/kg intravenous (IV) every 4 weeks lowered the rate of VOE and prolonged the median time to first and second VOE [31]. However, the phase 3 results did not show a significant difference in annualized VOE rates, leaving its efficacy uncertain [32]. It may have a role in men with SCD and priapism, as a small case series reported fewer episodes with treatment [33]. Real-world data are quite sparse and somewhat mixed [34]. Further research is needed to clarify the clinical utility of this newer therapy.

Voxelotor

Voxelotor was originally approved in 2019 for patients ages 12 years and older with SCD, with expanded approval in 2021 to include individuals 4 years and older; however, this medication was removed from the global market in late 2024 owing to concerning findings in international extension trials [35,36]. Voxelotor stabilizes hemoglobin S to prevent it from polymerizing, thus decreasing sickling and hemolysis and ultimately increasing hemoglobin (see Fig. 2D) [37]. Although reported benefits of voxelotor have included decreased frequency of VOE, fewer VOE-related hospitalizations, and decreased opioid usage, this medication is not currently available for use, although ongoing investigation of this drug is yet to be determined [38].

Chronic red cell transfusion therapy

Although chronic transfusions are typically indicated for secondary stroke prevention, some consider the use of chronic transfusions for patients with severe and recurrent sickle cell pain. In individuals with SCD who continue to experience recurrent pain episodes despite optimization with hydroxyurea and other disease-modifying therapies, a trial of monthly blood transfusion may be considered. Although the 2020 American Society of Hematology (ASH) guidelines for the management of acute and chronic pain in SCD do not offer a recommendation for or against monthly transfusion therapy as an option for pain management in refractory persistent SCD, some literature does suggest there may be benefit. Despite possible benefits, however, risks include iron overload, the burden of monthly visits and chelation therapy, IV access challenges, and high cost [21].

TRANSFORMATIVE TREATMENTS

Transformative therapies for people with SCD include hematopoietic stem cell transplant (HSCT) and gene therapy. HSCT has the best outcomes with an HLA-matched sibling; however, this is often not available [39]. Data are improving with haploidentical-related matched transplants [40]. These treatments are typically reserved for patients with severe disease–such as stroke or abnormal transcranial Doppler, frequent VOE, or acute chest syndrome [41]. Typical complications include graft failure, graft-versus-host disease, infection, and infertility [41]. In 2023, two different gene therapy technologies were FDA approved for use in people with SCD 12 years and older. One technique uses CRISPR-Cas9 gene editing to disrupt the BCL11A erythroid enhancer in the patient's hematopoietic stem cells, thereby reactivating HbF production. The other uses a lentiviral vector to insert a modified β-globin gene into the patient's stem cells, producing hemoglobin with antisickling properties [42]. Although exciting treatment options are on the horizon, they are not widely available or feasible for many patients with SCD, and there is still a lack of long-term data to determine the benefit and safety of these treatments.

PAIN MANAGEMENT

Although disease-modifying therapies have helped to reduce the frequency and severity of complications related to SCD, many individuals with SCD continue to experience both acute and chronic sickle cell pain, highlighting the importance of a comprehensive pain plan. In 2020, ASH released guidelines for the management of acute and chronic pain in SCD [21]. These guidelines emphasize the unique and individualized experience that each person with SCD will have when experiencing sickle cell–associated pain. As such, the management approach considered must be tailored to address the pain needs of the individual. Individualized care plans developed in collaboration with the primary care provider, pediatric hematologist, pain specialist, and mental health provider, which take into consideration prior effective pain strategies, can be a useful tool to ensure pain control is optimized and patient preferences are included. SCD acute and chronic pain management can be complex, but evolving treatment approaches seek to improve patient safety, clinical outcomes, and health care utilization [21] (Table 1).

Pharmacologic

Opioids

Opioids remain the mainstay of treatment of sickle cell pain. IV opioids via patient-controlled analgesia (PCA) are considered standard of care at many institutions caring for patients with SCD. Per ASH, a basal IV opioid infusion, in addition to on-demand dosing via PCA, is a widespread practice; however, owing to a lack of strong evidence, it remains unclear if there are advantages over intermittent opioid delivery alone [21]. As such, ASH does not offer a recommendation for or against a basal opioid infusion with on-demand PCA dosing. The 2014 NHLBI expert panel report for the management of SCD, however, cites low-quality evidence in recommending around-the-clock administration by PCA or frequently scheduled doses, rather than dosing only as needed [43]. The NHLBI recommendation was based on the American Pain Society guidelines and review of moderate- to low-quality evidence, including a prospective observational study in Saudi Arabia of 1154 patients, which found a higher discharge rate in patients who received continuous analgesics over an intermittent analgesic regimen [44].

Nonopioid analgesics

Although opioids remain the standard of care in acute pain management in children and adolescents with SCD, a short course of nonsteroidal anti-inflammatory drugs (NSAIDs) of 5 to 7 days is conditionally recommended for acute pain management in the absence of any contraindications [21]. Although NSAIDs are not first-line agents for sickle cell pain management, they should be included as part of a multimodal regimen, provided there are no renal concerns.

Table 1
Suggested pain medication dosing in pediatric sickle cell disease

Name		Dosing		Notes
Acetaminophen		10–15 mg/kg per dose po q4-6h		Not to exceed 75 mg/kg per day or 4000 mg per day, provided there are no contraindications
NSAIDs	Ibuprofen	5–10 mg/kg per dose po q6-8h		Maximum of 40 mg/kg per day or 2400 mg per day, provided there are no contraindications
	Ketorolac	0.5 mg/kg per dose IV q6h		Maximum of 30 mg per dose and 120 mg per day with maximum of 5-d duration. Requires careful monitoring for renal and gastrointestinal side effects
Opioids	Morphine	<50 kg	0.05–0.1 mg/kg IV q2-4h or PCA	Dose hydrophilic opioids (eg, morphine) by ideal body weight and lipophilic (eg, methadone) by total body weight [10]
		≥50 kg	2–4 mg IV q2-4h, titrated to effect	
	Hydromorphone	<50 kg	0.01–0.02 mg/kg IV q2-4h	
		≥50 kg	0.2–0.6 mg q2-4h, titrated to effect	
Ketamine		0.1–0.3 mg/kg per hour up to 1 mg/kg per hour		Used as infusion at subanesthetic doses. Reserved for settings with appropriate monitoring and expertise [21]
Gabapentin		5–10 mg/kg per day divided q8h		Adjunct for opioid-refractory pain, especially with neuropathic features [22]. Not to exceed maximum adult dosing (usually 3600 mg per day)
SNRIs, serotonin-norepinephrine reuptake inhibitors, and TCAs, tricyclic antidepressants		Not available		Potential option for opioid-refractory pain; limited pediatric data and may confer significant risks [23]
Buprenorphine		Not available		Potential option for patients with opioid-induced hyperalgesia, CS, or cyclical OWS

Other nonopioid pharmacologic therapies that have demonstrated promise for chronic pain management among adults with SCD include tricyclic antidepressants (TCAs) and serotonin-norepinephrine reuptake inhibitors (SNRIs). Although SNRIs are recommended for SCD-related chronic pain in adults that do not have an identifiable source, there is no recommendation for or against SNRI use among individuals with chronic pain secondary to avascular necrosis of the bone [21]. In addition, although TCAs are recommended for adults with chronic pain related to SCD without a known cause, no recommendation for or against TCA use is made for children given a lack of data in this age group [21]. As SNRIs and TCAs may increase the risk of suicidal ideation and suicidal behaviors in patients with major depressive disorder and other psychiatric disorders, ASH guidelines do not have a recommendation for or against their use in pediatric populations with SCD [21].

Neuropathic agents

Neuropathic pain is an often unrecognized contributor to sickle cell pain, and screening for the possibility of neuropathic pain through exploration of pain descriptors should be performed any time an increase in frequency of pain occurs or when increased opioid dosing is needed to achieve analgesia [12]. Symptoms of neuropathic pain, allodynia, or pain that presented in the setting of an acute temperature change should prompt consideration for neuropathic pain. Gabapentinoids, such as gabapentin and pregabalin, are first-line medications for neuropathic pain, and although the ASH guidelines recommend this class of medication for adults with SCD-related chronic pain without an identifiable cause, given a lack of data among pediatric populations, there is no recommendation for or against their use in children [12,21]. Many patients also experience coexisting depression and anxiety, which can amplify pain perception. When there is a suspected neuropathic component to a pain presentation, agents such as SNRIs and TCAs should be considered if there are no contraindications, and especially in the setting of coexisting depression or anxiety. It is important to note that neuropathic medications are not first-line treatment of acute VOE, but they may play a role as adjuncts within a broader pain management strategy. Ask the expert: guidance from a pain specialist

At our institution, opioids and PCA utilization is determined based on individual preferences and provider comfort. Oral and IV opioids are encouraged along with nonopioid multimodal medications, including acetaminophen, muscle relaxants, such as methocarbamol, neuropathic agents, and NSAIDs, provided there are no contraindications. If IV opioids are considered, then an as-needed administration is preferred over around-the-clock administration. Given the complexity of pain management with SCD, we typically see our patients using all 3 forms of these administration types.

Our institution preferentially uses hydromorphone as the opioid of choice given our experience with better pain control over morphine. When a hydromorphone PCA is considered, the usual demand dose ranges from 0.1 to 0.4 mg with an administration frequency every 10 to 20 minutes. PCA is only offered to patients who are alert, oriented, able to learn, and able to operate the PCA device independently.

The usual hydromorphone IV dosing range for those ≥20 kg or 7 to 12 years is 0.005 to 0.015 mg/kg IV as needed. Given the usual weight range of our patients, a PCA dosing range of 0.1 to 0.4 mg is generally safe in our experience. PCA is generally not offered to patients weighing less. When used, basal PCA rates are generally dosed at 0.001 to 0.004 mg/kg/hr with a maximum of 0.2 mg/hr for patients greater than 40 kg.

We often do not recommend a basal rate, as it is unlikely to significantly improve pain control during the acute period and may limit the demand doses the patient can safely receive. In select patients, however, a basal rate may be beneficial to maintain pain coverage during sleep and should be considered on a case-by-case basis. Although the use of PCA is not FDA approved for pediatric populations, in patients with acute sickle cell pain, benefits may outweigh the risk and should be considered when appropriate expertise is available (Table 1).

Subdissociative ketamine

Ketamine provides pain relief through *N*-methyl-D-aspartate receptor antagonism, which interrupts transmission of pain signals to the central nervous system (CNS). Subdissociative doses of ketamine starting at 0.1 to 0.3 mg/kg/h with a maximum of 1 mg/kg/h may be considered in patients with refractory or poorly controlled pain. It should be noted, however, that based on the studies available, there is no widely accepted definition of refractory pain [43]. Recent studies have demonstrated improvement in pain and reduced opioid utilization when ketamine was used as adjunctive analgesia for acute SCD pain [45]. Although studies have demonstrated ketamine to be a safe drug at subdissociative doses, administration should be reserved for settings in which appropriate expertise is available. Ask the expert: guidance from a pain specialist

We have found success with subdissociative doses of ketamine coupled with a multimodal pain regimen, which may include NSAIDs, acetaminophen, a muscle relaxant, SNRI or TCA, and gabapentin or pregabalin. Dosing ranges from 0.1 to 0.3 mg/kg of ketamine infused over a 1- to 3-hour duration with a repeat frequency tailored to individual needs. When the IV formulation is unavailable, success has also been observed with oral ketamine. Oral dosing is individualized and is typically 0.5 mg/kg per day divided into 3 to 4 doses. Uptitration is considered in increases of 5 mg per dose depending on pain goal and tolerability.

Regional anesthesia

Regional anesthesia describes the application of a single or continuous infusion of an analgesic agent, such as lidocaine, ropivacaine, or bupivacaine, through an epidural or peripheral nerve catheter, creating a blockade in the pain signal through inhibition of sodium ion influx into nerve fibers [45]. ASH guidelines conditionally recommend regional anesthesia (eg, epidural or peripheral nerve catheter-delivered analgesia for abdominal, hip, or leg pain) for localized pain that is refractory or not effectively treated with opioids alone [21]. Children and adolescents with VOE refractory to opioids that is localized to a single limb may be ideal candidates for regional anesthesia; however, because there is a dearth of high-quality data for use in patients with SCD, regional anesthesia should only be considered in centers with appropriate expertise. Optimal timing and indications for regional anesthesia in acute sickle cell pain among individuals with opioid refractory pain remain uncertain. Additional barriers to regional anesthesia include patient refusal, risk of limiting mobility, prophylactic use of anticoagulation, and the presence of diffuse, or migratory pain that cannot be adequately addressed by a localized block. In addition, among populations of children who experience prolonged episodes of VOE exceeding the typical 5- to 7-days' duration, an indwelling catheter may be suboptimal given safety concerns with prolonged use.

Nonpharmacologic Therapies

In addition to pharmacologic interventions, the 2020 ASH guidelines also sought to explore the use of nonpharmacologic therapies, including yoga, massage, transcutaneous electric nerve stimulation, virtual reality, and guided audio-visual relaxation. Based on multiple studies of children and adults with SCD, the use of nonpharmacologic therapies as an adjunct to pharmacologic therapies is encouraged, with benefits that include reduction in pain intensity and potential benefits of reduced opioid use, improved pain coping mechanisms, and decreased hospital length of stay. Although there is less literature to support their use, acupuncture, biofeedback, mindfulness, cognitive behavioral therapy, and meditation are also listed as therapies that can further improve pain experiences [21].

BARRIERS AND CHALLENGES IN PAIN MANAGEMENT

Despite the availability of multimodal treatment options for sickle cell pain, the reliance on opioids as first-line therapy poses significant challenges. Frequent opioid use places individuals at risk for physical dependence and opioid use disorder. It also increases risk for OIH, a paradoxic hyperalgesia that occurs when patients receive opioids [46,47]. OIH prevalence is unclear among patients with SCD, as there are no clear biomarkers, making it a diagnosis of exclusion [47]. A correlate of OIH is CS, which is another side effect in which the CNS amplifies pain signals despite minimal or absent peripheral input. Among sickle cell patients, CS varies greatly and has been described in 25% to 90% patients [48].

Although OIH and CS demonstrate how treatment with opioids can result in pain intensification, insufficient opioid dosing that follows initial pain control can contribute to cyclic opioid withdrawal syndrome (cyclic OWS). This frequently underrecognized complication can occur when an individual receives prolonged or high-dose opioid administration, such as during a hospital admission for an acute pain crisis, and there is a subsequent rapid decline in dosing or abrupt discontinuation of opioid administration that occurs when the individual is ready to transition home. This may occur after a transition from IV to oral opioids, with a higher risk when switching between opioid drugs or with abrupt discontinuation after achieving adequate pain control. During cyclic OWS, opioid withdrawal symptoms may include low-grade fevers, chills, nausea, vomiting, diarrhea, or gastrointestinal discomfort with progressive pain complaints concerning for recurrence of a VOE (Fig. 4) [11].

Beyond physiologic challenges in pain management among individuals with SCD, broader systemic barriers, such as structural racism in medicine and provider biases, continue to limit equitable care. Given a higher prevalence of SCD among individuals of sub-Saharan African ancestry, Black Americans are disproportionately more affected by SCD and are more likely to experience racial discrimination and stigma associated with their diagnosis [49]. Many individuals with SCD report feeling stigmatized by their diagnosis, with multiple studies demonstrating that health care providers overestimate the prevalence of opioid use and opioid use disorder among those with SCD, with frequent undertreatment of sickle cell pain at presentation and mislabeling of individuals presenting in pain crisis as drug seeking [49]. This is especially challenging given that opioids remain first-line therapy for individuals presenting with pain crisis.

FUTURE DIRECTIONS AND RESEARCH GAPS

Buprenorphine

Given the challenges associated with high levels of opioid use in individuals with chronic sickle cell pain, consideration of alternative treatments, such as

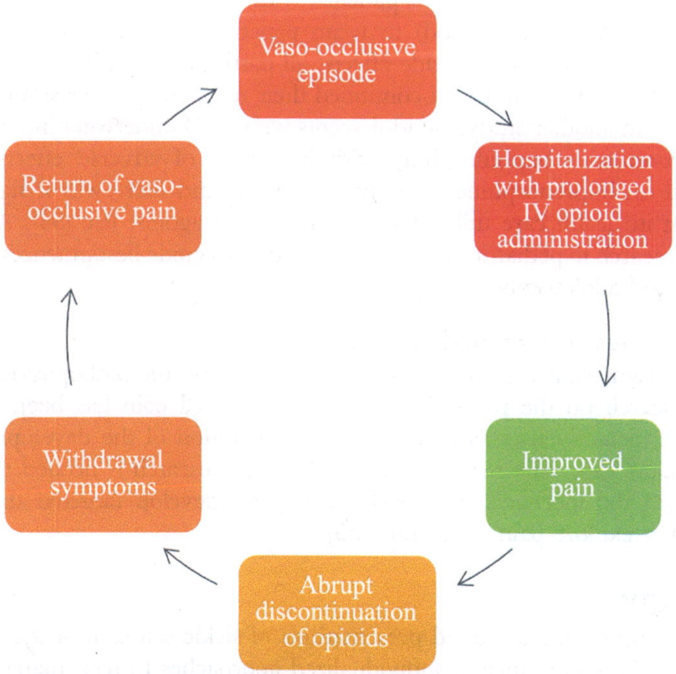

Fig. 4. Cyclic opioid withdrawal syndrome.

buprenorphine, may offer a promising alternative. Buprenorphine is a mixed opioid agonist-antagonist that produces analgesia by binding to opioid receptors in the CNS. It has been approved for use in acute and chronic pain in adult populations since 1981. Because of its unique partial mu-opioid receptor agonism, K-receptor antagonism, and lack of B-arrestin receptor recruitment, buprenorphine has shown promise in effectively treating chronic pain and opioid use disorder in adults, while avoiding harmful side effects like constipation, respiratory depression, and tolerance [50]. Buprenorphine has also proven helpful in avoiding the negative iatrogenic side effects of chronic high-dose opiates, including OIH, CS, and cyclical OWS. Although studies among adult populations have demonstrated that buprenorphine for the use of analgesia is associated with improved function and affect, while decreasing emergency department visits and hospitalization stay, literature on the utilization of buprenorphine for children and adolescents with SCD pain is scant and mostly based on case reports or low-powered studies [51–53].

Although initiation of buprenorphine may be a promising alternative to chronic opioid therapy, if it is administered too soon after a full opioid agonist in opioid-dependent individuals, it can trigger precipitated withdrawal. Historically, induction has required that patients be in mild opioid withdrawal and have discontinued full-opioid agonists for at least 24 hours. In a recent case report, however, alternative approaches to buprenorphine induction have been explored among adolescent patients, with the use of a microdose induction protocol (Bernese method) to wean patients off of large doses of full-agonist opioids with minimal side effects; all participants significantly reduced their health care utilization and continued their regimen for at least months after [52,53]. In another study, 14 adolescents with SCD underwent inpatient microinduction with buprenorphine with low rates of adverse effects. Most remained on buprenorphine over the next year, and there was a significant reduction in health care utilization and full-opioid agonist use [54]. As such, further research in pediatric populations is critical to guide best practices among children and adolescents.

Mechanistic research on sickle cell pain

Although significant research efforts have focused on the pathophysiology of SCD, research on the pathophysiology of sickle cell pain has been limited. This is particularly true as it relates to the evolution of the development of chronic pain, especially in pediatric populations. Research is needed to better understand the mechanisms of sickle cell pain, develop targeted therapies, and further explore pain perception [55].

SUMMARY

Given the complex and varied presentations of sickle cell pain, it is critical to appreciate the importance of individualized approaches to pain management. Patient- and family-centered discussions on acute and chronic pain management are critical to build trust, efficacy, and improved outcomes for patients with SCD. Education and shared decision making can help patients and families understand the potential benefits of current therapies available to address sickle cell pain, and multidisciplinary care teams can help best support the needs of patients.

Given a paucity of literature exploring many of the pain management modalities described above for children and adolescents with SCD, future research efforts are critical to assess the impact of varying pharmacologic and nonpharmacologic modalities on pain outcomes for pediatric patients.

DECLARATION OF AI AND AI-ASSISTED TECHNOLOGIES IN THE WRITING PROCESS

During the preparation of this work, the authors used ChatGPT in order to organize topic content and improve readability. After using this service, the authors reviewed and edited the content as needed and take full responsibility for the content of the publication.

Acknowledgments

Thank you to Jeremy Uglow for the creation of the artwork in Fig. 2.

Disclosure

The authors have nothing to disclose.

References

[1] National Academies of Sciences, Engineering, and Medicine. In: Martinez RM, Osei-Anto HA, McCormick M, editors. Addressing sickle cell disease: a strategic plan and blueprint for action. Washington, DC: The National Academies Press; 2020.
[2] Bou-Maroun LM, Meta F, Hanba CJ, et al. An analysis of inpatient pediatric sickle cell disease: incidence, costs, and outcomes. Pediatr Blood Cancer 2018;65(1):e26758.
[3] Payne JN, Gee BE. Management of acute sickle cell disease pain. Pediatr Rev 2024;45(1): 26–38.
[4] Sundd P, Gladwin MT, Novelli EM. Pathophysiology of sickle cell disease. Annu Rev Pathol 2019;14(1):263–92.
[5] Darbari DS, Sheehan VA, Ballas SK. The vaso-occlusive pain crisis in sickle cell disease: definition, pathophysiology, and management. Eur J Haematol 2020;105(3):237–46.
[6] Nazaire H. Life is a PAINting. Lancet Haematol 2020;7(11):e787–8.
[7] Field JJ, Ballas SK, Campbell CM, et al. AAAPT diagnostic criteria for acute sickle cell disease pain. J Pain 2019;20(7):746–59.
[8] Takaoka K, Cyril AC, Jinesh S, et al. Mechanisms of pain in sickle cell disease. Br J Pain 2021;15(2):213–20.
[9] Dampier C, Palermo TM, Darbari DS, et al. AAPT diagnostic criteria for chronic sickle cell disease pain. J Pain 2017;18(5):490–8.
[10] Hadland SE, Agarwal R, Raman SR, et al. Opioid prescribing for acute pain management in children and adolescents in outpatient settings: clinical practice guideline. Pediatrics 2024;154(5):e2024068752.
[11] Osunkwo I, O'Connor HF, Saah E. Optimizing the management of chronic pain in sickle cell disease. Hematology 2020;2020(1):562–9, 2014, the American Society of Hematology Education Program Book.
[12] Glaros A, Brandow AM. Neuropathic pain in sickle cell disease: measurement and management. Hematology 2020;2020(1):553–61, 2014, the American Society of Hematology Education Program Book.

[13] Kenney MO, Wilson S, Shah N, et al. Biopsychosocial factors associated with pain and pain-related outcomes in adults and children with sickle cell disease: a multivariable analysis of the GRNDaD multicenter registry. J Pain 2024;25(1):153–64.
[14] Shapiro BS. The management of pain in sickle cell disease. Pediatr Clin 1989;36(4): 1029–45.
[15] Brandow A.M., DeBaun M.R., Key components of pain management for children and adults with sickle cell disease, *Hematology/Oncology Clinics*, **32** (3), 2018, 535 - 550.
[16] Levenson JL, McClish DK, Dahman BA, et al. Depression and anxiety in adults with sickle cell disease: the PiSCES project. Biopsychosocial Science and Medicine 2008;70(2): 192–6.
[17] Osunkwo I, Andemariam B, Minniti CP, et al. Impact of sickle cell disease on patients' daily lives, symptoms reported, and disease management strategies: results from the international Sickle Cell World Assessment Survey (SWAY). Am J Hematol 2021;96(4):404–17.
[18] Yates AM, Aygun B, Nuss R, et al. Health supervision for children and adolescents with sickle cell disease: clinical report. Pediatrics 2024;154(2):e2024066842.
[19] Yawn BP, Buchanan GR, Afenyi-Annan AN, et al. Management of sickle cell disease: summary of the 2014 evidence-based report by expert panel members. JAMA 2014;312(10): 1033–48.
[20] Kavanagh PL, Fasipe TA, Wun T. Sickle cell disease: a review. JAMA 2022;328(1): 57–68.
[21] Brandow AM, Carroll CP, Creary S, et al. American Society of Hematology 2020 guidelines for sickle cell disease: management of acute and chronic pain. Blood Adv 2020;4 (12):2656–701.
[22] Puri L, Nottage K, Hankins JS, et al. Gabapentin for acute pain in sickle cell disease: a randomized double-blinded placebo-controlled phase II clinical trial. EJHaem 2021;2(3): 327–34.
[23] Brandow AM, Farley RA, Dasgupta M, et al. The use of neuropathic pain drugs in children with sickle cell disease is associated with older age, female sex, and longer length of hospital stay. J Pediatr Hematol Oncol 2015;37(1):10–5.
[24] Walden J, Creary S. Practical guide for disease-modifying medication management of children and adolescents with sickle cell disease. Hematology 2024;2024(1):604–10.
[25] McGann PT, Ware RE. Hydroxyurea therapy for sickle cell anemia. Expet Opin Drug Saf 2015;14(11):1749–58.
[26] McGann PT. Sickle cell anemia: an underappreciated and unaddressed contributor to global childhood mortality. J Pediatr 2014;165(1):18–22.
[27] Niihara Y, Miller ST, Kanter J, et al. A phase 3 trial of l-glutamine in sickle cell disease. N Engl J Med 2018;379(3):226–35.
[28] Wu H-W, Gannon M, Hsu LL. Evaluation of glutamine utilization in patients with sickle cell disease. J Pediatr Hematol Oncol 2023;45(1):e52–5.
[29] Gotesman M, Elgar G, Santiago LH, et al. Pediatric patients with sickle cell disease at a public hospital: nutrition, compliance and early experience with L-glutamine therapy. in vivo 2022;36(4):1761–8.
[30] FDA approves crizanlizumab-tmca for sickle cell disease. 2019. Available at: https://www.fda.gov/. Accessed September 15, 2025.
[31] Ataga KI, Kutlar A, Kanter J, et al. Crizanlizumab for the prevention of pain crises in sickle cell disease. N Engl J Med 2017;376(5):429–39.
[32] Novartis A. Novartis provides update on Phase III STAND trial assessing crizanlizumab. 2023.
[33] Idowu M, Garcia RL, Sule OB. Successful treatment of SCD-related priapism with crizanlizumab: a case series. Journal of Investigative Medicine High Impact Case Reports 2023;11:23247096231191873.
[34] Cheplowitz H, Block S, Groesbeck J, et al. Real-world data of crizanlizumab in sickle cell disease: a single-center analysis. Journal of Hematology 2023;12(3):105.

[35] FDA approves drug to treat sickle cell disease in patients aged 4 up to 11 years. 2021. Available at: https://www.fda.gov/drugs/news-events-human-drugs/fda-approves-drug-treat-sickle-cell-disease-patients-aged-4-11-years. Accessed September 15, 2025.
[36] FDA is alerting patients and health care professionals about the voluntary withdrawal of oxbryta from the market due to safety concerns. 2024. Available at: https://www.fda.gov/drugs/drug-safety-and-availability/fda-alerting-patients-and-health-care-professionals-about-voluntary-withdrawal-oxbryta-market-due. Accessed September 15, 2025.
[37] Vichinsky E, Hoppe CC, Ataga KI, et al. A phase 3 randomized trial of voxelotor in sickle cell disease. N Engl J Med 2019;381(6):509–19.
[38] Shah N, Lipato T, Alvarez O, et al. Real-world effectiveness of voxelotor for treating sickle cell disease in the US: a large claims data analysis. Expert review of hematology 2022;15(2):167–73.
[39] Gluckman E, Cappelli B, Bernaudin F, et al. Sickle cell disease: an international survey of results of HLA-identical sibling hematopoietic stem cell transplantation. Blood, The Journal of the American Society of Hematology 2017;129(11):1548–56.
[40] Rostami T, Rad S, Rostami MR, et al. Hematopoietic stem cell transplantation in sickle cell disease: a multidimentional review. Cell Transplant 2024;33:09636897241246351.
[41] Stenger EO, Shenoy S, Krishnamurti L. How I treat sickle cell disease with hematopoietic cell transplantation. Blood, The Journal of the American Society of Hematology 2019;134(25): 2249–60.
[42] Sharma A. How I treat sickle cell disease with gene therapy. Blood 2024;144(26): 2693–705.
[43] Evidence-based management of sickle-cell disease: Expert Panel Report 2014. 2014.
[44] Udezue E., Girshab A.M., Observations on the management of acute pain crisis in adult sickle cell disease in eastern Saudi Arabia, *Ann Saudi Med*, **25** (2), 2005, 115 - 119.
[45] Azul M, Brandow AM. Beyond IV push: alternative methods for management of acute pain in SCD. Hematology 2024;2024(1):611–7.
[46] Lee M, Silverman SM, Hansen H, et al. A comprehensive review of opioid-induced hyperalgesia. Pain Physician 2011;14(2):145.
[47] Sagi V, Mittal A, Tran H, et al. Pain in sickle cell disease: current and potential translational therapies. Transl Res 2021;234:141–58.
[48] Campbell CM, Moscou-Jackson G, Carroll CP, et al. An evaluation of central sensitization in patients with sickle cell disease. J Pain 2016;17(5):617–27.
[49] Anderson D, Lien K, Agwu C, et al. The bias of medicine in sickle cell disease. J Gen Intern Med 2023;38(14):3247–51.
[50] Spreen LA, Dittmar EN, Quirk KC, et al. Buprenorphine initiation strategies for opioid use disorder and pain management: a systematic review. Pharmacotherapy 2022;42(5): 411–27.
[51] Davis MP. Twelve reasons for considering buprenorphine as a frontline analgesic in the management of pain. J Support Oncol 2012;10(6):209–19.
[52] Irwin M, Gunther W, Keefer P, et al. Buprenorphine for chronic pain in a pediatric patient with sickle-cell disease. J Pain Symptom Manag 2021;62(5):1086–91.
[53] Buchheit BM, Joslin T, Turner HN, et al. Ambulatory microdose induction of buprenorphine-naloxone in two adolescent patients with sickle cell disease. Pediatr Blood Cancer 2021;68(1):e28766.
[54] Patel A, Kalmus G, Dampier C, et al. Treatment experience using a micro-induction buprenorphine protocol for chronic pain in pediatric sickle cell disease. Pediatr Blood Cancer 2025;72:e31731.
[55] Belfer I, Chen W, Weber W, et al. Unmet need: mechanistic and translational studies of sickle cell disease pain as a whole-person health challenge. J Pain 2024;25(10):104603.

Advances in Pediatrics 73 (2026) 83–105

ADVANCES IN PEDIATRICS

Reducing Restraint Use in the Pediatric Agitated Patient

A Review of Approaches and Best Practices

Desmond L. Green, MD, MPH[a], Neil G. Uspal, MD[b,*]

[a]Department of Child and Adolescent Psychiatry and Behavioral Sciences, Children's Hospital of Philadelphia, Philadelphia, PA, USA; [b]Division of Pediatric Emergency Medicine, Department of Pediatrics, University of Washington, Seattle, WA, USA

Keywords

• Aggression • Agitation • Physical • Chemical • Restraints • Seclusion • De-escalation • Advocacy

Key points

- Review dangers of restraint use and opportunities for early detection and treatment of underlying cause of agitation to minimize their use.
- Review evidence-based approaches to patient de-escalation and other non-pharmacologic means of managing agitation.
- Explain best practices for managing agitation, including safe ways of utilizing medications and physical restraints when needed.
- Identifying further opportunities for advocacy to reduce short-term and long-term consequences of restraint use in pediatric populations.

INTRODUCTION

The behavioral and mental health needs of children have greatly increased over the past few years [1]. According to data from the Centers for Disease Control and Prevention, up to 20% of all children have a mental health disorder [2]. Between 2016 and 2021, the percentage of children in the United States with mental, behavioral, and developmental disorders increased from 25.3% to 27.7% [3]. Emergency department (ED) visits for behavioral complaints have also risen, with the proportion of pediatric ED visit for mental health

*Corresponding author. 4400 Sand Point Way NE, Mail-stop MB.7.520, Seattle, WA 98105. *E-mail address:* Neil.uspal@seattlechildrens.org

https://doi.org/10.1016/j.yapd.2026.02.001

Abbreviations

ASD	autism spectrum disorder
CK	creatine kinase
CT	computed tomography
ED	emergency department
EEG	electroencephalogram
EMS	Emergency Medical Services
EPS	extrapyramidal symptoms
FDA	Food and Drug Administration
ICU	intensive care unit
IM	intramuscular
IV	intravenous
PO	oral

emergencies doubling between 2011 and 2020 [4]. Numerous stressors may be contributory to this increase, including the effects of the coronavirus disease 2019 pandemic [5], ongoing systemic racism [6], homophobia [7] and transphobia [8], and the ubiquity of cell phones and social media [9].

The child mental health crisis has become so concerning that, in 2021, the American Academy of Pediatrics, American Academy of Child and Adolescent Psychiatry, and Children's Hospital Association declared a National State of Emergency in Child and Adolescent Mental Health [10]. One year later, these organizations sent a letter to the Biden administration urging it to make a National Emergency Declaration to address the needs of child mental health. In response, President Biden put forth a comprehensive national strategy for supporting public mental health in the United States, as outlined in his State of the Union Address in 2022 [11,12].

Concomitant with the overall increase in mental health disorders in children has been an increase in mental health conditions associated with externalizing behaviors [13]. Externalizing behaviors are outward, acting-out actions directed at the environment or others, such as aggression, defiance, impulsivity, hyperactivity, and rule-breaking [14]. In the United States, rates of mental health disorders associated with externalizing behaviors in school-aged children vary from 10.1% to 24.3% depending on state of residence [15]. Autism spectrum disorder (ASD) diagnoses, which can be associated with externalizing behaviors, increased 4 fold in children between 2000 and 2020 [16]. Children with externalizing behaviors frequently seek behavioral care in EDs [17] and often have behavioral escalations while in the ED environment [18]. These escalations often include agitation, defined as increased psychomotor activity, restlessness, and emotional distress, and aggression, characterized by behaviors that pose a risk to self, others, or property [19].

Restraint is frequently used in children presenting to EDs with mental health complaints [20,21], The Center for Medicare and Medicaid Services defines a restraint as "any manual method, physical or mechanical device, material, or equipment that immobilizes or reduces the ability of a patient to move his or her arms, legs, body, or head freely; or a drug or medication when it is used as a restriction to manage the patient's behavior or restrict the patient's freedom of movement and is not a standard treatment or dosage for the patient's condition." [22] Restraint use in the clinical management of children with agitation and aggression is controversial. Restraint use is considered necessary when the safety of patients, families, providers, and staff is at imminent risk. However, substantial concern exists that restraint use is inequitable [23], associated with significant harms [23], and is often avoidable [24].

When restraint is used, clinicians should employ the least restrictive restraint modality, and restraint should be used for as brief a time as possible. The goal of restraint should be to keep patients, staff, and families safe while simultaneously providing care, balancing between safety and compassion [22]. Knowledge of best practices around restraints can reduce their use and minimize their harms when they are necessary.

EPIDEMIOLOGY/DISPARITIES IN RESTRAINT USE

Restraint use among children in ED settings has grown in frequency, outpacing increases in overall pediatric ED encounters. One study found that between 2009 and 2019, mental health visits to pediatric EDs increased by 268%, yet chemical restraint use increased by 370% [25]. Among children presenting to US EDs with behavioral complaints, 1.9% to 2.0% are subjected to physical restraint [21,26], while 3.5% to 4.8% were described as receiving chemical restraint [20,25].

Certain patients have been shown to be disproportionately exposed to restraint. In one psychiatric facility, 5% of patients accounted for 50% of overall restraint use [24]. Frequency of exposure to restraint is also associated with a patient's diagnosis. Disruptive disorders (alcohol-related disorders, ASD, conduct disorder, and intermittent explosive disorder) are associated with an increased risk of restraint use [27]. Patients with ASD are 2.3 times more likely to be restrained than children without ASD [28]. Patients with ASD in children's hospital inpatient units were described as experiencing chemical restraint on approximately 8% of patient days, the highest rate of exposure of any diagnostic group [29].

Multiple studies have shown that black race is also associated with higher rates of restraint use independent of patient diagnosis. The largest of these studies, examining over 500,000 pediatric mental health visits at children's hospitals, found Black patients were 22% more likely to be restrained than White patients [30]. In a New England health care system, Black patients were found to be 80% more likely to be restrained relative to their White counterparts. Interpersonal racism, institutional racism, and systemic racism were identified as possible drivers of this disparity [31]. Additional risk factors for restraint use include being a male individual [30,31] and having public insurance [27,31].

Restraint is also used frequently in the prehospital setting; 9.5% to 12.3% of children with mental health complaints are physically restrained during Emergency Medical Services (EMS) transport [32,33]. Black race and transport from a higher economic disadvantage neighborhood are associated with a higher likelihood of handcuffing by law enforcement during transport [34]. Additionally, children who are male individuals, aged less than 12 years, and transported from school settings are at higher risk of requiring physical restraint.

SEQUELAE OF EXPOSURE TO RESTRAINT

Being restrained against one's will is universally distressing. A concomitant disruptive disorder or related condition may worsen the distress of restraint, increasing feelings of fear, anger, confusion, and emotional instability [35]. Restraint use is particularly harmful for children, who are still growing physical, mentally, socially, and emotionally. Restraint use can have lasting effects on pediatric patient's sense of self, overall feelings of security, and larger relationship with the health care system. Especially when coupled with discrimination and bias faced in other settings, restraint can have permanent deleterious effects [36,37]. While both chemical and physical restraints are associated with physical and psychological harm, physical restraint is particularly associated with deleterious effects [38].

In the school setting, higher rates of restraint use carry an increased risk of not completing high school, need to remediate school years, and involvement with the legal system [39]. Adults have been shown to experience posttraumatic stress disorder after restraint in either inpatient psychiatric facilities or intensive care unit (ICU) settings [40,41]. A review of research articles examining children's experiences of physical restraint found it led to feelings of "anger, fear, loneliness, distress, powerlessness, not being listened to, sadness, tiredness, pain, regret, punishment, suicidal, humiliation, [and] loss of autonomy." [42]

Restraint is also associated with physical harm. Physical restraints carry significant risks including asphyxia, strangulation, sudden death, abrasions, skin breakdown, contusions, extremity fractures, joint dislocations, neurovascular compromise, and rhabdomyolysis leading to acute renal failure [22]. A seminal 1998 article documented 142 deaths during or shortly after restraint or seclusion over the previous decade in mental health facilities and group homes [43]. Nunno and colleagues [44] has since documented 79 restraint-related deaths of children between 1993 and 2018, including 22 in psychiatric care centers. In adults, rates of patient injury are estimated to occur in 0.8% to 4.0% of clinical events where physical restraint was used [45].

IDENTIFICATION AND PREVENTION OF AGITATION AND AGGRESSION

The best strategy for the management of agitation is to identify at-risk patients and implement mitigation strategies to reduce restraint use on both individual and systems levels. Risk factors for agitation include prior history of acute agitation (especially in the last 24 hours), personal history of abuse or being a victim of violence or trauma, communication barrier such as neurodivergence or developmental delay, male sex, predisposing mental and behavioral health conditions, and transient living situations such as foster care, group homes, and incarceration [46].

EDs and other settings that take care of patients at risk for agitation can take steps to reduce the risk of patient escalation. While a medical evaluation is occurring, clinicians should obtain history to evaluate risk factors for agitation. The care environment for identified high-risk patients should be modified to remove anything in the milieu that the patient could use to harm themselves or others. Having a trusted caregiver to whom patients are relatively securely attached to can also be a helpful mitigation strategy for escalation [46]. Caregivers can also be helpful in identifying both triggers for agitation and the best means of patient de-escalation. Note that sometimes caregivers themselves can be a trigger for agitation and thus should be removed, if appropriate, even if for a brief period during de-escalation efforts [47]. Creating schedules for patients and giving anticipatory guidance of expectations can help reduce anxiety around evaluation or hospitalization [48]. For patients with ASD, minimizing wait times, rooming patients in low stimulus spaces, and offering comfort items can also reduce the risk of agitation [48].

In the ED, it is also important to recognize early signs of agitation and aggression, which can help to avoid further escalation and more invasive interventions. Presentation of agitation can vary, but includes difficulty calming, pacing or restlessness, paranoia or incredulousness, irritability, hostility, confusion, disorientation, difficulty communication, and vital sign changes [49]. Predicting which patients are at an increased risk for requiring restraint allows preemptive measures and appropriate resource allocation. Predictive modeling shows promise in allowing for early identification of patients at risk for aggression. The Brief Rating of Aggression by Children and Adolescents–Short version is a 5 question screening tool that has been shown to effectively stratify children with behavioral health complaints into low-risk, moderate-risk, and high-risk tiers, though it has not been prospectively validated [50]. Other tools have either shown poor sensitivity [51] or have limited evidence of efficacy [52] in the ED setting.

APPROACH TO THE MANAGEMENT OF AGGRESSIVE PATIENTS IN EMERGENCY DEPARTMENT AND INPATIENT SETTINGS

Most patients who present with behavioral health emergencies are initially evaluated in the ED, where knowledge of past medical and psychiatric history is often limited, at least initially. In these situations, it is important to consider organic etiologies of agitation. This is particularly salient for patients with neurodevelopment differences who may perceive and communicate their symptoms differently [53]. Thorough medical investigation in patients with ASD often finds physical pain as causative of agitation in these patients [54].

Close attention to history, physical examination findings, and vital signs, including presence of fever, which can indicate an organic cause of their aggression such as intoxication, infection, or thyrotoxicosis, are crucial [46]. Conditions that could cause agitation include electrolyte derangements (eg, uremia, hypo/hypernatremia, and hypo/hyperglycemia), infection, thyroid dysfunction, withdrawal (either from scheduled medications or from substance use), intoxication and ingestions, head trauma, postictal states, and pain (Table 1) [55].

In the management of agitated patients, the use of physical restraint and/or pharmacologic interventions should be considered only after other nonrestraint options have been considered and attempted. In general, pharmacologic interventions are preferred over physical restraint. It is vital to have staff training and policies in place for managing patients with agitation and restraint use.

Verbal de-escalation

The first step in the management of any agitated patient is de-escalation. De-escalation can be described as a set of interwoven communication strategies and actions that aim to eliminate or reduce patient aggression/agitation irrespective of cause, while minimizing patient coercion or restriction [56]. De-escalation respects patient autonomy and is the safest means of addressing agitation and aggression. It can be effectively used even on the most agitated patients [57]. Goals of this approach include both calming the patient and determining and addressing the etiology of the agitation to prevent future occurrences [22].

There are several techniques that can be utilized in de-escalation. The American Association for Emergency Psychiatry describes 10 domains of de-escalation (Table 2) [58]. Similarly, the ERASER mnemonic, used by Los Angeles County EMS, can also be helpful to recall steps of verbal de-escalation, particularly in prehospital settings: *E*yeball the patient, *R*espect the patient's space, *A* single member of EMS personnel does the talking and builds rapport, *S*ensible listening, *E*stablish expectations and set boundaries, *R*easonable choices are given to the patient [59].

When using verbal de-escalation, it is important to use a calm and neutral tone when speaking and communicate via nonthreatening body language [46]. Showing acceptance, support, and warmth for another person (or oneself) without judgment or conditions, known as positive regard and empathy, has benefit in all settings of mental health care, from psychotherapy to de-escalation events [60,61].

Successful implementation of de-escalation strategies requires a multidisciplinary approach. Mental health professionals, security officers, child life specialists, nurses, and physicians are all key in facilitating successful verbal de-escalation strategies, and all should be familiar with and/or trained in de-escalation management, working together as a team [62]. Free online training resources in de-escalation are available online [63,64], though they are not specific to pediatrics. Behavioral response teams can also be utilized for advanced de-escalation support at the bedside [62].

Pharmacologic Interventions

Pharmacologic interventions are warranted when de-escalation techniques are not effective and there is no immediate danger to the patient or staff. When there is immediate danger, pharmacologic restraint can be used concomitantly with or after immediate physical restraint. Pharmacologic interventions should be used in concert with ongoing nonpharmacologic de-escalation.

Table 1
Selected organic etiologies of agitation and recommended evaluation

Etiologic	Clinical presentation	Suggested workup
Electrolyte derangements (eg, uremia, hypo/hypernatremia, and hypo/hyperglycemia)	Altered mental status, nausea, vomiting, fluid retention, seizures, and blood pressure changes	Basic metabolic panel and urine studies
Bloodstream infection/Sepsis	Altered mental status, fever, tachycardia, and hypotension	Blood culture, complete blood count, C-reactive protein and/or erythrocyte sedimentation rate, and lactate
Meningitis	Altered mental status, fever, seizure, tachycardia, and hypotension (sepsis)	MRI, lumbar puncture, and electroencephalogram (EEG)
Thyroid dysfunction	Fever, tachycardia, arrythmias, hypertension, confusion, heat/cold intolerance, edema, nausea, and vomiting	Thyroid studies (thyroid-stimulating hormone [TSH], free T4), chest radiography or computed tomography (CT) scan (to assess for thymoma), and EKG
Postictal state	Confusion, preceding seizure-like activity on examination or by history	EEG, obtain thorough history
Opioid withdrawal	Lacrimation, rhinorrhea, piloerection, myalgia, diarrhea, nausea, vomiting, pupillary dilation, photophobia, insomnia, autonomic hyperactivity, yawning, and irritability	Medication reconciliation, obtain thorough history Clinical Opioid Withdrawal Scale
Benzodiazepine and alcohol withdrawal	Sleep disturbances, irritability, increased anxiety/panic attacks, hand tremors, shaking, sweating, confusion, nausea, vomiting, diarrhea, headaches, seizures, delirium tremens (alcohol use), and alcoholic hallucinosis (alcohol use)	Medication reconciliation, obtain thorough history, Clinical Institute Withdrawal Assessment for Alcohol or Benzodiazepines, ethanol level
Alcohol intoxication	Walking difficulties, agitation, slurred speech, nausea, and vomiting	Ethanol level/blood alcohol content measurement

(*continued on next page*)

Table 1
(*continued*)

Etiologic	Clinical presentation	Suggested workup
Phencyclidine (PCP), methamphetamine intoxication	Hypertension, tachycardia, nystagmus (primary care physician [PCP] only), sweating, behavioral changes often with retrograde amnesia (PCP only), paranoia, dissociation, tactile hallucinations (methamphetamines only), and repetitive uncontrollable movements (methamphetamines only)	Urine drug screen, creatine kinase (CK) to assess for rhabdomyolysis
Head trauma	History of recent injury, physical injury at site of collision, ± altered mental status	CT scan, MRI
Pain	Grimacing, relentlessness, hypertension, tachycardia, irritability, and guarding	Obtain history, appropriately treat pain and monitor for resolution of agitation
Sympathomimetic toxicity	Tachycardia, hypertension, hyperthermia, mydriasis (dilated pupils), diaphoresis (sweating), and seizure	Medication reconciliation, obtain thorough history, acetaminophen and salicylate level, EKG, complete metabolic panel, urine drug screen, and CK
Serotonin syndrome	Tachycardia, hypertension, hyperthermia, diaphoresis, neuromuscular hyperactivity, gastrointestinal symptoms, and seizure	Medication reconciliation, obtain thorough history, acetaminophen and salicylate level, EKG, complete metabolic panel, and urine drug screen
Anticholinergic toxicity	Anhidrosis (dry skin), hyperthermia, mydriasis, urinary retention, decreased bowel sounds, seizure, and arrythmia	Medication reconciliation, obtain thorough history, acetaminophen and salicylate level, EKG, complete metabolic panel, and urine drug screen
Cholinergic toxicity	Bronchorrhea, bronchospasm, bradycardia, miosis, hypersalivation, lacrimation, urination, diarrhea, vomiting, and diaphoresis, and seizure arrythmia	Medication reconciliation, obtain thorough history, acetaminophen and salicylate level, EKG, complete metabolic panel, and urine drug screen
Acute mania and psychosis	Assess for Mania via DIGFAST (*D*istractibility, *I*ndiscretion/Impulsivity, *G*randiosity, *F*light of ideas, *A*ctivity increase, *S*leep deficit, and *T*alkativeness), paranoia, delusions, disorganized thinking and speech, and auditory/visual hallucinations (psychosis)	Consult psychiatry

Adapted from Refs [87,100,101].

Table 2
The 10 domains of verbal de-escalation

Domain	Explanation
Respect Personal Space	Maintaining at least 2 arm's length distance respects the patient's space, keeps clinicians safe, and minimizes patient retraumatization
Do Not Be Provocative	Clinicians should assume a relaxed posture, keeping hands visible to the patient and avoiding challenging statements
Establish Verbal Contact	Have one trained clinician communicate with the patient who introduces themselves and states they are present to help the patient
Be Concise	Avoid confusion by making simple statements and repeating key messages
Identify Wants and Feelings	Listen for and ask about the stressors that have led to the patient's dysregulation
Listen Closely to What the Patient Is Saying	Convey empathy and understanding in your words and posture. Attempt to understand the situation from the patient's perspective
Agree or Agree to Disagree	Find areas of agreement between yourself and the patient. This may be in facts, principles, or that others would share the patient's feelings in their situation. Agree to disagree when there is no honest way to agree with the patient
Lay Down the Law and Set Clear Limits	Establish where firm boundaries exist, such that patients hurting themselves or others, and the consequences of crossing those boundaries. Establish that mutual respect will allow the patient to be helped
Offer Choices and Optimism	Offer choice to give patients a sense of control. This may be in provision of nonpharmacologic aids (ie, blankets and food) or, where applicable, the means of receiving medication. Remind patients that things will improve and be positive but realistic in your ability to help patients solve problems
Debrief the Patient and Staff	Once the patient is de-escalated, discuss the reasons for intervention with them. Work with patients to discuss alternative ways of handling stressors. Debriefing should also occur with staff to discuss thing that went well and could have been improved in the care of the patient

Adapted from Richmond JS, Berlin JS, Fishkind AB, et al. Verbal De-escalation of the Agitated Patient: Consensus Statement of the American Association for Emergency Psychiatry Project BETA De-escalation Workgroup. West J Emerg Med 2012;13(1):17–25. https://doi.org/10.5811/westjem.2011.9.6864.

The term "chemical restraint" is controversial. Chemical restraint had previously defined as the "involuntary use of psychoactive medication in a crisis situation to help a patient contain out-of-control aggressive behavior." [65] More recently, this terminology has fallen out of favor [38]. As discussed previously, definition of restraint includes "restriction to manage the patient's behavior or restrict the patient's freedom of movement." [22] However, in most cases medications are administered to calm dangerous behaviors, thereby allowing more freedom to interact with the environment. Therefore, in general, the term "pharmacologic treatment of agitation" is preferable [38].

The first step when considering the use of pharmacologic interventions is to review the patient's medication list if possible and ensure timely administration of scheduled home medications. Medications prescribed as needed at home for agitation or anxiety should also be considered, as it is likely that these medications are known to be effective and well tolerated. Additional doses of these same home medications can also be considered [46]. Home medication administration reduces the risk of patients having a paradoxic medication reaction, defined as a medication causing the opposite of its intended effect, particularly in patients with ASD [66]. It will also address the possibility of medication withdrawal as a cause of agitation [67].

Unless unsafe to do so, oral (PO) medications should be prioritized over intramuscular (IM) or intravenous (IV) medications to reduce risk of adverse events [47]. If the initial dose of a medication is ineffective, the clinician should administer a second dose of the same medication [68], unless the patient has reached the total daily limit of that medication or is having an adverse reaction [47]. Repeating a medication rather than trying a new one decreases the risk of drug–drug interactions and associated adverse events.

There is no single class of medication that serves as the gold standard when managing pediatric patients with agitation [69]. The choice of medication should be based on a variety of factors including prior medication use, patient age, and the reason for patient agitation (Table 3). Many medications used for the management of agitation can prolong corrected QT interval (QTc). Thus, obtaining a baseline electrocardiogram (EKG) and any history of susceptibility to arrythmias is important when selecting medications with this effect. It is also best practice to consider obtaining a urine drug screen and pregnancy test (for all persons with a uterus) when able, given the teratogenic effect that many of these medications can have on a developing fetus.

Antihistamines

When agitation is of unclear etiology, hydroxyzine and diphenhydramine can be used for first-line treatment, as they have both PO and IM options and are generally well tolerated. These medications have good anxiolytic properties [70] and are frequently used in younger patients [68]. Antihistamines can have anticholinergic side effects so patients should be monitored for delirium and delirium agitation [71]. Antihistamines can also cause paradoxic reactions and should be used cautiously in children with ASD or a history of these reactions [71]. Hydroxyzine can cause QTc interval prolongation and arrhythmias in susceptible individuals [72].

Benzodiazepines

Benzodiazepines are used to treat a broad spectrum of agitation causes, including substance-induced agitation and withdrawal, mania, and psychosis. They are powerful anxiolytics without QTc prolongation risk [69]. Benzodiazepines carry risks of paradoxic reactions, delirium, respiratory depression, and dependence and long-term cognitive effects with ongoing use [69]. The most commonly used benzodiazepines for agitation are midazolam, lorazepam,

Table 3
Common medications for pediatric agitated patients [4]

Medication (drug class)	Benefits	Drawbacks
Diphenhydramine (antihistamine)	• PO, IM, and IV options • No QTc prolongation • Anxiolytic properties	• Strongly anticholinergic so can increase risk of delirium • Can cause paradoxic reactions, particularly in neuro-divergent patients
Hydroxyzine (antihistamine)	• PO and IM options • Significantly less anticholinergic than diphenhydramine • Anxiolytic properties	• Can prolong QTc • Somewhat anticholinergic so can still increase risk of delirium
Diazepam, lorazepam, midazolam (benzodiazepines)	• PO, IM, and IV options • Varying half-lives and onsets of action for several clinical situations • Treats a broad spectrum of agitation causes • No QTc prolongation • Anxiolytic properties	• Can cause paradoxic reactions, particularly in neuro-diverse patients • Should *not* be given within 1 h of IM olanzapine given risk of respiratory depression • Carry risk of chemical dependence and long-term cognitive effects with ongoing use
Risperidone, aripiprazole, quetiapine (second-generation antipsychotic)	• Less EPS risk compared to first-generation antipsychotics • Aripiprazole and risperidone have FDA indications for management of irritability in children with ASD	• PO option only • Increased risk of akathisia • Can somewhat increase QTc (lowest risk with aripiprazole) • Longer onset of action
Olanzapine (second-generation antipsychotic)	• PO and IM options • Noted to be more sedating • Less EPS risk compared to first-generation antipsychotics	• IM olanzapine should *not* be given within 1 h of IM/IV benzodiazepine given risk of respiratory depression • Can somewhat increase QTc • PO option has longer onset of action than benzodiazepines • IV option not available for use given poor tolerance

(*continued on next page*)

Table 3
(*continued*)

Medication (drug class)	Benefits	Drawbacks
Ziprasidone (second-generation antipsychotic	• PO and IM options • Less EPS risk compared to first-generation antipsychotics	• Significantly increases QTc • Theoretic risk of worsening agitation • Need for significant food intake when given orally
Haloperidol (first-generation antipsychotic)	• PO, IM, and IV options • Long history of safe and effective use for agitation	• Significant increased QTc • Increased risk of EPS (to reduce risk, use concomitant anticholinergic or benzodiazepine)
Droperidol (first-generation antipsychotic)	• PO, IM, and IV options • Specifically effective for management of nausea and vomiting	• Significant increased QTc (more than Haldol) • Increased risk of EPS (to reduce risk, use concomitant anticholinergic or benzodiazepine) • Not technically indicated for psychiatric use
Chlorpromazine (first-generation antipsychotic)	• PO and IM options • More sedating than other first-generation antipsychotics	• Significant increased QTc • Increased risk of EPS (to reduce risk, use concomitant anticholinergic or benzodiazepine) • Increased risk of hypotension • Significantly anticholinergic • Lowers seizure threshold • IV option not available for use given poor tolerance
Clonidine, guanfacine (alpha-2 agonist)	• Well tolerated, low side effect profile • Sedating (clonidine more so) • No QTc prolongation • Anxiolytic properties	• PO option only • Guanfacine not very sedating
Dexmedetomidine (alpha-2 agonist)	• Very effective in managing agitation • No QTc prolongation • Anxiolytic properties	• Requires ICU monitoring given significant effects on blood pressure and heart rate • Typically run via continuous infusion
Ketamine (N-methyl-D-aspartate [NMDA] receptor antagonist)	• PO, IM, and IV options • Rapid onset of sedation	• Causes significant sedation requiring ongoing monitoring in ED or ICU • In rare cases can cause QTc prolongation and heart arrhythmias

From Refs [46,68,69,71–73,76,77,81,82,84–86].

and diazepam, all of which have PO and IM/IV options. Benzodiazepine selection is primarily based on medication half-life and onset of action. Diazepam has the longest half-life and onset of action, followed by lorazepam, then midazolam [73].

Antipsychotics

While antipsychotics have shown benefit in the treatment of agitation, clinicians should be mindful of their longer time to onset of action and side effect profile (eg, acute dystonic reactions, neuroleptic malignant syndrome, and other extrapyramidal symptoms [EPS]) [68]. Antipsychotics are frequently used to treat agitation caused by psychosis, characterized by the presence of delusions, hallucinations, or disorganized speech or behavior and delirium, characterized by cognitive dysfunction and agitation caused by intoxication or medical conditions [47,74,75]. Aripiprazole and risperidone have Food and Drug Administration (FDA) indications for the management of irritability in children with ASD. Clinicians should preferentially use second-generation antipsychotics, such as risperidone, olanzapine, ziprasidone, aripiprazole, and quetiapine, over first-generation antipsychotics, such as haloperidol, chlorpromazine, and droperidol [76]. Second-generation antipsychotics are better tolerated with lower rates of QTc prolongation and EPS, including acute dystonic reactions and neuroleptic malignant syndrome, than first-generation medications [69].

If a patient requires IM or IV antipsychotic administration options include olanzapine (IM only), ziprasidone, haloperidol, chlorpromazine, and droperidol. Olanzapine is a good initial choice because it is generally considered safer than its first-generation counterparts and is found to be more sedating than haloperidol [77]. Ziprasidone is probably best avoided even though it has similar efficacy to olanzapine and haloperidol because of the risk of QTc prolongation and theoretic risk of worsening agitation [68]. Coadministration of antipsychotics with benzodiazepines, diphenhydramine, or benztropine (anticholinergic medication) should strongly be considered to reduce the risk of EPS and for better synergistic sedative effects, especially if using a first-generation antipsychotic medication [69]. The exception to this is that olanzapine should *not* be given within an hour of lorazepam, particularly if both medications are administered intramuscularly, as this has been associated with an increased risk of respiratory depression [78].

The literature on relative efficacies of pharmacologic agents for agitation management of pediatric patients in the ED is limited. The recent randomized PEACHy-O study comparing oral olanzapine to oral diazepam found no difference in de-escalation at 1 hour between groups (61% vs 57%, $P = .43$) [79]. The study also found no difference in need for restraint or adverse events across groups. In a single-center, retrospective study in an inpatient psychiatric unit, olanzapine was more likely to lead to de-escalation within 30 minutes than lorazepam or chlorpromazine [80]. A meta-analysis in adult patients looking primarily at IM medication administration found one of the following: (1)

olanzapine, or (2) haloperidol plus promethazine or (3) droperidol to be most effective and safe for agitation treatment, while midazolam had the fastest onset of effect [74]. This study further indicates that choice of pharmacologic intervention should be made on an individual and case-by-case basis, taken into account the patient's medical history and clinical needs at the time of intervention.

As previously discussed, there is no single medication that has superior efficacy in the treatment of acute agitation. One approach would be to use diphenhydramine for younger (prepubescent) patients, lorazepam for patients with agitation associated with intoxication or anxiety or in patients at risk of QTc prolongation. Ultimately, however, individual patient experiences and characteristics need to be considered in treatment decisions.

Alpha-2 agonists

Alpha-2 agonists can treat agitation while having minimal impact on QTc. Clonidine can be used to treat agitation, as it is both safe and is effective in reducing agitation [46]. Unfortunately, there is no IM/IV option of this medication. Guanfacine is also another medication from this drug class, and there is some evidence to support its use in patients with delirium, but is less sedating than clonidine, limiting its use [81]. Dexmedetomidine is effective in treating agitation and hyperactive delirium, but does require monitoring in a critical care unit, given its significant effects on both blood pressure and heart rate [82]. When weaning dexmedetomidine, a clonidine taper should be considered to reduce the risk of rebound agitation from withdrawal [83].

Ketamine

In children with violent agitation at imminent risk of harm to self or others, IM ketamine has been used to achieve rapid sedation [84,85]. It has been shown to achieve more rapid sedation than more traditional agents in adults [86], but its use results in high levels of sedation and risk for ketamine-associated emergence phenomena, which may mimic delirium or psychosis [85]. Given these risks, ketamine use should be limited to situations of highly imminent threat.

Physical restraint

When there is an imminent risk of danger to the patient, family, or staff and all other interventions are unsuccessful, physical restraints may be indicated. While there exists many forms of physical restraints, the primary forms of physical restraint used in the pediatric settings are locked seclusion, 2 point limb restraints (eg, wrists are wrapped in padded material and then secured via ties to the gurney frame to prevent movement of the arms), and 4 point limb restraints. The last 2 are considered mechanical restraints as a subclass of physical restraint. Another form of physical restraint is physically restraining or holding an individual without the use of mechanical restraint. When using physical restraints, the goal should be to use the least restrictive option possible to be effective while maintaining safety [22]. As stated prior, physical restraint carry significant physical and psychological risks. Clinicians should be especially mindful of the risk of rhabdomyolysis in intoxicated patients, and preferentially treat these patients with pharmacologic interventions when possible [87]. Use of restraints should be in combination with ongoing verbal de-escalation techniques as well as pharmacologic interventions, when appropriate. Ongoing evaluation should occur to ensure that restraints are discontinued as quickly and safely as possible.

Including caregivers in discussions of physical restraint use is important. It can be incredibly distressing for families to watch their child be restrained; many, when offered, may prefer not to witness their child in restraints. However, it is important to educate family and the patient on the reasons for physical restraints, the type of restraint being used, and risks and benefits associated with restraint, monitoring protocols while in restraints, and conditions needed for restraint removal [22]. Afterward, families and patients, either separately or together, should be debriefed on the restraint event to reduce psychological harm and help identify mitigation strategies to prevent the need for future physical restraint [22].

Locked seclusion

Of available options, locked seclusion, considered a physical restraint, is the least restrictive. According to the World Health Organization, seclusion is defined as the "practice of isolating an individual by physically restricting their ability to leave a designated area" and should be used for therapeutic intervention only [88]. Locked seclusion is thought to be advantageous by providing an alternative safe environment to de-escalate after violent and/or self-destructive behavior [22]. Most inpatient psychiatric units are required to have "quiet rooms" where patients can self-report when needing time alone; these spaces may not be available in EDs.

While in locked seclusion, the pediatric patient needs continuous monitoring by staff via video or through a window. There is an increased risk of self-harm when patients go into locked seclusion [45]. Locked seclusion also should not be utilized if patients require close medical monitoring, are medically unstable, or are unable to be visualized during seclusion [22].

Nonmechanical physical restraint

Although not rigidly defined, nonmechanical physical restraint refers to individuals using bodily contact to hold a child in place without the use of a mechanical device. The Joint Commission considers physical restraint equivalent to mechanical restraint for regulatory purposes, as nonmechanical physical restraint has similar risk of patient harm [89]. A study of restraint-associated fatalities in medical and nonmedical care setting over a 26 year period found that 63 of 79 deaths were during physical holds, emphasizing the significant risk of this form of restraint [44]. Physical holds may be especially retraumatizing for patients, particularly those with a history of sexual abuse [65]. In the ED and inpatient psychiatric settings, physical restraint may be briefly necessary while patients are transitioned to mechanical restraint; if a patient needs prolonged restraint, mechanical restraint is preferable for the safety of the patient and staff.

"Spit hoods" are masks placed over a patient's face to prevent the spread of salvia or other bodily fluid. Spit hoods should not be employed, as their use has been associated with a number of deaths [90]. If there are concerns about a patient spitting on staff, staff should wear face shields.

Mechanical restraint

In 2 point restraint, both wrists are tied to an immobile, sturdy apparatus, typically the frame of a bed, while in 4 point restraint, all limbs are tied to the apparatus [22]. In the vast majority of cases, 2 point restraints should be utilized over 4 point restraints, as prolonged restraint application and increased movement restriction is associated with an increased risk of psychological and physical harm [38,45].

When using limb-restraints, it is important that an appropriate number of trained professionals assist in placement to perform the act as smoothly and safely as possible [87]. Ideally, 5 people, one for each limb and a fifth for the head, are present for restraint placement [91]. Patient should be placed in mechanical restraints preferably when in the supine position with the head of the bed elevated and the patient allowed cervical movement [87]. Prone positioning may be necessary when supine positioning is not feasible due to patient noncompliance, though this is associated with increased patient risk [87]. Hospitals are required by accreditation bodies to have detailed policies on the use of physical restraints and seclusion [89].

Removal of restraints should be done in a calm, organized manner. Patients should be talked through the steps of restraint removal in a calm tone. Whether restraints are removed stepwise (eg, 4 point to 2 point) or all at once is situation-dependent and clinician-dependent. However, patients should never be left alone with only one wrist retrained or have wrists freed before their feet. This creates potential for patient injury, especially if they become agitated upon restraint removal [92].

Medico-legal requirements

Given the safety risk of physical restraint, the Joint Commission on Accreditation of Healthcare Organizations (JCAHO) has detailed patient monitoring and assessment requirements. When a patient is placed in any form of physical restraint, an order must be placed and a face-to-face evaluation performed by a licensed practitioner within 1 hour of restraint initiation [38]. Ongoing evaluation by a staff member is required every 15 minutes to assess for physical safety and patient's readiness to have restraints discontinued [22]. Restraint orders are time limited based on age: 4 hours for adults aged 18 years or older, 2 hours for youth aged 9 to 17 years, and 1 hour for children aged younger than 9 years [89]. After this time has elapsed, the licensed practitioner must reassess the patient to determine the need for continued restraint use prior to reordering restraint.

It is important that clear documentation occurs in the EMR after every restraint event. While each hospital has their respective policies on information required for documentation, documentation detailing the state of the emergency requiring the physical restraint, benefits of treatment of the patient necessitating restraints, and inability to obtain consent provides legal protection [91].

OPPORTUNITIES FOR ADVOCACY

Given the potential for marked physical and psychological harms and inequity of restraint use, it is imperative that all of us who care for children seek ways to reduce restraint use. The first step in this process is reaching a standardized consensus on what is considered pharmacologic restraint. What is the threshold between giving a medication to allow children more freedom to interact with their environment and giving that same medication to restrain them? [29] While the former is the ideal goal of treatment, the latter may be the be the safest alternative in children at risk of imminent harm to self or others. Additionally, the variable effects of these medications make the outcomes of their use hard to predict. Often the primary goal of treatment may be to eliminate dangerous behaviors irrespective of the patient's subsequent ability to interact with their environment.

The inequitable use of restraints in minoritized children who are racial, ethnic, sexual, or gender minorities necessitates interventions to recognize and address implicit bias that may lead to inequitable use of restraint in these patients. All staff involved in restraint application should receive training in awareness of and mitigation of implicit bias, institutions should actively track restraint use for inequity, and institutions should utilize restraint checklists that ensure other nonrestraint interventions are equitably considered and employed before resorting to restraint [93].

Encouragingly, there are several studied interventions that have reduced restraint use. A large children's hospital's inpatient unit, where patients boarded awaiting psychiatric disposition, used team-based quality improvement methodology to reduce physical restrained use from 2.6% to 0.9% over a 2 year period without additional harm to staff [94]. Interventions included systems to recognize early signs of escalation, a new order set, restructure of clinical teams, and development of individualized care plans. Another study showed that implementation of a clinical debriefing program following behavioral events was associated with a 67% decrease in recurrence of restraint use for ED patients and an 82% reduction in time patients spent in restraints. Other strategies to reduce restraint use include environmental modification, specialized behavioral response teams, and improved patient and family involvement in care planning [65,89]. Borrowing from school data, Hodgkiss and Harding indicates that use of Positive Behavioral Interventions and Supports to promote positive interactions with the child's environment also can help minimize restraint use [95].

Standardization of care through pathways and order sets has also shown promise in reducing the need for physical restraint. A dedicated quality improvement intervention to improve care of agitation that included a standard care pathway and order set and personalized care plan among other interventions showed both improved adherence to recommended medication and a median decrease in patient time in restraints [96]. A number of pathways for agitation are either published or readily available online [68,97–99].

SUMMARY

Patient restraint remains a necessary component of care for patients who are in imminent danger of harming themselves or others. Yet restraint use has been demonstrated to be inequitable, physically and psychologically harmful, and, in rare cases, fatal. Through knowledge of signs of early escalation, techniques for de-escalation, methods of restraint, and individual and systems changes to reduce the use of restraint, clinicians may provide the best, most humane care for these high-risk patients.

CLINICS CARE POINTS

- Early signs of agitation, such as difficulty calming, pacing, irritability, hostility, and difficulty communicating, should be recognized and addressed with verbal deescalation techniques to reduce the risk of more severe agitation and aggression.
- Clinicians should priortize the use of home and orally administered medications when pharmacologically treating agitation.
- Physical restraint should only be utilized when there is imminent danger to patients, family or staff. The least restrictive option should be used for physical restraint, and restraint should be discontinued as soon as safely possible.

Disclosure

The authors have nothing to disclose.

References

[1] Child and Adolescent Mental Health. 2022 national healthcare quality and disparities report [internet]. Agency for Healthcare Research and Quality (US); 2022. Available at: https://www.ncbi.nlm.nih.gov/books/NBK587174/. Accessed November 30, 2025.
[2] Weitzman C, Guevara J, Curtin M, et al. Promoting optimal development: screening for mental health, emotional, and behavioral problems: clinical report. Pediatrics 2025;156 (3):e2025073172; https://doi.org/10.1542/peds.2025-073172.
[3] Leeb RT, Danielson ML, Claussen AH, et al. Trends in mental, behavioral, and developmental disorders among children and adolescents in the US, 2016–2021. Prev Chronic Dis 2024;21; https://doi.org/10.5888/pcd21.240142.
[4] Bommersbach TJ, McKean AJ, Olfson M, et al. National trends in mental health-related emergency department visits among youth, 2011-2020. JAMA 2023;329(17):1469–77.
[5] Hillis SD, Blenkinsop A, Villaveces A, et al. COVID-19-Associated orphanhood and caregiver death in the United States. Pediatrics 2021;148(6):e2021053760; https://doi.org/10.1542/peds.2021-053760.
[6] Lazaridou FB, Heinz A, Schulze D, et al. Racialised identity, racism and the mental health of children and adolescents. Int Rev Psychiatry 2023;35(3–4):277–88.
[7] Feinstein BA, van der Star A, Dorrell KD, et al. Sexual orientation and mental health in a US cohort of children: a longitudinal mediation study. J Child Psychol Psychiatry 2024;65(2): 188–98.

[8] Becerra-Culqui TA, Liu Y, Nash R, et al. Mental health of transgender and gender nonconforming youth compared with their peers. Pediatrics 2018;141(5):e20173845; https://doi.org/10.1542/peds.2017-3845.
[9] Fassi L, Thomas K, Parry DA, et al. Social media use and internalizing symptoms in clinical and community adolescent samples: a systematic review and meta-analysis. JAMA Pediatr 2024;178(8):814–22.
[10] AAP-AACAP-CHA declaration of a national emergency in child and adolescent mental health. Available at: https://www.aap.org/en/advocacy/child-and-adolescent-healthy-mental-development/aap-aacap-cha-declaration-of-a-national-emergency-in-child-and-adolescent-mental-health/. Accessed November 30, 2025.
[11] Health organizations urge the biden administration to declare a federal national emergency in children's mental health. Available at: https://www.aap.org/en/news-room/news-releases/aap/2022/health-organizations-urge-the-biden-administration-to-declare-a-federal-national-emergency-in-childrens-mental-health/. Accessed November 30, 2025.
[12] FACT SHEET: Biden-harris administration highlights strategy to address the national mental health crisis I the American presidency project. Available at: https://www.presidency.ucsb.edu/documents/fact-sheet-biden-harris-administration-highlights-strategy-address-the-national-mental. Accessed January 15, 2026.
[13] Momen NC, Beck C, Lousdal ML, et al. Mental health disorder trends in Denmark according to age, calendar period, and birth cohort. JAMA Psychiatry 2025;82(2):161–70.
[14] Liu J. Childhood externalizing behavior: theory and implications. J Child Adolesc Psychiatr Nurs 2004;17(3):93–103.
[15] Danielson ML, Bitsko RH, Holbrook JR, et al. Community-based prevalence of externalizing and internalizing disorders among school-aged children and adolescents in four geographically dispersed school districts in the United States. Child Psychiatry Hum Dev 2021;52(3):500–14.
[16] Maenner MJ, Warren Z, Williams AR, et al. Prevalence and characteristics of autism spectrum disorder among children aged 8 years - autism and developmental disabilities monitoring network, 11 sites, United States, 2020. MMWR Surveill Summ 2023;72(2):1–14.
[17] Waseem M, Moustafa AF, Esposito KD, et al. Characteristics of young children presenting to the emergency department for psychiatric evaluation. J Emerg Med 2025;80:104–11.
[18] Garrick A, Lee ML, Scarffe C, et al. An Australian cross-sectional survey of parents' experiences of emergency department visits among children with autism spectrum disorder. J Autism Dev Disord 2022;52(5):2046–60.
[19] Salvi V, Orsolini L, Martino LM, et al. Recognizing, managing and treating acute agitation in youths. Curr Pharm Des 2022;28(31):2554–68.
[20] Tang AS, Shieh MS, Pekow PS, et al. Treatment of pediatric behavioral health patients with intravenous and intramuscular chemical restraints: results from a nationwide sample of emergency departments. Acad Emerg Med 2023;30(10):1029–38.
[21] Agraharkar S, Horwitz S, Lewis K, et al. Agitation and restraint in a pediatric psychiatric emergency program: clinical characteristics and diagnostic correlates. Pediatr Emerg Care 2021;37(12):e836–40.
[22] Haywood M, Patel L. Physical restraint use in the pediatric emergency department. Pediatr Emerg Care 2023;39(10):807.
[23] Eswaran V, Molina MF, Hwong AR, et al. Racial disparities in emergency department physical restraint use: a systematic review and meta-analysis. JAMA Intern Med 2023;183(11):1229–37.
[24] Wong AH, Ray JM, Cramer LD, et al. Design and implementation of an agitation code response team in the emergency department. Ann Emerg Med 2022;79(5):453–64.
[25] Foster AA, Porter JJ, Monuteaux MC, et al. Pharmacologic restraint use during mental health visits in pediatric emergency departments. J Pediatr 2021;236:276–83.e2.
[26] Rolison MJ, Adu M, Faustino IV, et al. 5.1 identifying drivers of physical restraint use in a pediatric emergency department. J Am Acad Child Adolesc Psychiatr 2024;63(10):S7–8.

[27] Luccarelli J, Kalluri AS, Kalluri NS, et al. Pediatric physical restraint coding in US hospitals: a 2019 kids inpatient database study. Hosp Pediatr 2024;14(5):337–47.
[28] Calabrese ME, Sideridis G, Weitzman C. Physical and pharmacologic restraint in hospitalized children with autism spectrum disorder. Pediatrics 2023;153(1):e2023062172; https://doi.org/10.1542/peds.2023-062172.
[29] Dalton EM, Doupnik SK. Envisioning zero: a path to eliminating restraint use in children's hospitals. Pediatrics 2024;153(1):e2023064054; https://doi.org/10.1542/peds.2023-064054.
[30] Foster AA, Porter JJ, Monuteaux MC, et al. Disparities in pharmacologic restraint use in pediatric emergency departments. Pediatrics 2023;151(1):e2022056667; https://doi.org/10.1542/peds.2022-056667.
[31] Nash KA, Tolliver DG, Taylor RA, et al. Racial and ethnic disparities in physical restraint use for pediatric patients in the emergency department. JAMA Pediatr 2021;175(12):1283–5.
[32] Foster AA, Watkins K, Trivedi TK, et al. Physical restraint use in children with mental and behavioral health emergencies in the prehospital setting. J Am Coll Emerg Physicians Open 2023;4(4):e13016; https://doi.org/10.1002/emp2.13016.
[33] Cummings C, Babcock L, Zhang Y, et al. Prehospital restraint use in pediatric patients with mental and behavioral health emergencies. Pediatr Emerg Care 2025;41(1):30.
[34] Watkins K, Glomb NW, Trivedi TK, et al. Race, neighborhood disadvantage, and prehospital law enforcement handcuffing in children with behavioral health emergencies. JAMA Netw Open 2024;7(11):e2443673; https://doi.org/10.1001/jamanetworkopen.2024.43673.
[35] Specialist JT EMT P, Balancing safety and compassion: mechanical restraints in pediatric mental health crises. JEMS: EMS, Emergency Medical Services - Training, Paramedic, EMT News. 2025. Available at: https://www.jems.com/patient-care/mechanical-restraints-in-pediatric-mental-health-crises/. Accessed December 4, 2025.
[36] Forsner M, Cyrén M, Gerdin A, et al. It hurts to get forced: children's narratives about restraint during medical procedures. Paediatric and Neonatal Pain 2023;5(4):110–8.
[37] Stephens G. Impact of seclusion and restraint on post high school outcomes - opening doors to safer and more inclusive schools. 2024. Available at: https://endseclusion.org/2024/01/12/impact-of-seclusion-and-restraint-on-post-high-school-outcomes/. Accessed December 4, 2025.
[38] APA resource document on seclusion or restraint. Available at: https://www.psychiatry.org/getattachment/e9b21b26-c933-4794-a3c4-01ad427eed91/Resource-Document-Seclusion-Restraint.pdf. Accessed December 19, 2025.
[39] 07-23-Beyond-Suspensions.pdf. Available at: https://www.usccr.gov/files/pubs/2019/07-23-Beyond-Suspensions.pdf. Accessed December 19, 2025.
[40] Chieze M, Hurst S, Kaiser S, et al. Effects of seclusion and restraint in adult psychiatry: a systematic review. Front Psychiatry 2019;10:491.
[41] Berger S, Grzonka P, Amacher SA, et al. Adverse events related to physical restraint use in intensive care units: a review of the literature. Journal of Intensive Medicine 2024;4(3):318–25.
[42] Cramer AM, Virgin AS, Barnard-Brak L. Perceptions of the use of restraint with children and young adults with disabilities and mental health disorders: a review of the literature. Child Youth Serv Rev 2024;161:107666; https://doi.org/10.1016/j.childyouth.2024.107666.
[43] Hundreds of the nation's most vulnerable have been killed by the system intended to care for them. – Hartford Courant. Available at: https://www.courant.com/1998/10/11/hundreds-of-the-nations-most-vulnerable-have-been-killed-by-the-system-intended-to-care-for-them/. Accessed December 4, 2025.
[44] Nunno MA, McCabe LA, Izzo CV, et al. A 26-Year study of restraint fatalities among children and adolescents in the United States: a failure of organizational structures and processes. Child Youth Care Forum 2022;51(3):661–80.

[45] Kersting XAK, Hirsch S, Steinert T. Physical harm and death in the context of coercive measures in psychiatric patients: a systematic review. Front Psychiatry 2019;10:400.
[46] Saidinejad M, Foster AA, Santillanes G, et al. Strategies for optimal management of pediatric acute agitation in emergency settings. J Am Coll Emerg Physicians Open 2024;5(4): e13255; https://doi.org/10.1002/emp2.13255.
[47] Gerson R, Malas N, Mroczkowski MM. Crisis in the emergency department: the evaluation and management of acute agitation in children and adolescents. Child Adolesc Psychiatr Clin N Am 2018;27(3):367–86.
[48] Wolpert KH, Kodish I, Kim SJ, et al. Behavioral management of children with autism in the emergency department. Pediatr Emerg Care 2023;39(1):45–50.
[49] Sharma NP, Huecker MR. Agitation. In: StatPearls. StatPearls Publishing; 2025. Available at: http://www.ncbi.nlm.nih.gov/books/NBK493153/. Accessed December 23, 2025.
[50] Ketabchi B, Babcock L, Zhang Y, et al, Cincinnati Children's Hospital Medical Center Prehospital Care Committee. Predicting agitation in the emergency department. Pediatrics 2025;156(1):e2024068727; https://doi.org/10.1542/peds.2024-068727.
[51] Mitra B, Settle K, Koolstra C, et al. Introduction of the broset violence checklist in the emergency department: a retrospective cohort study. Emerg Med Australas 2025;37(1): e14546; https://doi.org/10.1111/1742-6723.14546.
[52] Sund G, Kirkpatrick T, Choi KR. Applying the DASA-YV for aggression risk reduction in pediatric acute care. J Pediatr Nurs 2025;82:e23–30.
[53] Stenning A, Bertilsdotter-Rosqvist H. Neurodiversity studies: mapping out possibilities of a new critical paradigm. Disabil Soc 2021;36(9):1532–7.
[54] Guinchat V, Cravero C, Diaz L, et al. Acute behavioral crises in psychiatric inpatients with autism spectrum disorder (ASD): Recognition of concomitant medical or non-ASD psychiatric conditions predicts enhanced improvement. Res Dev Disabil 2015;38:242–55.
[55] Foster AA, Saidinejad M, Li J. Approach to acute agitation in the pediatric emergency department. Curr Opin Pediatr 2024;36(3):245.
[56] Hallett N, Dickens GL. De-escalation of aggressive behaviour in healthcare settings: concept analysis. Int J Nurs Stud 2017;75:10–20.
[57] Georgadarellis AG, Baum CR. De-escalation techniques for the agitated pediatric patient. Pediatr Emerg Care 2023;39(7):535.
[58] Richmond JS, Berlin JS, Fishkind AB, et al. Verbal De-escalation of the agitated patient: consensus statement of the American Association for emergency psychiatry Project BETA De-escalation workgroup. West J Emerg Med 2012;13(1):17–25.
[59] 1129222_1307.2-VerbalDe-Escalation.pdf. Available at: https://file.lacounty.gov/SDSInter/dhs/1129222_1307.2-VerbalDe-Escalation.pdf. Accessed December 4, 2025.
[60] How to manage acute agitation in children. ACEP now. Available at: https://www.acepnow.com/article/how-to-manage-acute-agitation-in-children/. Accessed December 4, 2025.
[61] Farber BA, Suzuki JY, Lynch DA. Positive regard and psychotherapy outcome: a meta-analytic review. Psychotherapy 2018;55(4):411–23.
[62] Lelonek G, Crook D, Tully M, et al. Multidisciplinary approach to enhancing safety and care for pediatric behavioral health patients in acute medical settings. Child Adolesc Psychiatr Clin N Am 2018;27(3):491–500.
[63] Creating safe scenes training course. 2024. Available at: https://www.samhsa.gov/technical-assistance/dtac/training/safe-scenes. Accessed December 15, 2025.
[64] Verbal De-escalation for Healthcare Professionals. CU psych learning. 2025. Available at: https://cupsychlearning.org/courses/verbal-de-escalation-for-healthcare-professionals/. Accessed December 15, 2025.
[65] Masters KJ, Bellonci C, Bernet W, et al. Practice parameter for the prevention and management of aggressive behavior in child and adolescent psychiatric institutions, with special reference to seclusion and restraint. J Am Acad Child Adolesc Psychiatr 2002;41(2, Supplement):4S–25S.

[66] Persico AM, Ricciardello A, Lamberti M, et al. The pediatric psychopharmacology of autism spectrum disorder: a systematic review - part I: the past and the present. Prog Neuro Psychopharmacol Biol Psychiatr 2021;110:110326.
[67] Storck W, de Laportalière TT, Yrondi A, et al. Withdrawal syndrome after antipsychotics discontinuation: an analysis of the WHO database of spontaneous reports (Vigibase) between 2000 and 2022. Psychopharmacology (Berl) 2024;241(6):1205–12.
[68] Gerson R, Malas N, Feuer V, et al. Best practices for evaluation and treatment of agitated children and adolescents (BETA) in the emergency department: consensus statement of the American Association for emergency psychiatry. WestJEM 2019;20(2):409–18.
[69] Wilson MP, Pepper D, Currier GW, et al. The psychopharmacology of agitation: consensus statement of the American Association for emergency psychiatry Project BETA psychopharmacology workgroup. West J Emerg Med 2012;13(1):26–34.
[70] Sonnier L, Barzman D. Pharmacologic management of acutely agitated pediatric patients. Pediatr Drugs 2011;13(1):1–10.
[71] Curry A, Malas N, Mroczkowski M, et al. Updates in the assessment and management of agitation. Focus 2023;21(1):35–45.
[72] Schlit A, Delaunois A, Colomar A, et al. Risk of QT prolongation and torsade de pointes associated with exposure to hydroxyzine: re-evaluation of an established drug. Pharmacol Res Perspect 2017;5(3):e00309.
[73] Griffin CE, Kaye AM, Bueno FR, et al. Benzodiazepine pharmacology and central nervous system–mediated effects. Ochsner J 2013;13(2):214–23.
[74] Malas N, Brahmbhatt K, McDermott C, et al. Pediatric delirium: evaluation, management, and special considerations. Curr Psychiatry Rep 2017;19(9):65.
[75] Expert Panel on Neurological Imaging, Soares BP, Shih RY, Utukuri PS, et al. ACR appropriateness criteria® altered mental status, coma, delirium, and psychosis: 2024 update. J Am Coll Radiol 2024;21(11S):S372–83.
[76] Allen MH, Currier GW, Carpenter D, et al, Expert Consensus Panel for Behavioral Emergencies 2005. Introduction: methods, Commentary, and Summary. J Psychiatr Pract 2005;11:5.
[77] Chan EW, Lao KSJ, Lam L, et al. Intramuscular midazolam, olanzapine, or haloperidol for the management of acute agitation: a multi-centre, double-blind, randomised clinical trial. eClinicalMedicine 2021;32; https://doi.org/10.1016/j.eclinm.2021.100751.
[78] Food and Drug Administration. Zyprexa (olanzapine) [package insert]. Silver Spring, MD: US Department of Health and Human Services; 2014. Available at: https://www.accessdata.fda.gov/drugsatfda_docs/label/2014/020592s062021086s040021253s048 lbl.pdf (Accessed 20 March 2026).
[79] Bourke EM, Kochar A, Shellshear D, et al. PEAChY-O: pharmacological emergency management of agitation in children and young people: a randomized controlled trial of oral medication. Ann Emerg Med 2025;86(1):1–11.
[80] Swart GT, Siman E, Stewart SL. The use of pro re nata or statim medications for behavioral control: a summary of experience at a tertiary care children's mental health center. J Child Adolesc Psychopharmacol 2011;21(1):67–78.
[81] Pattamin N, Phongphithakchai A, Spano S, et al. Efficacy and safety of guanfacine in hospitalized patients with delirium: a scoping review. Crit Care Resusc 2024;26(4):286–94.
[82] Ng KT, Shubash CJ, Chong JS. The effect of dexmedetomidine on delirium and agitation in patients in intensive care: systematic review and meta-analysis with trial sequential analysis. Anaesthesia 2019;74(3):380–92; https://doi.org/10.1111/anae.14472.
[83] Nguyen TL, Lam WM, Orr H, et al. Clonidine for the treatment of agitation after dexmedetomidine discontinuation in pediatric patients: a retrospective cohort study. J Pediatr Pharmacol Therapeut 2021;26(8):821–7.
[84] Kowalski JM, Kopec KT, Lavelle J, et al. A novel agent for management of agitated delirium: a case series of ketamine utilization in the pediatric emergency department. Pediatr Emerg Care 2017;33(9):e58.

[85] Sandoval S, Goyal A, Frawley J, et al. Prehospital use of Ketamine versus benzodiazepines for sedation among pediatric patients with behavioral emergencies. Prehosp Emerg Care 2023;27(7):908–14.
[86] Barbic D, Andolfatto G, Grunau B, et al. Rapid agitation control with ketamine in the emergency department: a blinded, randomized controlled trial. Ann Emerg Med 2021;78(6):788–95.
[87] Chun TH, Mace SE, Katz ER, American Academy of Pediatrics, Committee on Pediatric Emergency Medicine, and American College of Emergency Physicians, Pediatric Emergency Medicine Committee. Evaluation and management of children and adolescents with Acute mental health or behavioral problems. Part I: common clinical challenges of patients with mental health and/or behavioral emergencies. Pediatrics 2016;138(3): e20161570; https://doi.org/10.1542/peds.2016-1570.
[88] Hawsawi T, Power T, Zugai J, et al. Nurses' and consumers' shared experiences of seclusion and restraint: a qualitative literature review. Int J Ment Health Nurs 2020;29(5):831–45.
[89] R3 Report Issue 44: New and revised restraint and seclusion requirements for behavioral health care and human services organizations I Joint Commission. Available at: https://www.jointcommission.org/en-us/standards/r3-report/r3-report-44. Accessed December 19, 2025.
[90] Furfaro H. When medical workers cover patients' heads with hoods, no one is watching. The Seattle Times. 2026. Available at: https://www.seattletimes.com/seattle-news/mental-health/when-hospitals-use-spit-hoods-on-patients-no-one-is-watching/. Accessed February 16, 2026.
[91] Dorfman DH. The use of physical and chemical restraints in the pediatric emergency department. Pediatr Emerg Care 2000;16(5):355.
[92] Chapter 194. Physical Restraints I Emergency Medicine Procedures, 2e I AccessEmergency Medicine I McGraw Hill Medical. Available at: https://accessemergencymedicine.mhmedical.com/content.aspx?bookid=683&sectionid=45343845. Accessed December 19, 2025.
[93] Jin RO, Anaebere TC, Haar RJ. Exploring bias in restraint use: four strategies to mitigate bias in care of the agitated patient in the emergency department. Acad Emerg Med 2021;28(9):1061–6.
[94] Dalton EM, Herndon AC, Cundiff A, et al. Decreasing the use of restraints on children admitted for behavioral health conditions. Pediatrics 2021;148(1):e2020003939.
[95] Hodgkiss B, Harding E. Reducing physical restraint in educational settings: a systematic literature review. Available at: https://nasenjournals.onlinelibrary.wiley.com/doi/10.1111/1471-3802.12598. Accessed December 19, 2025.
[96] Hoffmann JA, Pergjika A, Liu L, et al. Standardizing and improving care for pediatric agitation management in the emergency department. Pediatrics 2023;152(1):e2022059586; https://doi.org/10.1542/peds.2022-059586.
[97] Philadelphia TCH of. Behavioral health issues clinical pathway – emergency department I children's Hospital of Philadelphia. Available at: https://www.chop.edu/clinical-pathway/behavioral-health-issues-clinical-pathway. Accessed December 17, 2025.
[98] CSW Agitation & Aggression Management pathway. Available at: https://www.seattlechildrens.org/globalassets/documents/healthcare-professionals/clinical-standard-work/agitation-aggression-mgmt-org-pathway.pdf. Accessed December 17, 2025.
[99] PED Agitation Pathway .pdf. Available at: https://www.med.unc.edu/pediatrics/cccp/wp-content/uploads/sites/1156/2020/04/PED-Agitation-Pathway-1.pdf. Accessed December 17, 2025.
[100] Marzullo LR. Pharmacologic management of the agitated child. Pediatr Emerg Care 2014;30(4):269–75 [quiz: 276–78].
[101] Schneider S, Jennings A. Medical causes of patients with agitation: systemic illness. In: Nordstrom KD, Wilson MP, Zeller SL, editors. The diagnosis and management of agitation. Cambridge University Press; 2017. p. 48–73; https://doi.org/10.1017/9781316556702.007.

Advances in Pediatrics 73 (2026) 107–120

ADVANCES IN PEDIATRICS

Trauma-Informed Screening and Intervention for Trauma, Adverse Childhood Experiences, and Resilience in the Pediatric Inpatient Medical Setting

Maggie Kozman, MD, FAAP, FACP[a,b,*]

[a]David Geffen School of Medicine, at University of California Los Angeles; [b]Internal Medicine, Pediatrics, Harbor-UCLA Medical Center, Torrance, CA, USA

Keywords

• Trauma-informed care • Trauma screening
• Adverse childhood experiences screening • Inpatient • Hospital

Key points

- Screening and intervention for trauma, adverse childhood experiences, and resilience in the inpatient medical setting are in their early stages, predominantly in pediatric patients.
- There is ample time during medical hospitalization for trauma-informed screening and efficient mobilization of multidisciplinary resources desired by patients and families.
- Successful implementation in varied inpatient medical settings has demonstrated feasibility despite distinct challenges and has enabled early identification of vulnerable patients/families for whom targeted interventions can improve outcomes.

INTRODUCTION

Background

Screening medically hospitalized patients for a history of trauma and adverse childhood experiences (ACEs), followed by intervention during their inpatient medical stay, has emerged and come a long way in the last several years. While

*1000 West Carson Street, Building N25, Box 491, Torrance, CA 90502. *E-mail address:* mkozman@dhs.lacounty.gov

https://doi.org/10.1016/j.yapd.2025.12.006
0065-3101/26/Published by Elsevier Inc.

Abbreviations

ACEs	adverse childhood experiences
NICU	neonatal intensive care unit
PEARLS	Pediatric ACEs and Related Life-events Screener
PICU	pediatric intensive care unit
PROMIS	Patient-Reported Outcomes Measurement Information System
STEPP	Screening Tool for Early Predictors of PTSD (Post-Traumatic Stress Disorder)
STS	secondary traumatic stress
TIC	trauma-informed care

the concept of trauma-informed care (TIC) has been discussed and implemented in psychology since at least the 1990s, the concept seems to have arrived to the field of medicine later, in part through the Substance Abuse and Mental Health Services Administration's effort to create a shared understanding across all service sectors in its concept article in 2014 [1]. Implementation of trauma-informed principles has now become widespread in both outpatient and inpatient settings, and in both behavioral/psychiatric and medical settings.

Historically, however, the actual screening and intervention on trauma history and ACEs have taken place in inpatient psychiatric units, outpatient mental health clinics, or outpatient primary care pediatric or adult clinics. Many studies describe a range of screening methods in those settings and demonstrate their efficacy. But screening and intervening for patients while they are acutely hospitalized for a *medical* indication is currently making its debut, and it has largely begun in the pediatric world.

History and Definitions

Clear definitions of the terms used in the literature are essential, as they are more nuanced than the use of these words in daily speech. The landmark study of ACEs by Felitti and colleagues [2] in 1998 first described ACEs as 7 categories of childhood exposures to abuse (psychological, physical, and sexual) and household dysfunction (mother being threatened or physically abused; household member with substance use, mental illness, history of suicide attempt, or imprisonment). The study found a dose–response relationship between the number of ACEs and 10 risk factors for the leading causes of death, and between ACEs and several disease conditions, which was particularly pronounced with 4 or greater ACEs. Several iterations of the ACEs questionnaire have been developed since then, including the currently common 10 item ACEs questionnaire and the World Health Organization's ACE-International Questionnaire [3]. From nearly 40 years of literature, ACEs are generally understood as specifically studied childhood adversities with negative health consequences, and some have expanded their ACEs list beyond the widely known 10. But these lists are by no means the only adversities that children experience, hence the need to screen for more than just ACEs [4].

SAMHSA's concept article provides a particularly helpful definition of individual *trauma*, stating that it "results from an event, series of events, or set of circumstances that is experienced by an individual as physically or emotionally harmful or life threatening, and that has lasting adverse effects on the individual's functioning and mental, physical, social, emotional, or spiritual well-being." [1].

TIC is a framework that guides the response of individuals and systems to trauma. The concept of having a trauma-informed approach and system was first described in 2001 by Harris and Fallot [5], licensed clinical psychologists, after they had begun the process of becoming trauma-informed in their work in the mid-1990s. One of the most representative definitions is the consensus-based description from Hopper and colleagues [6]: "a strengths-based framework that is grounded in an understanding of and responsiveness to the impact of trauma, that emphasizes physical, psychological, and emotional safety for both providers and survivors, and that creates opportunities for survivors to rebuild a sense of control and empowerment." SAMHSA also highlights that TIC should resist retraumatization, meaning avoid the creation of environments that are stressful or triggering for the clients being served, or that are toxic to the well-being of staff or to the fulfillment of the organization's mission [1].

SAMHSA also built on the principles of TIC that Harris and Fallot [7] had identified in their subsequent 2001 study, highlighting SAMHSA's 6 key principles:

1. Safety
2. Trustworthiness and transparency
3. Peer support
4. Collaboration and mutuality
5. Empowerment, voice, and choice
6. Cultural, historical, and gender issues [1].

Rather than asking "What is wrong with you?," as health care practitioners are so often trained to think when diagnosing a patient's pathology, TIC reframes the conversation to "What happened to you?" and "What is *strong* with you?," which leads to the next key definition [8].

Resilience is "the capacity of a system to adapt successfully to challenges that threaten its function, survival, or future development" [9]. Rather than being an inherent quality one is either born with or not, it is a skill that can be cultivated by the "ordinary magic" of safe, stable, secure relationships and experiences [10]. There are numerous individual-level, family-level, and community-level resilience factors that enable a person to buffer the traumas they experience, which clinicians and systems can come alongside to support. *Individual* resilience factors include secure attachment to a safe, stable, nurturing caregiver (the most important foundational factor and most effective buffer to adversity), a sense of oneself and their relation to others, physical health, internal motivation, age-appropriate development, self-efficacy, self-regulation, and maintaining hope/optimism/faith. *Family* factors include authoritative (not authoritarian) parenting style, supportive and positive parent–child interactions, family structure and cohesion, a stimulating home environment, and adequate income. *Community* factors include neighborhood safety, adequate health services, religious/spiritual organizations, early prevention/intervention programs, libraries, recreational facilities, economic opportunities, and protective cultural beliefs and practices [8].

When left unbuffered, trauma can embed itself biologically as the *toxic stress response*. This results from "the prolonged activation of the stress response when a child experiences strong, frequent, and/or prolonged adversity in childhood without adequate buffering factors, leading to disruptions in neurologic, endocrine, immune, metabolic, and/or genetic systems" [11]. Fig. 1 illustrates how early life adversity in critical periods of development can lead to biological changes in multiple systems, sometimes mediated by one's genetic endowment, and can result in altered adult outcomes and behaviors [12].

Trauma-Informed Care Strategies

Resources for TIC strategies abound in the form of best practices, training modules, and toolkits. The National Child Traumatic Stress Network was created by Congress in 2000 and is administered by SAMHSA, and it offers a wealth of resources for the public and clinicians to learn trauma-informed practices [13]. The American Academy of Pediatrics offers online courses for basic and advanced skills in trauma-informed care implementation and resilience promotion [14]. Among the most robust state-led efforts are California's ACEs Aware initiative, which was the first of its kind in the nation, and New Jersey's ACEs Collaborative, Statewide Action Plan, and first-in-the-nation Office of Resilience [4,15]. The Karyn Purvis Institute of Child Development at Texas Christian University also offers extensive resources for its evidence-based, attachment-focused model called Trust-Based Relational Intervention,

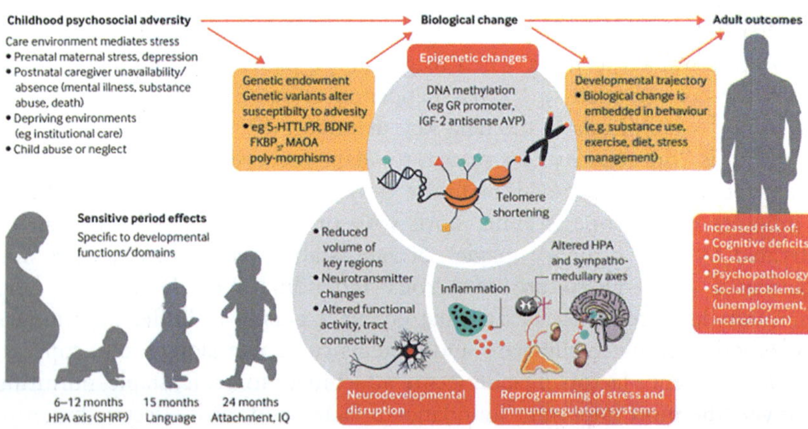

Fig. 1. Toxic stress response. *From* Nelson et al. Adversity in childhood is linked to mental and physical health throughout life. BMJ. 2020;371:m3048 (Berens, A.E., Jensen, S.K.G. & Nelson, C.A. Biological embedding of childhood adversity: from physiological mechanisms to clinical implications. BMC Med 15, 135 (2017). https://doi.org/10.1186/s12916-017-0895-4.), with permission from BMJ.

designed to guide adults working in any setting with children with complex needs due to trauma histories. The institute features a self-guided course for the public, including foster and adoptive parents, and specialized training courses for clinical practitioners, teachers, and camp staff [16]. Equipped with growing resources, health care practitioners can implement trauma-informed practices into any health care setting to respond to patients' trauma by bolstering their resilience to buffer their adversity, mitigate toxic stress, avoid retraumatization, and give patients control that facilitates their healing. This is the foundation upon which screening and intervention must be built.

DISCUSSION

Why Inpatient?

The inpatient medical environment can be traumatizing in and of itself, even for a patient with 0 ACEs or trauma history. On top of their being acutely ill, their normal routines are completely interrupted, sleep is disrupted, they are having repeated physical examinations and blood draws, and they may be getting imaging studies that require them to lay immobile for prolonged periods in a small tube while a loud machine takes pictures of them. Strangers are constantly entering their room. They are given food that is different from what they typically like. They do not have their toys or other coping tools they normally use when stressed. They cannot see all their family and friends as usual. They do not know how long they will have to stay in this unfamiliar place or how much better they will feel when they leave. This environment is substantially more triggering and even retraumatizing for patients who have already experienced trauma or ACEs. This is not just true of children; hospitalized older adults with a history of psychological trauma can be retraumatized by the aforementioned factors and practices like assisted toileting/bathing and locked wards for those with dementia [17]. Screening inpatients of any age for a history of trauma and ACEs can provide a wealth of insight to providers that can guide them in a trauma-informed approach to each patient that considers their unique triggers and needs.

The inpatient medical setting is also a place where patients and families spend significant time waiting in their rooms for additional tests or results, consultants, and for their treatment to bring enough improvement that they can be discharged. There is ample time in the hospital to screen patients and efficiently mobilize the multidisciplinary resources concentrated in that space. The alternative of establishing care with all those separate resources as an outpatient is typically lengthy and disjointed, if those resources are even accessible in the outpatient setting.

Furthermore, trauma centers are in fact now *required* to perform inpatient mental health screenings for all patients admitted for traumatic injury. In early 2022, the American College of Surgeons released its *Resources for Optimal Care of the Injured Patient*, detailing the requirements that all trauma centers must meet to be verified trauma centers. In addition to already-required substance misuse screening, level I and II trauma centers are required to have a "protocol to screen patients at high risk for psychological sequelae with subsequent referral to a mental health provider," while level III trauma centers are only required to have "a process for referral to a mental health provider… should a problem or risk be identified during inpatient admission" [18].

Evidence Supporting Inpatient Screening and Intervention

A review of the literature revealed multiple examples of screening *sub*populations in the inpatient medical setting, using a wide array of screeners.

Trauma Services

The earliest published studies of inpatient medical unit screening were conducted on trauma services with patients admitted for acute physical traumatic injury, starting in 2018. When the ACS released its 2022 *Resources for Optimal Care of the Injured Patient*, it did not specify which mental health issues must be screened for and did not mandate the use of particular screeners. The *ACS Trauma Quality Program Best Practices Guidelines* released later in 2022 note that besides posttraumatic stress, other postinjury mental health sequelae that can be screened for include suicidality, medical trauma, anxiety, and posttraumatic grief. The guidelines provide a list of examples of validated tools that can be used. They also note the utility of hospital-based violence intervention programs with a mental health component [19]. But individual trauma centers have flexibility in implementing their own processes.

Four published studies were found of inpatient screening for pediatric patients admitted to a trauma service for injury, with one study including adults up to the age of 94 years. In a 2018 retrospective chart review study of children aged 8 to 17 years and their parents who were administered the 12 item Screening Tool for Early Predictors of PTSD (STEPP) by advanced practice nurses, if either the child or parent STEPP score was positive, the intervention was inpatient psychology consultation. This involved 1 to 2 meetings with the family for assessment and brief educational intervention. One-quarter of screens triggered a psychology consultation, and over 68% of consultations were completed, a significant increase in completed consultations from 0.85% of those not eligible for STEPP to 15.12% of those who completed STEPP [20].

In another trauma center's 2023 quality improvement effort, a posttrauma consultation service with a dedicated therapist was created to screen, treat, and refer pediatric trauma service patients for acute stress symptoms. The therapist screened with the 4 item Child Stress Disorder Checklist-Short Form, 33 item Mood and Feelings Questionnaire, and 27 item Child PTSD Symptom Scale. Any patient not screened in the hospital because of weekend admission or rapid turnover was screened after discharge via phone. Of 147 screened 3 to 15 year old patients, 32.7% were positive for acute stress symptoms so received at least 1 therapy session while inpatient, and 29.2% of them were provided with additional community mental health resources. No families declined screening, resources, or therapy [21].

In 2025, a quality improvement longitudinal cohort pilot study was done on routine inpatient screening with the Acute Stress Checklist-3 for 205 pediatric patients with trauma aged 8 to 18 years. The 23.9% who screened positive had outpatient PTSD and quality-of-life screening 1 month later, with positive PTSD screens (18.4%) correlating with lower emotional/school/psychosocial functioning and triggering referral to behavioral health services [22].

These studies did not screen for things beyond acute psychological symptoms in the hospital after a specific physical trauma. Overall, their emphasis was on early detection of mental health issues resulting from acute injury, which has proven highly effective for improving future outcomes.

However, noting that nearly 25% of hospitalized postinjury patients who screen negative on bedside screens may develop depression or PTSD after discharge, another 2025 study assessed 15 to 94 year old patients deemed low risk by the bedside 9 item Injured Trauma Survivor Screen. Using the bedside 5 item Medical Outcomes Survey Social Support questionnaire and outpatient screeners for PTSD and depression, they found that 30 days after injury, violent injuries and lower levels of social support were associated with greater PTSD symptoms, and lower social support was also linked to higher risk of depressive symptoms. This raised awareness that these metrics should be included in screenings and that mental health referral has utility even for those who screen low risk with some tools [23].

Longer standing issues like ACEs and any lifetime history of trauma have not yet been routinely screened for in the published trauma literature. Neither have resilience factors or patient-desired/caregiver-desired multidisciplinary resources. This is being pioneered in other subpopulations.

Adult Burn Units

After pediatric patients with trauma, the next group in which screening began was adults hospitalized in burn units. One study in 2019 screened 53 hospitalized adult burn patients with the ACE-18 questionnaire, 16 item Individual and Family Strengths and Needs Assessment, and 6 item Brief Resiliency Scale during admission. After discharge, they were asked to complete a 3 item pain assessment, patient health questionnaire-9 (PHQ-9), 5 item Primary Care PTSD Screen, and 60 item Life Impact Burn Recovery Evaluation Profile. This showed that ACEs were correlated with lower preburn resilience and higher preburn needs, and with greater postburn depressive symptoms and positive PTSD screens and less positive postburn Family and Friends interactions, all of which complicate burn recovery [24].

In the United Kingdom, a 2022 retrospective chart review study of the methods of screening for psychosocial difficulties (per recommendations from the National Burn Care Standards for England and Wales) in 891 hospitalized adult burn unit patients revealed that different tiers of screening had occurred. These tiers were screening by a weekly multidisciplinary team's discussion, a graduate-level assistant psychologist, a clinical psychologist, or a liaison psychiatrist for patients with preinjury mental health problems or suicidality. The authors suggested a tiered approach could be a cost-effective way of utilizing resources and protecting the time of more highly qualified professionals for the most distressed, complex patients. They also suggest tiered screening facilitates tiered intervention, by which an assistant psychologist can offer low-level interventions (relaxation, social skills training, and so forth), while a clinical psychologist or psychiatrist can offer more intensive interventions [25].

Pediatric Ward

The next place where inpatient screening started was the ward, with a single published study in the pediatric ward found. The 2020 cross-sectional study of 265 parents of children admitted to a hospitalist service used a newly created 26 item survey adapted from existing social screening tools in the literature to assess social risk factors, including ACEs, financial stress (food insecurity, difficulty paying for rent or utilities), medical bill or insurance concerns, and caregiver mental health issues. When the results were analyzed with demographic and medical complexity data, the study showed that screening on the pediatric ward was feasible, social risk factors were highly prevalent, and children with chronic conditions were more likely to have any ACEs than those without such conditions. In terms of intervention, caregivers who indicated on their survey that they wanted a social work consult received one during the admission [26].

The pediatric ward is also the setting in which work at the author's institution is ongoing, described later [27].

Pediatric Intensive Care Unit

A 2022 prospective observational study of 84 pediatric intensive care unit (PICU) patients aged 0 to 17 years was conducted by screening with the 8 item ACEs questionnaire and Patient-Reported Outcomes Measurement Information System (PROMIS) short forms containing 44 items about life satisfaction, meaning and purpose, positive affect, anxiety, depressive symptoms, psychological stress experiences, family and peer relationships, and sleep disturbances. PICU patients were more likely than the general population to report ACEs in general, especially parental/guardian separation or divorce, parental incarcerations, neighborhood violence, and living with someone with mental illness. Those who had 2 or greater ACEs had worse PROMIS scores than those with 1 or less ACE in the domains of anxiety and family relationships. While the study did not evaluate interventions, the authors reference the Centers for Disease Control and Prevention's National Center for Injury Prevention and Control, noting that pediatric intensivists can refer at-risk patients and families to services like enhanced primary care programs, home visitation programs, mentorship programs, and trauma-focused cognitive behavioral therapy and multisystemic therapy [28,29].

A 2023 cross-sectional feasibility study of 400 PICU patients whose parents were screened for patients' ACEs with the 10 item ACEs screener did not find an association between ACEs and respiratory illness severity or length of stay, but the authors attributed this to their exclusion criteria and parent unavailability, and they still concluded that the study provided precedent for screening in the PICU [30].

Also in 2023, a prospective observational study of 145 PICU parents using demographic questions, 10 item ACEs questionnaire, 4 item Brief Resilient Coping Scale, and 7 item Abbreviated Parental Stressor Scale for PICU (with additional posttraumatic stress questionnaires 30 days after discharge) showed that *parents* with 4 or greater ACEs had 10 times greater odds of parental PTSD, with no correlation to the children's risk of PTSD. Children whose parents had low resilient coping had 83% higher odds of scoring at-risk for PTSD. The authors concluded that screening in the PICU allows identification of those needing additional support for positive parental coping and resilience, which inevitably impacts their children's coping and resilience during and after a PICU stay [31].

A qualitative study published in 2024 with semistructured interviews of 11 PICU parents showed that 10 of them felt being screened for social determinants of health and ACEs in the PICU was acceptable, valuable, and provided useful context for their child's medical team, *even* if there was no specific tangible resource for a particular endorsed issue. Most parents recommended screening be done after patient stabilization, with a preface that screening is universal, and that resources be available if desired or needed by the participants [32].

A 2024 prospective pilot cohort study of 60 PICU parents who were administered the 39 item Parental Stressors Scale and 20 item State-trait Anxiety Inventory during PICU admission (and then SAI plus 10 item Perceived Stress Scale at 1 month follow-up) showed that *parental* ACEs were linked to higher parental stress during the admission and higher parental perceived stress at 1 month follow-up. This highlights the need for targeted psychological interventions and resources for the distinct needs of vulnerable parents, like cognitive reappraisal of stressors, stress management techniques, journal writing, and nurse-led listening visits during which nurses attentively listen to parents' experiences [33].

Neonatal Intensive Care Unit

A 2023 cross-sectional survey study of inpatient screening of 119 neonatal intensive care unit (NICU) mothers in their first month of hospitalization utilized the 10 item ACEs questionnaire, 22 item Impact of Events Scale-Revised (acute stress disorder), 2 item Generalized Anxiety Disorder (postpartum anxiety), Patient Health Questionnaire-2 (postpartum depression), 46 item NICU Parental Stressor Scale (perceived stress in various domains), and questions asking mothers to identify the single most distressing aspect of their infant's progression to the NICU (index trauma) and any other subsequent traumatic aspects. Many mothers (37%) had 4 or greater ACEs. Mothers' cumulative ACEs and peripartum trauma scores were significantly correlated with acute stress disorder, postpartum anxiety, and postpartum depression. The authors emphasized that these symptoms were present in mothers within the first month in the NICU, highlighting the importance of early identification, intervention, and treatment, ideally built into the NICU [34]. Examples of NICU interventions that can assist mothers in real-time to buffer their infants' first toxic stress (from the NICU hospitalization itself) include seeing their baby 3 hours or less of delivery, skin-to-skin, breastfeeding, facilitated tucking, and greater caregiver involvement in infant cares that enable the infant to coregulate with the parent [35].

Challenges

While the earlier studies all demonstrate inpatient screening and intervention are feasible, there are several barriers to successful completion. Patients or caregivers may be uncomfortable with screening due to the sensitive nature of their experiences, or due to stigma they feel about their experiences or the services being offered to them, especially Social Work and mental health services. Providers may avoid screening in fear of retraumatizing patients, especially in a system without accessible interventions.

Logistics may also pose significant obstacles. Multiple studies noted the need for appropriate staff with capacity and training to screen patients, as well as limitations in screening due to staff schedules. Repeated screening attempts may be needed since patients may be indisposed due to feeling unwell, testing or procedures, or parent unavailability. Language barriers and lack of available translators or screeners in patients'/parents' primary language are further challenges. Importantly, buy-in from the multidisciplinary team is crucial as they will need to support and participate in screening, intervention, documentation, and hand-off to outpatient providers.

Which Screener?

Choosing which of the many screeners for various indications to use in a particular setting requires intentional thought and planning. In the discussion of studies earlier, a point was made to include the screener titles and number of items in each. Longer screeners are challenging to complete between conversations with providers, testing, and patients' attempts to sleep. The lengthier the screener may mean the less willing a patient or caregiver is to participate.

Based on cognitive qualitative interviews with parents of recently or concurrently hospitalized children, Shah and colleagues [36] created the 6 item Collaborate to Optimize Parent Experience tool. It includes a primer for parents about how stress from a hospitalization may manifest, a visual stress thermometer for parents to mark how they feel, questions about transportation and food insecurity, resilience, whether staff could help, and a menu of support services for parents to select if desired.

Ongoing quality improvement efforts led by the author of this study include an independently developed 6 item questionnaire with similar components. After eliciting whether the child/adolescent has a history of physical/sexual/medical trauma, the questionnaire asks if this history is causing current distress during the hospitalization, based on the Trauma and Resilience-informed Inquiry for Adversity, Distress, and Strengths Framework from the UCSF Center to Advance Trauma Informed Health Care [37]. The questionnaire then asks for the child's strengths and coping strategies and offers a menu of inpatient and outpatient services the patient/caregiver can choose if desired, rather than paternalistically forcing resources on them. The screener concludes with the Bay Area Research Consortium on Toxic Stress and Health's Pediatric ACEs and Related Life-events Screener (PEARLS) Part 1 (10 item ACEs) and Part 2 (7–9 items depending on age, screening for additional adversities, and socio-behavioral determinants of health) [27].

Secondary Traumatic Stress

A final challenge to address is secondary traumatic stress (STS), also known as compassion fatigue, in staff. This describes symptoms caused by indirect exposure to others' traumatic experiences, which can resemble PTSD, including anxiety, dissociation, physical symptoms, sleep disturbances, confusion, isolation, helplessness, poor work performance, and strained personal relationships. STS is distinct from and often additional to burnout, and burnout may predispose one to STS. Just as for patients, individual and corporate resilience factors are vital for staff who provide care for trauma survivors [8].

DISSENTING OPINIONS

It is worth noting that some disagree that routine ACEs screening should be done in *any* setting. Their concern is that the questionnaire's limitations are not being critically evaluated: limited inclusion of items, collapsing multiple items and response options into single multifaceted yes/no questions, simplistic scoring system, lack of psychometric assessment to test validity and reliability, and inappropriately applying population-level associations of ACEs with health to individuals [38,39]. With no randomized control trials of ACEs screening programs, the argument is that resources should instead go toward high-quality trials of interventions to prevent ACEs and evidence-based treatments for health and psychosocial issues, whether or not they are attributable to ACEs [39].

FUTURE DIRECTIONS

There is a gap in the literature when it comes to screening and intervention for all-comers in pediatric medical/surgical units who are admitted for *any* medical indication, not just acute physical injury. Further studies are also needed in medically hospitalized adults, whether in the medical/surgical ward or intensive care unit. Additionally, the varied inpatient medical unit screening and intervention algorithms discussed here serve as proof of concept, not a one-size-fits-all formula to apply to every inpatient medical setting in the same way. Just as each individual patient's experience of trauma and ACEs is distinct, so is each institution's unique combination of patient demographics, provider training, and available resources. Some settings are conducive to the use of already validated screeners, while others may require tools uniquely created or adapted for their setting that can then be assessed for their utility and generalizability. But the success of the distinct approaches mentioned earlier sets precedent that screening and intervention in inpatient medical settings are feasible, beneficial, and replicable. Incorporating this into the inpatient setting offloads screening from outpatient providers in time-constrained clinic visits. It also provides supporting evidence that governmental reimbursement to health systems for completing outpatient screenings (like that provided by Medi-Cal in California for PEARLS screening) should also be provided for inpatient screenings.

SUMMARY

Screening and intervention for trauma, ACEs, and resilience in the inpatient medical setting has been proven to be feasible and to unearth high levels of adversity in patients and caregivers that impact their hospitalization and post-discharge outcomes. Further study is needed for screening all-comers admitted to any pediatric or adult units for any indication. Clinical practice settings should adapt their screening and intervention approach to the population they serve and the resources available in their system, with the goal of supporting patients' resilience factors by efficiently mobilizing desired multidisciplinary resources in the hospital to buffer their adversity and facilitate patients' holistic recovery.

CLINICS CARE POINTS

- Health care practitioners and systems should expand their implementation of TIC to include the inpatient medical setting and utilize hospitalizations for screening and intervention.
- Supporting patients'/families' resilience factors and avoiding retraumatization are essential components of these efforts.
- Interventions should be targeted to the needs and desires of patients/families.
- Each practice setting must adapt its approach to its unique combination of patient demographics, provider training, and available resources.

Disclosure

The author has a grant from the University of California Los Angeles / University of California San Francisco ACEs Aware Family Resilience Network (UCAAN), which has funded the inpatient screening and intervention quality improvement project and TIC efforts in Harbor-UCLA Medical Center's Pediatric Ward.

References

[1] Substance Abuse and Mental Health Services Administration, SAMHSA's concept of trauma and guidance for a trauma-informed approach. 2014. HHS Publication No. (SMA) 14-4884, Available at: https://www.nctsn.org/sites/default/files/resources/resource-guide/samhsa_trauma.pdf. (Accessed 7 October 2025), 2014.

[2] Felitti VJ, Anda RF, Nordenberg D, et al. Relationship of childhood abuse and household dysfunction to many of the leading causes of death in adults: the adverse childhood experiences (ACE) study. Am J Prev Med 1998;14(4):245–58.

[3] World Health Organization. Adverse childhood experiences international questionnaire (ACE-IQ). 2020. Available at: https://www.who.int/publications/m/item/adverse-childhood-experiences-international-questionnaire-(ace-iq)/. Accessed October 7, 2025.

[4] ACEs Aware. The science of ACEs and toxic stress. 2025. Available at: https://www.acesaware.org/ace-fundamentals/the-science-of-aces-toxic-stress/. Accessed October 7, 2025.
[5] Harris M, Fallot RD. Envisioning a trauma-informed service system: a vital paradigm shift. New Dir Ment Health Serv 2001;(89):3–22.
[6] Hopper EK, Bassuk EL, Olivet J. Shelter from the storm: trauma-informed care in homelessness services settings. Open Health Serv Pol J 2010;3(1).
[7] Harris M, Fallot RD. Using trauma theory to design service systems. In: Harris M, Fallot RD, editors. San Francisco (CA): Jossey-Bass; 2001.
[8] Forkey HC, Griffin JL, Szilagyi M. Childhood trauma and resilience: a practical guide. American Academy of Pediatrics 2021;p1(12):179–82.
[9] Masten AS, Barnes AJ. Resilience in children: developmental perspective. Children 2018;5(7):98.
[10] Masten AS. Ordinary magic: resilience processes in development. Am Psychol 2001;56(3):227–38.
[11] Gilgoff R, Schwartz T, Owen M, et al. Opportunities to treat toxic stress. Pediatrics 2023;151(1):e2021055591.
[12] Nelson CA, Scott RD, Bhutta ZA, et al. Adversity in childhood is linked to mental and physical health throughout life. BMJ 2020;371:m3048.
[13] The National Child Traumatic Stress Network. Creating trauma-informed systems. Available at: https://nctsn.org/trauma-informed-care/creating-trauma-informed-systems. Accessed October 7, 2025.
[14] American Academy of Pediatrics. Trauma-Informed Care: Self-Directed Learning. Available at: https://www.aap.org/en/patient-care/national-center-for-relational-health-and-trauma-informed-care/trauma-informed-care-education-self-directed-learning (Accessed 5 January 2026).
[15] Gears H, Schulman M. Center for Health Care Strategies. From coast to coast: state strategies to address adverse childhood experiences. 2022. Available at: https://www.chcs.org/from-coast-to-coast-state-strategies-to-address-adverse-childhood-experiences. Accessed October 7, 2025.
[16] Karyn Purvis Institute of Child Development. Trust-based relational intervention. Available at: https://child.tcu.edu/about-us/tbri/#sthash.spy4Qdqe.dpbs. Accessed October 7, 2025.
[17] Couzner L, Spence N, Fausto K, et al. Delivering trauma-informed care in a hospital ward for older adults with dementia: an illustrative case series. Front Rehabil Sci 2022;3:934099.
[18] American College of Surgeons. Resources for optimal care of the injured patient, 7th edition. 2022. Available at: https://www.facs.org/quality-programs/trauma/tqp/center-programs/vrc/standards. Accessed September 22, 2025.
[19] American College of Surgeons Trauma Programs. Best practices guidelines: screening and intervention for mental health disorders and substance use and misuse in the acute trauma patient. 23-65. Available at: https://www.facs.org/media/nrcj31ku/mental-health-guidelines.pdf (Accessed 7 October 2025), 2022.
[20] Price J, Genuario K, Romeo D, et al. Implementation of a standardized screening program for risk of posttraumatic stress disorder among youth hospitalized with injury. Psychol Serv 2019;16(1):48–57.
[21] Fuchs J, Zwemer E, Gillespie A, et al. Making trauma less traumatic: implementing inpatient pediatric screening of acute stress symptoms. Hosp Pediatr 2023;13(8):702–9.
[22] Liang NE, Alvarez K, Dalusag K, et al. Beyond physical injury: routine screening for acute stress disorder and posttraumatic stress disorder in pediatric trauma patients – a longitudinal cohort pilot study. J Pediatr Surg 2025;60(2):1–6.
[23] Brier ZMF, Ruggiero KJ, deRoon-Cassini TA, et al. Bedside mental health risk screening of traumatic injury patients is enhanced by measurement of injury mechanism and social support. Injury 2025;56(5):112078.

[24] Fassel M, Grieve B, Hosseini S, et al. The impact of adverse childhood experiences on burn outcomes in adult burn patients. J Burn Care Res 2019;40(3):294–301.
[25] Shepherd L, Beveridge A. A tiered approach to inpatient psychosocial screening in an adult UK burns service. Burns 2022;48(3):698–702.
[26] Vaz LE, Wagner DV, Ramsey KL, et al. Identification of caregiver reported social risk factors in hospitalized children. Hosp Pediatr 2020;10(1):20–8.
[27] Kozman M, Gomez P. Trauma-informed care on the pediatric ward: a novel application of ACEs/trauma screening and intervention in the inpatient medical setting. Poster presented at: Pediatric Academic Societies Meeting 2025; April 26, 2025; Honolulu (HI).
[28] Rodenbough A, Opolka C, Wang T, et al. Adverse childhood experiences and patient-reported outcome measures in critically ill children. Front Pediatr 2022;10:923118.
[29] Centers for Disease Control and Prevention. Preventing adverse childhood experiences: leveraging the best available evidence. Atlanta, GA: National Center for Injury Prevention and Control, Centers for Disease Control and Prevention; 2019.
[30] Derck JE, Livingston JD, Zhang A, et al. Feasibility and challenges with measuring adverse childhood experiences in the pediatric intensive care unit. J Child Adolesc Trauma 2023;16:477–80.
[31] Pryce P, Gangopadhyay M, Edwards JD. Parental adverse childhood experiences and post-PICU stress in children and parents. Pediatr Crit Care Med 2023;24(12):1022–32.
[32] Asp RA, Paquette ET. Parent perspectives on social risk screening in the pediatric intensive care unit. Pediatr Crit Care Med 2024;25(1):953–8.
[33] Alzawad Z, Weiss JM, Lee J, et al. Exploring factors affecting parental psychological vulnerability during their child's PICU admission: a prospective pilot cohort study. J Pediatr Health Care 2024;38(3):323–36.
[34] Williams A, Parlier-Ahmad AB, Thompson E, et al. Peripartum traumas and mental health outcomes in a low-income sample of NICU mothers: a call for family-centered, trauma-informed care. Children 2023;10(9):1477.
[35] Sanders MR, Hall SL. Trauma-informed care in the newborn intensive care unit: promoting safety, security and connectedness. J Perinatol 2018;38(1):3–10.
[36] Shah AN, Goodman E, Lawler J, et al. Inpatient screening of parental adversity and strengths. Hosp Pediatr 2023;13(10):922–30.
[37] University of California San Francisco Center to advance trauma informed health care. What is TRIADS. 2025. Available at: https://cthc.ucsf.edu/triads/what-is-triads. Accessed October 7, 2025.
[38] McLennan JD, MacMillan HL. Afifi TO. Questioning the use of adverse childhood experiences (ACEs) questionnaires. Child Abuse Negl 2020;101:1–4.
[39] McLennan JD, Gonzalez A, MacMillan JL, et al. Routine screening for adverse childhood experiences (ACEs) still doesn't make sense. Child Abuse Negl 2025;168(1):1–7.

Advances in Pediatrics 73 (2026) 121–144

ADVANCES IN PEDIATRICS

Recent Advances in the Management of Type 1 Diabetes in Children

Nancy L. Beck, MD

Department of Pediatrics, Texas Tech University Health Sciences Center, 3601 4th Street, Stop 9406, Lubbock, TX 79430, USA

Keywords

• Type 1 diabetes screening and staging • Autoantibodies • Immunomodulation
• B-cell replacement • Continuous glucose monitoring
• Automated insulin delivery systems • Closed-loop systems

Key points

- Type 1 diabetes is a chronic autoimmune disease with etiology derived from both genetic factors and environmental inputs.
- Autoantibody screening of individuals at high risk for the development of type 1 diabetes can identify the presence of the autoimmune process before the frank onset of the disease.
- Teplizumab, a monoclonal antibody, is the first disease-modifying treatment shown to delay clinical onset of type 1 diabetes in high-risk individuals and is in on-label clinical use.
- Research regarding β-cell replacement and regeneration is rapidly advancing, with an allogeneic stem cell-derived, fully differentiated, insulin-producing islet cell therapy, which is now in a phase 3 trial.
- Continuous glucose monitoring and automated insulin delivery system technologies have provided for improved glycemic control and enhanced quality of life for individuals with diabetes.

INTRODUCTION

Type 1 diabetes mellitus (T1D) is a chronic autoimmune disease with etiology derived from both genetic factors and environmental inputs. The autoimmune process progresses through 3 sequential stages, ultimately leading to the loss of pancreatic β-cell mass and function and resulting in lifelong dependence on exogenous insulin therapy [1–3].

E-mail address: nancy.beck@ttuhsc.edu

https://doi.org/10.1016/j.yapd.2025.12.012

Abbreviations

ADA	American Diabetes Association
CGM	continuous glucose monitoring
CGMS	continuous glucose monitoring system
CRISPR	Clustered regularly interspaced short palindromic repeat
DKA	diabetic ketoacidosis
FDA	Food and Drug Association
GMI	glucose management indicator
HCL	hybrid closed-loop system
PLGS	predictive low glucose suspend
sBLA	supplemental biologics license application
T1D	type 1 diabetes mellitus
TIR	time-in-range

In 2015, publication of a Scientific Statement by the Juvenile Diabetes Research Foundation, the Endocrine Society, and the American Diabetes Association (ADA), proposed a staging classification system for presymptomatic type 1 diabetes. Adoption of this system was endorsed by the American Association of Clinical Endocrinologists and the International Society for Pediatric and Adolescent Diabetes [4].

- In *stage 1*, β-cell autoimmunity exists, with *two or more islet autoantibodies* present. The blood glucose is in the normal range (*fasting plasma glucose 70–99 mg/dL*). This stage is *presymptomatic.*
- In *stage 2*, β-cell autoimmunity exists, with *two or more islet autoantibodies* present; this stage is *presymptomatic.* However, *dysglycemia* is now present (*fasting plasma glucose 100–125 mg/dL*).
- In *stage 3*, β-cell autoimmunity exists, with *two or more islet antibodies* present; this stage is characterized by the onset of symptomatic disease; *hyperglycemia* exists (*fasting plasma glucose* $\geq$*126 mg/dL*).

The 2025 ADA Standards of Care in Diabetes provides essentially the same staging criteria, with the inclusion of dysglycemia in stage 2 having 3 options for definition: fasting plasma glucose 100 to 125 mg/dL, or a plasma glucose of 140 to 199 mg/dL at 2 h on an oral glucose tolerance test, A1c 5.7% to 6.4% or a $\geq$10% in A1c [5].

Since type 1 diabetes is still associated with a notable degree of morbidity, and with the advent of the first disease-modifying therapy approved by the Food and Drug Association (FDA) and the opportunity to now treat diabetes as an immunologic disease rather than just a metabolic disease, the Endocrine Society sought to address the challenges and opportunities for understanding the pathogenesis of type 1 diabetes in their Scientific Statement [6].

In the Scientific Statement, notation was made that with the 100th anniversary of the discovery of insulin in 2021, we are reminded that millions of lives were saved by this historic scientific breakthrough [7]. However, there is still a great need to reduce the daily burden of care and comorbidities associated with T1D [6].

The Endocrine Society authors added a "Stage 0" to the classical schematic model of Stages 1, 2, and 3 in the development of T1D [8]. The purpose of this modification was to highlight that there is little knowledge regarding the factors present prior to stage 1, which impedes our understanding of the processes that incite the autoimmune process. In Stage 0, we have little understanding of (1) islet mass and function at birth; (2) pancreatic islet immune cells after birth, and (3) factors initiating islet autoimmunity seroconversion [6].

The Endocrine Society Scientific Statement above identified genetics of T1D, heterogeneity of T1D, pathology of the pancreas, immunologic biomarkers in peripheral blood, the exocrine pancreas in T1D, and screening to identify individuals at risk for T1D as areas to focus present and future efforts on understanding the pathogenesis of T1D [6].

IMMUNOMODULATION AND PREVENTION

Screening for type 1 diabetes mellitus

One of the main benefits of screening for T1D is to diagnose T1D as early as possible and thereby avoid the development of diabetic ketoacidosis (DKA). Up to 60% of children present with DKA at the time of diagnosis. Children who have been screened for T1D present in DKA less than 5% of the time [9,10].

Regarding the establishment of screening programs for presymptomatic type 1 diabetes, a detailed report provides guidance for endocrinology providers within their practices, institutions, communities, and health care networks [11]. Key steps in this regard include:

- Nominating a program champion.
- Building a team to implement the screening program.
- Developing processes for the screening program.
  - Communicating with at-risk individuals about autoantibody (Aab) testing.
  - Ordering Aab tests.
  - When to screen.
  - Diagnostic codes.
  - Processes following positive/negative screening test results.
- Educating and motivating providers to participate in the screening program.
- Communicating the value of screening to decision-makers [11].

Other guidelines for screening patients for T1D are available for medical practitioners [12–15].

In previous years, screening relatives of people with T1D was beneficial in terms of identifying that the autoimmune process involved in T1D was transpiring. That knowledge afforded affected individuals the ability to be clinically monitored, to initiate appropriate medical care as soon as they were diagnosed, and to hopefully avoid the development of ketoacidosis. Presently, there is another rationale for screening, which is treatment to slow the rate of progression of the autoimmune process.

Immunomodulatory therapies

Investigations and usage of immunomodulating therapies are progressing along the full developmental continuum, from basic laboratory studies, through clinical trials, and to implementation in clinical practice.

Teplizumab

Teplizumab, an anti-CD3 monoclonal antibody, was the first disease-modifying treatment shown to slow down the clinical onset of type 1 diabetes in high-risk individuals. Anti-CD3 therapy targets the chain of the CD3 receptor on the T-cell surface. The mechanism may involve partial agonistic signaling and deactivation of pancreatic β-cell T lymphocytes [16–19].

Under the commercial name TZIELD, teplizumab is the first FDA-approved, and currently, the only drug used in clinical practice to delay progression of the autoimmune process involved in the development of type 1 diabetes. Teplizumab became FDA-approved in November 2022 in the United States. It is indicated to delay the onset of stage 3 type 1 diabetes in adults and pediatric patients aged 8 years and older with Stage 2 type 1 diabetes [20].

Medical evaluation prior to starting Tzield requires confirming Stage 2 type 1 diabetes by documenting:

- At least 2 positive pancreatic islet cell autoantibodies.
  - Glutamic acid decarboxylase 65 autoantibodies.
  - Insulin autoantibody.
  - Insulinoma-associated antigen 2 autoantibody.
  - Zinc transporter 8 autoantibody.
  - Islet cell autoantibody.
- Dysglycemia without overt hyperglycemia using an oral glucose tolerance test.
- The clinical history should not suggest type 2 diabetes [21].

Tzield is administered as a 30 min intravenous infusion every day for 14 consecutive days, with the process repeated in 6 months.

Warnings and precautions relate to:

- Cytokine release syndrome.
- Serious infections.
- Lymphopenia.
- Hypersensitivity reactions.
- Vaccinations [21].

In a Phase 2 randomized placebo-controlled trial (TrialNet TN-10) with 76 participants (72% under age 18 years) who were relatives of individuals with type 1 diabetes and who had at least 2 autoantibodies and abnormal glucose tolerance test results were treated with a single course of teplizumab and followed with oral glucose tolerance tests every 6 months. The mean age thereafter for diagnosis of diabetes was 2 years. At the conclusion of the trial, 57% of the treatment group were disease-free, double that of the placebo group (28%) [22].

The PROTECT trial (Provention Bio's Type 1 Diabetes Trial Evaluating C-Peptide with Teplizumab) evaluated whether 2 courses of teplizumab would preserve β-cell function. Patients were randomized in a 2:1 ratio to receive teplizumab or placebo, intravenously, for two 12 day courses. Patients were male and female, ages 8 to 17 years, who had been diagnosed with type 1 diabetes within

6 weeks according to ADA criteria. Patients had at least one autoantibody associated with type 1 diabetes and a peak stimulated C-peptide level ≥0.2 pmol per milliliter. Patients in the teplizumab group received the drug in two 12 day courses, 26 weeks apart. 328 children and adolescents were enrolled [23].

Patients treated with teplizumab had significantly higher stimulated C-peptide levels (≥0.2 pmol per milliliter) (94.9%) than patients receiving placebo (79.2%) at week 78. Occurrence of adverse events (which were usually mild and transient) was not significantly different between groups. The groups did not differ significantly in terms of insulin doses required to meet glycemic goals, A1c, time in target glucose range, hypoglycemia, or quality of life data [23].

TZIELD does not currently have an FDA-approved indication for new-onset type 1 diabetes. However, on October 20, 2025, a press release from the manufacturer, Sanofi, announced that the FDA has accepted for expedited review the supplemental biologics license application (sBLA) for Tzield (teplizumab-mzwv) to delay the progression of stage 3 T1D in adults and pediatric patients 8 years of age and older, recently diagnosed with stage 3 T1D. The sBLA is supported by the results from the PROTECT phase 3 study [24].

β-CELL REPLACEMENT AND REGENERATION

Historically, β-cell replacement with islet or pancreas transplant reduces or eliminates the need for insulin therapy, as well as decreasing the frequency of severe hypoglycemia since exogenous insulin is not being administered [25]. However, barriers exist to this practice, due to organ availability, as well as variability and the quality of islets. Challenges also occur with the requirement of immunosuppressive drugs to avoid rejection of the transplants. The need for multiple transplants from multiple donors, and the requirement for multiple cadavers to retrieve enough cells for one patient, is also a limitation to achieving consistently appropriate clinical outcomes [26–30].

Pluripotent stem cell-derived islet therapies

Pluripotent stem cells can be differentiated into therapeutic cells to replace damaged or diseased cells. Studies have demonstrated that stem cells can be differentiated into insulin-producing β-cells and glucagon-producing α-cells [31,32].

Using an approach based on this finding, zimislecel (VX-880) was developed. The investigators hypothesized that administering zimislecel by methods used in the transplantation of islets from a deceased donor [33,34] would result in regulated secretion of endogenous insulin, improved glycemic control, and cessation of severe hypoglycemic events, and insulin independence in humans [35].

- *FORWARD Trial (VX-880. Zimislecel, Vertex Pharmaceuticals).*
    - Zimislecel is an allogeneic stem cell-derived, fully differentiated, insulin-producing islet cell therapy, which is now in a Phase 3 trial [35].
    - It is infused into the hepatic portal vein of individuals with type 1 diabetes, with the aim to restore islet cell production of insulin in response to glucose.
    - Since the therapy involves transplanted cells, immunosuppressive drugs must be taken lifelong.

- During the Phase 1 to 2 trial:
- Part A: Participants were adults with type 1 diabetes, with impaired hypoglycemia awareness (defined as a reduced ability to perceive the onset of hypoglycemia) and severe hypoglycemia with at least 2 severe hypoglycemic events in the previous year, and insulin dependence for at least 5 years. A severe hypoglycemic event was defined by the presence of symptoms of hypoglycemia during which the participant needed assistance with treatment and by either blood glucose less than 54 mg/dL or prompt recovery after the receipt of oral carbohydrate, intravenous glucose, or glucagon. Participants received a half dose of Zimislecel as a single infusion, with the option to receive a second half dose within 2 years.
- In Parts B and C, participants received a full dose of zimislecel as a single infusion.
- All participants also received glucocorticoid-free immunosuppressive therapy.
- Primary endpoints were
  - Part A—Safety.
  - Parts B and C—Freedom from severe hypoglycemic events during days 90 through 365, A1c less than 7% or a decrease of at least 1 point from baseline at least once between days 180 through 365.
  - The secondary endpoint for Part C was
    Safety and insulin independence between days 180 and 365.
  - Assessment of primary and secondary endpoints in Part C involved participants who received the full dose of the infusion in Parts B or C.
  - To assess engraftment and islet function, a mixed meal tolerance test, with detection of C-peptide, was used.

- *Results were*
  - 14 participants completed (2 in Part A and 12 in Parts B and C) at least 12 months of follow-up.
  - C-peptide was undetectable at baseline in all 14 participants.
  - After Zimislecel infusion, all participants had enough engraftment and islet cell function.
  - The most common serious adverse event was neutropenia (3 participants).
  - 2 deaths—not thought to be related to the study treatment.
  - All 12 participants in Parts B and C had no further hypoglycemia episodes, had an A1c less than 7%, and spent greater than 70% TIR (70–180 mg/dL).
  - 10 of the 12 participants had insulin independence and were not using exogenous insulin on day 365.
  - The investigators concluded that Zimislecel can restore physiologic islet function and warrants further investigation [35–38].

Encapsulation and immunoprotection

One of the long-term challenges of most cell-based therapies is the protection of transplanted cells from immune attack [39].

Macroencapsulation devices have evolved to provide a protective barrier for transplanted cells while still allowing nutrients, oxygen, and insulin to diffuse into the cells [40,41].

Microencapsulation methods have moved forward in terms of materials science and manufacturing techniques. Novel hydrogel formulations with adaptable properties allow for more control over capsule size, permeability, and mechanical stability. Other developments include the use of nanoparticles and bioactive molecules within the capsules to make a more supportive environment for encapsulated cells [42].

Allotransplantation and islet transplant evolution

- Gene-Edited Allogeneic Islet Cells (CRISPR Technology).

Clustered regularly interspaced short palindromic repeats (CRISPR) and its related Cas proteins have been used in the treatment of an increasing number of genetic diseases [43].

Multiple genetic diseases are being targeted by CRISPR technology currently. They are being addressed through a variety of CRISPR-based therapies [44].

The first FDA-approved CRISPR-based therapy, in 2023, was Casgevy (exagamglogene autoemcel), for the treatment of sickle cell disease and transfusion-dependent beta-thalassemia [45]. Casgevy is a one-time gene therapy that works by using CRISPR/Cas9 technology to edit a patient's own blood-forming stem cells. It deactivates a gene that suppresses fetal hemoglobin, allowing the edited cells to produce more healthy fetal hemoglobin. An individual's blood stem cells are collected and separated from their blood. The cells are then edited *ex vivo* using CRISPR-Cas9 to disrupt the BCL11A gene (the gene that turns off fetal hemoglobin). After a conditioning regimen of chemotherapy, the edited cells are reinfused into the patient, where they are expected to engraft in the bone marrow and produce healthy red blood cells [45,46].

Hereditary transthyretin amyloidosis is being treated with CRISPR/Cas9 therapies delivered via nanoparticles to reduce the production of a disease-causing protein. Other genetic disorders, including Duchenne muscular dystrophy, hereditary angioedema, Leber congenital amaurosis, cancer, and hemophilia, human immunodeficiency virus/acquired immunodeficiency syndrome (HIV/AIDS), Huntington's disease, and hepatitis B virus, are also targets of CRISPR technologies [47–54].

CRISPR technology has found a place in ongoing type 1 diabetes research. A man with long-standing type 1 diabetes was the recipient of transplantation of genetically modified allogeneic donor islet cells, which were transplanted into his forearm muscle. He received no immunosuppressive drugs. CRISPR-associated protein 12b gene editing was used to genetically modify the cells to avoid rejection. At 12 weeks posttransplantation, he showed no immune response against the cells. He maintained stable C-peptide measurements and glucose-responsive insulin secretion [55].

DIABETES TECHNOLOGY: CONTINUOUS GLUCOSE MONITORING AND AUTOMATED INSULIN DELIVERY

Continuous glucose monitoring

The first continuous glucose monitor (CGM) ever marketed was the MiniMed Continuous Glucose Monitoring System (CGMS), which was granted FDA approval in 1999. It did not provide real-time readings. The sensor was worn for 3 days, then the data were downloaded in the clinic setting for review [56].

Continuous glucose monitors have significantly improved the quality of life for individuals with diabetes and have repeatedly shown improvement in blood glucose control over insulin injections. When paired with insulin pumps as a component of automated insulin delivery/hybrid closed-loop system (AID/HCL) or a fully closed-loop system, more precise tailoring of insulin delivery throughout the day can occur [57]. Parents of young children whose diabetes is managed with a closed-loop system spend less time performing diabetes activities. They thus state that their children have a better quality of life due to the utilization of these devices and systems [58,59].

Updates in terms of FDA approval, days of wear, age indications, manufacturer discontinuation of products, and changes in compatibility with other devices are constantly occurring. Therefore, the status of any CGM product in terms of these factors is not static, and compiling a list of CGM options for patients that will remain accurate for a reasonable length of time is difficult. At this writing, the CGM devices that are currently on the market in the United States and that are indicated for children with type 1 diabetes are listed below [60].

1. Abbott Freestyle Libre 2, indicated for age 4 years or more, 14 days wear.
2. Abbott Freestyle Libre 2 Plus, indicated for age 2 years or more, 15 days wear.
3. Abbott Freestyle Libre 3, indicated for age 4 years or more, 14 days wear.
4. Abbott Freestyle Libre 3 Plus, indicated for age 2 years or more, 15 days wear.
5. Dexcom G6, indicated for age 2 years or more, 10 days wear (this product is being discontinued).
6. Dexcom G7, indicated for age 2 years or more, 10 days wear ± 12 h grace period.
7. Abbott Freestyle Libre 14 day, indicated for age 18 years or more, 14 day wear.
8. Medtronic Guardian 4, indicated for age 7 years or more, 7 days wear (this product is being discontinued). The newer Minimed sensors being developed are listed in Table 1.

Automated insulin delivery/closed loop and hybrid closed-loop systems

There are currently 5 AID/HCL systems commercially available in the United States. One of the current trends in these systems is that there is greater compatibility between multiple brands of CGMS and insulin pumps, so individuals can choose each element of their system independently based on their personal needs.

1. Minimed 780G insulin pump.

The Minimed 780G is an AID combining a tubed insulin pump with a CGM. It is approved for individuals aged 7 years and older with type 1 diabetes. It has a smart algorithm called "SmartGuard," and the system adjusts and delivers insulin every 5 minutes based on information from the CGM readings. Features include automatic correction boluses and meal detection

Table 1
Minimed insulin pumps and compatible devices

MiniMed product	Category	User base	Pivotal studies	Number of patients	Time in range (TIR)	Time below range (TBR)	Compatible devices
Minimed™ 780 G Approved for people age 7 y and older. Employs a smart algorithm called "SmartGuard"	Insulin pump with tubing	Est >700,000	Carlson AL, Sherr JL, Shulman DI, et al. Safety and Glycemic Outcomes During the MiniMed™ Advanced Hybrid Closed-Loop System Pivotal Trial in Adolescents and Adults with Type 1 Diabetes. Diabetes Technol Ther. 2022;24 (3):178-189.	157	75%	2.3%	*Instinct™* (Abbott CGM that lasts up to 15 d) Designed exclusively for the 780G system. 1 h warm-up period Factory-calibrated (no fingersticks needed in closed-loop mode but may be needed in manual mode or to start the system *Simplera Sync™* See description in box below.
			Real World Data Presented at *ADA 2025* (Medtronic data on file: *Minimed™* 780 G data uploaded voluntarily by 374,548 users globally to CareLink Personal from 02 January 2020 to 30 April 2025)	374,548	72%	1.4%	
Minimed™ Flex Under development Tubed pump 7-d wear time Controlled by smart phone Half the size of current 780G Will have no screen Will utilize the current infusion set Will have an improved algorithm	Insulin pump with tubing	N/A	N/A	N/A	N/A	N/A	*Instinct™* *Simplera SyncTM* Disposable all-in-one CGM that works with the Minimed 780G system 2-step insertion process and 6 d wear time with 24 h grace period Requires no fingerstick calibrations when paired with Smart Guard technology Transmits glucose data wirelessly to a smartphone app or smartwatch. Data can be uploaded to CareLink cloud

(*continued on next page*)

Table 1
(*continued*)

MiniMed product	Category	User base	Pivotal studies	Number of patients	Time in range (TIR)	Time below range (TBR)	Compatible devices
Minimed™ Fit (8-series) Under development Tubeless patch style pump 7-d wear time. Expected FDA submission by late 2026.	Patch insulin pump	N/A	N/A	N/A	N/A	N/A	*Instinct™* *Simplera Sync™*

to help with blood glucose stabilization. For the best results, though, user-initiated meal notification is required. Studies have shown superior blood glucose control compared to insulin injections [61]. Notifications and data can be sent through the mobile phone application, Minimed mobile app.

The current Guardian sensors utilized with the 780G pump will be discontinued in the future.

The *Minimed Fit* is a tubeless, patch-style insulin pump under development by Medtronic/Minimed. It is designed to be worn on the body. Wear time is 7 days. Its insulin capacity is 300 units. It has a rechargeable component combined with a rechargeable battery. It is expected to be submitted to the FDA soon. It has a modular design, unlike single-piece patch pumps.

The *Minimed Flex* is another tubed pump under development, which will be controlled by a smartphone and is half the size of the current 780G model. It will have no screen. It is likely to be called "Minimed 8-Series." It will use the same 7 day infusion set and other supplies associated with the 780G pump.

The *Instinct CGM* is manufactured by Abbott. It is FDA-approved for individuals aged 7 years and older. It was designed exclusively to work with the Minimed 780G system. It lasts up to 15 days. It has a 1 hour warm-up period. It is factory-calibrated, so fingersticks are not required in the closed-loop mode, though they may be needed in manual mode or to start the system. The sensor can be started with the MiniMed mobile app.

Simplera Sync is a disposable all-in-one CGM sensor that works with the Medtronic 780G system. It has a simple 2 step insertion process, a 6 day wear time with a 24 h grace period, and requires no fingerstick calibrations when it is paired with SmartGuard technology. It transmits glucose data wirelessly to a smartphone app. It is compatible with smart watches, and data can also be uploaded to the CareLink cloud. It is in a single, disposable unit, and no overtape is needed. It is water-resistant up to 8 feet for 30 minutes [62].

The Minimed 780G system has gained widespread use in various parts of the world, as evidenced by a report celebrating the benchmarking of 100,000 Minimed 780G system users in Europe, the Middle East, and Africa. CareLink personal data CGM-based endpoints were aggregated for 2 cohorts, one being the full cohort, and a second 12 month longitudinal cohort. Subanalyses were done for users with optimal settings. Data from 101,629 users in 34 countries were analyzed. Mean time in range was 72.3%, glucose management indicator (GMI) was 7%, and time below range of 70 mg/dL was 2.0%. 59% of users had a GMI less than 7%. In the longitudinal cohort, time in range was 75.5% in the first month and remained at 73.3% or higher over the 12 month period [63].

Medtronic/Minimed pumps are described further in Table 1.

2. *Omnipod 5* is a patch insulin pump manufactured by Insulet that integrates with Dexcom G6 and Dexcom G7 CGMS, as well as the Freestyle Libre 3 Plus glucose sensor. It is approved for children aged 2 years and older with type 1 diabetes [64].

In a clinical trial in which 112 children and 129 adults followed a 2 week standard therapy phase, followed by 3 months of AID. A1c was significantly reduced by 0.71% and time in range improved from standard therapy by 15.6% or 3.7 hours per day [65].

A retrospective study of the device and person-reported datasets of Omnipod 5 system users (individuals with type 1 diabetes, ages 2 years and older) as of July 2023 was conducted. 31.7% of the users in the group were children and adolescents (ages 2–17 years). Data from a total of 69,902 users were included. Findings include

a. Multiple and higher glucose targets were commonly used in younger age groups.
b. Median percentage time in range (70–180 mg/dL) was:
   i. 68.8% for users with average glucose target of 110 mg/dL.
   ii. 61.3% for users with average glucose target of 120 mg/dL.
   iii. 53.6% for users with average glucose target of 130 to 150 mg/dL.
c. Median for all users less than 1.3% of time less than 70 mg/dL.

Of note, 6.6% of the users were children and adolescents (age 2–17 years) with their primary insurance coverage being Medicaid. Medicaid users (all ages) had a median GMI of less than 8.0% across all glucose targets [66].

Omnipod 5 pumps are described further in Table 2.

3. Tandem Pumps.
   a. *Tandem t:slim X2 insulin pump*—this tubed pump is larger than the Mobi pump, is controlled through its built-in color touch screen, and has a mobile app for data access (compatible with both iOS and Android). It has a rechargeable battery [67].
   b. *Tandem Mobi system*—this tubed pump is less than half the size of the t:slim X2. It is fully controlled by a compatible iPhone mobile application and has an on-pump button for quick boluses. There is no built-in screen. It employs inductive (wireless) charging, with a cartridge lasting about 4 to 5 days. The cartridge holds 200 units of insulin [68].

Both Tandem pumps are components of an AID system and use the same Control-IQ technology to automatically adjust insulin based on data from a CGM. It can deliver automatic correction boluses if glucose is predicted to rise above 180 mg/dL, as well as decrease or stop basal insulin to prevent low blood glucose. The system makes decisions based on CGM readings, the user's weight, and total daily insulin use, which must be entered into the pump.

The International Diabetes Closed Loop trial, a 6 month randomized, multicenter trial of 168 patients, assigned in a 2:1 ratio to receive treatment with a closed-loop system (closed-loop group) or a sensor-augmented pump (control group), with the primary outcome measure being the percentage of time that the blood glucose was in the target range of 70 to 180 mg/dL. Patient ages ranged from 14 to 71 years. A1c level ranged from 5.4% to 10.6% [69].

The findings were as follows:

- The mean percentage of time that the glucose was in the target range in the closed-loop group was 61 ± 17% at baseline; at 6 months, the time in target range was 71 ± 12%.

Table 2
Omnipod and Tandem pumps and compatible devices

Product	Category	User base	Pivotal studies	Number of patients	Time in range (TIR)	Time below range (TBR)	Compatible devices
Omnipod 5	Insulin patch pump	Est 365,000	Brown SA, Forlenza GP, Bode BW, et al. Multicenter Trial of a Tubeless, On-Body Automated Insulin Delivery System With Customizable Glycemic Targets in Pediatric and Adult Participants With Type 1 Diabetes. *Diabetes Care*. 2021;44 (7):1630-1640. https://doi.org/10.2337/dc21-0172	235 total 111 children A1c was reduced by 0.71% in children.	74% (adults) TIR improved from standard therapy by 15.6% in children.	1.3% in adults	Dexcom G6 & G7 glucose sensor (G6 is being discontinued). Freestyle Libre 3 Plus glucose sensor Compatible with select smartphones (list on website of compatible devices) or with Insulet controller
			Real-World Data: Forlenza GP, DeSalvo DJ, Aleppo G, et al. Real-World Evidence of Omnipod® 5 Automated Insulin Delivery System Use in 69,902 People with Type 1 Diabetes. *Diabetes Technol Ther*. 2024;26 (8):514-525. https://doi.org/10.1089/dia.2023.0578	69,902	TIR in children 65.0%		
Tandem t:slim X2 Has a Touchscreen interface.	Insulin pump with tubing Both pumps use	Est 320,000	Brown SA, Kovatchev BP, Raghinaru D, et al. Six-Month Randomized,	168	67%	2.1%	*t:slim X2 Pump Compatibility:* Dexcom G6 and G7

(continued on next page)

Table 2
(*continued*)

Product	Category	User base	Pivotal studies	Number of patients	Time in range (TIR)	Time below range (TBR)	Compatible devices
Rechargeable pump. *Tandem Mobi* Significantly smaller than t:slim X2 200-unit cartridge. Can be worn with adhesive or clipped on. Inductive wireless charging Controlled by iPhone app	Control-IQ technology for automated insulin delivery with predictive algorithms, basal insulin adjustments, and automatic correction boluses		Multicenter Trial of Closed-Loop Control in Type 1 Diabetes. *New England Journal of Medicine*. 2019;381(18):1707-1717. doi: https://doi.org/10.1056/nejmoa1907863				FreeStyle Libre 2 Plus & 3 Plus
			Real World Data: Kovatchev BP, Singh H, Mueller L, Gonder-Frederick LA. Biobehavioral Changes Following Transition to Automated Insulin Delivery: A Large Real-life Database Analysis. *Diabetes Care*. 2022;45(11):2636-2643. https://doi.org/10.2337/dc22-1217	20,000	71%	1.5%	*Mobi Pump Compatibility:* Dexcom G6 and G7 FreeStyle Libre 3 Plus: Expected in 2026 in the US.

- The mean percentage of time in the target range for the control group remained unchanged at 59 ± 14%.
- Regarding safety outcomes, there were no serious hypoglycemic events in either group. There was one DKA episode in the closed-loop group.
- Secondary outcomes were
  - Percentage of time glucose was greater than 180 mg/dL.
  - Mean glucose concentration.
  - A1c.
  - Percentage of time the glucose was less than 70 mg/dL.
  - Percentage of time the glucose was less than 54 mg/dL.

Statistical analyses for all secondary outcomes favored the closed-loop system [69].

The closed-loop system used in this study was a t:slimX2 with Control-IQ technology.

This trial was pivotal in demonstrating the potential for achieving greater precision in blood glucose control with closed-loop systems compared with sensor-augmented pumps [69].

A later study compared CGM data and insulin therapy data for 19,354 individuals with type 1 diabetes, during 1 month of predictive low glucose suspend (PLGS) use, in which their pump would be suspended when their glucose was predicted to be under 80 mg/dL, followed by a 3 month period in which they changed to AID use. During the 3 months of AID use, their hybrid closed-loop system not only reacted to predicted hypoglycemia but also increased basal rate of insulin delivery for predicted high blood glucose, as well as delivering automatic correction doses. Time-in-range (TIR) increased from 58.4% during the PLGS period to 70.5% during the AID period [70]. The AID in the second phase of this study was the Control-IQ technology used in both tandem pumps currently.

Tandem pumps are described in more detail in Table 2.

4. The *twiist insulin pump* is a tubed insulin pump that uses the Tidepool Loop algorithm, which is the software that acts as the glycemic controller, adjusting insulin delivery based on CGM readings and predicted glucose values. The algorithm started as an initiative within the diabetes community that was later steered through FDA clearance by Tidepool, a nonprofit organization. It is approved for individuals aged 6 years and older. It utilizes iiSure technology, which is a hardware feature found specifically in this pump. It uses sound waves to precisely measure every pulse of insulin given. This feature provides for highly accurate dosing and the ability to detect occlusions nine times faster than other pumps. It holds up to 300 units of insulin. It has a target glucose range of 87 to 180 mg/dL and provides flexible wear options (fits in pocket, clips to belt, and there are adhesive options being developed for wearing it on the body) [71].

The Loop Do-It-Yourself AID system was tested in an observational study, with 558 individuals with type 1 diabetes, ages 171 years, who initiated Loop either on their own or through community resources and provided data for

Table 3
twiist and iLet bionic pancreas insulin pumps and compatible devices

Product	Category	User base	Pivotal studies	Number of patients	Time in range (TIR)	Time below range (TBR)	Compatible devices
twiist Utilizes Tidepool Loop algorithm.	Tubed insulin pump	Est 2000	Lum JW, Bailey RJ, Barnes-Lomen V, et al. A Real-World Prospective Study of the Safety and Effectiveness of the Loop Open Source Automated Insulin Delivery System *Diabetes Technol Ther.* 2021; 23(5):367-375. https://doi.org/10.1089/dia.2020.0535 Data presented at ADA2025 by Sequel Med Tech	558	73% 70%–80%	2.8% 2.9%–3.0%	Freestyle Libre 3 Plus
iLet Bionic Pancreas 3 components: CGM Algorithm software Insulin pump Uses body weight to start along with meal announcements (small, medium, large) Uses "lifelong learning algorithms" to adapt and	Tubed insulin pump	Est 24,000	Bionic Pancreas Research Group, Russell SJ, Beck RW, et al. Multicenter, Randomized Trial of a Bionic Pancreas in Type 1 Diabetes. *N Engl J Med.* 2022;387(13): 1161-1172. https://doi.org/10.1056/NEJMoa2205225	219	65%	1.8%	Dexcom (G6 or G7) glucose sensors Freestyle Libre 3 Plus

Box 1: Other current advances and areas for future development in type 1 diabetes (part 1)Advance or Area for Future Development

- Immunotherapy vaccine for type 1 diabetes

  Singer M, Kandeel F, Husseiny MI. *Salmonella*-Based Vaccine: A Promising Strategy for Type 1 Diabetes. *Vaccines (Basel)*. 2025;13 (4):405. Published 2025 Apr 14. https://doi.org/10.3390/vaccines 13040405.

- Verapamil to preserve β-cell function

  Degroote L, Martens PJ, Viaene M, et al. Verapamil and low-dose anti-mouse thymocyte globulin combination therapy stably reverses recent-onset type 1 diabetes in NOD mice by acting on the beta cell and immune axes. *Diabetologia*. 2025;68(10):2263-2276. https://doi.org/10.1007/s00125-025-06490-8.

- Screening T1D autoantibodies in individuals with autoimmune disorders (Hashimoto thyroiditis, Graves disease, celiac disease) without a family history of T1D

  Edelman SV, Agardh D, Cui N, Hao L, Wieloch M, Meneghini L. Risk of new-onset type 1 diabetes in individuals with celiac disease and thyroid disease—An observational study. *Diabetes Obesity and Metabolism*. Published online May 28, 2025. doi:https://doi.org/10.1111/dom.16454

- Machine learning and testing individuals who were diagnosed with type 2 diabetes in childhood for possible misdiagnosis of type 1 diabetes

  Cheheltani R, King N, Lee S, et al. Predicting misdiagnosed adult-onset type 1 diabetes using machine learning. *Diabetes Res Clin Pract*. 2022;191:110029. https://doi.org/10.1016/j.diabres.2022.110029.

- Electronic medical record algorithms to detect laboratory results and other medical findings to identify patients with possible unidentified type 1 diabetes

  Brusini I, Lee S, Hollingsworth J, et al. Deploying machine learning models in clinical settings: a real-world feasibility analysis for a model identifying adult-onset type 1 diabetes initially classified as type 2. *JAMIA Open*. 2025;8(5):ooaf133. Published 2025 Oct 26. https://doi.org/10.1093/jamiaopen/ooaf133.

- Glucose-responsive "smart insulin" systems

  Rege NK, Phillips NFB, Weiss MA. Development of glucose-responsive 'smart' insulin systems. *Curr Opin Endocrinol Diabetes Obes*. 2017;24 (4):267-278. https://doi.org/10.1097/MED.0000000000000345.

- Dual hormone pumps that deliver both insulin and glucagon

  El-Khatib FH, Balliro C, Hillard MA, et al. Home use of a bihormonal bionic pancreas versus insulin pump therapy in adults with type 1 diabetes: a multicentre randomised crossover trial. *Lancet*. 2017;389(10067):369-380. https://doi.org/10.1016/S0140-6736(1632567-3).

- Non-insulin drugs for treatment of T1D (GLP-1 receptor agonists, SGLT-2 inhibitors)

  Koike Y, Terauchi Y. Are current SGLT2 Inhibitors efficacious treatment options for Type 1 diabetes?. *Expert Opin Pharmacother.* 2021;22(9):1079-1081. https://doi.org/10.1080/14656566.2021.1900824.

- Low dose anti-thymocyte globulin to preserve β-cell function

  Foster TP, Jacobsen LM, Bruggeman B, et al. Low-Dose Antithymocyte Globulin: A Pragmatic Approach to Treating Stage 2 Type 1 Diabetes. *Diabetes Care.* 2024;47(2):285-289. https://doi.org/10.2337/dc23-1750.

- Oral insulin

  Sosenko JM, Skyler JS, Herold KC, et al. Slowed Metabolic Decline After 1 Year of Oral Insulin Treatment Among Individuals at High Risk for Type 1 Diabetes in the Diabetes Prevention Trial-Type 1 (DPT-1) and TrialNet Oral Insulin Prevention Trials. *Diabetes.* 2020;69(8):1827-1832. https://doi.org/10.2337/db20-0166.

- Mesenchymal stromal cell treatment to promote regulatory T cells (Tregs) to restore immune tolerance

  Carlsson PO, Schwarcz E, Korsgren O, Le Blanc K. Preserved β-cell function in type 1 diabetes by mesenchymal stromal cells. *Diabetes.* 2015;64(2):587-592. https://doi.org/10.2337/db14-0656.

- Autologous hematopoietic stem cell transplantation

  Nikoonezhad M, Lasemi MV, Alamdari S, et al. Treatment of insulin-dependent diabetes by hematopoietic stem cell transplantation. *Transplant Immunology.* 2022;75:101682. doi:https://doi.org/10.1016/j.trim.2022.101682

- JAK-STAT pathway inhibition (such as baricitinib, ritlecitinib, abrocitinib)

  ClinicalTrials.gov USNLoM. Janus kinase (JAK) inhibitors to preserve c-peptide production in new onset type 1 diabetes (T1D). https://clinicaltrials.gov/study/NCT05743244. Accessed November 30, 2025.

- Combination therapies to suppress autoimmunity (such as liraglutide and immunotherapy based on tolerogenic liposomes)

  Villalba A, Rodriguez-Fernandez S, Perna-Barrull D, et al. Antigen-specific immunotherapy combined with a regenerative drug in the treatment of experimental type 1 diabetes. *Sci Rep.* 2020;10(1):18927. Published 2020 Nov 3. https://doi.org/10.1038/s41598-020-76041-1.

- Cytokine-directed therapy (TNFα and IL-12/IL-23 inhibition)

  Mastrandrea L, Yu J, Behrens T, et al. Etanercept treatment in children with new-onset type 1 diabetes: pilot randomized, placebo-controlled, double-blind study. *Diabetes Care.* 2009;32(7):1244-1249. https://doi.org/10.2337/dc09-0054.

  Tatovic D, Marwaha A, Taylor P, et al. Ustekinumab for type 1 diabetes in adolescents: a multicenter, double-blind, randomized phase 2 trial. *Nat*

Med. 2024;30(9):2657-2666. https://doi.org/10.1038/s41591-024-03115-2.

- Xenotransplantation

  Mourad NI, Gianello P. Enhanced Insulin Production From Porcine Islets: More Insulin, Less Islets. *Transpl Int.* 2024;37:13954. Published 2024 Dec 18. https://doi.org/10.3389/ti.2024.13954.

6 months. In that study period, TIR (70–180 mg/dL) increased from 67 ± 16% at baseline to 73 ± 13% during the 6 months [72].

Additionally, real-world data presented at ADA2025, by Joanna Mitri, Chief Medical Officer of Sequel Med Tech, showed that 54 persons with type 1 diabetes wearing the twiist system had TIR 70%–80%, and TBR 2.9%–3.0% [73].

5. *iLet Bionic Pancreas* is a closed-loop system, approved for individuals ages 6 years and older. It utilizes an ACE pump, either a Dexcom glucose sensor or a Freestyle Libre 3 Plus sensor, and is initialized based on body weight. The user provides simple meal announcements (small, medium, or large), and autonomous dosing decisions are made using the iLet Dosing Decision Software. Carbohydrate counting and other decision-making processes are eliminated for the wearer, which enhances quality of life [74].

In a 13 week, multicenter, randomized trial, 219 participants, ages 6 to 79 years, were randomly assigned in a 2:1 ratio, persons at least 6 years of age with type 1 diabetes to receive bionic pancreas treatment with aspart or lispro or to receive standard care with CGM. The primary outcome was A1c level at 13 weeks. The secondary outcome was the percentage of time that the glucose level by CGM was below 54 mg/dL. At 13 weeks, the A1c level decreased from 7.9% to 7.3% in the bionic-pancreas group, and the A1c did not change in the standard-care group. The percentage of time that the glucose was below 54 mg/dL did not differ significantly between the two groups. Severe hypoglycemia rate was also not significantly different between the two groups, and neither group experienced any episodes of DKA [75].

The twist and iLet Bionic Pancreas systems are described further in Table 3.

OTHER CURRENT ADVANCES AND AREAS FOR FUTURE DEVELOPMENT IN TYPE 1 DIABETES

A myriad of strategies for prevention, amelioration of disease, and cure, not discussed herein, are underway, including, which are listed in Box 1.

The list in Box 1 highlights the multitude of avenues of ongoing investigation that will hopefully lead to further improvements in care and eventually, a cure for, T1D.

SUMMARY

T1D is a chronic autoimmune disease, with origins that are not fully elucidated. Genetic predisposition is a factor in the etiology of the illness. An unknown trigger of the immune system incites pancreatic islet autoantibody production, resulting in eventual lifelong exogenous insulin dependence. Several professional societies have endorsed a staging classification for the development of presymptomatic T1D, which is based upon the number of autoantibodies present and measures of glycemic control.

Utilization of the T1D staging classification system has directed points of entry in the disease process, wherein routes of investigation have been targeted. Advancements in both understanding of the pathogenesis of T1D, as well as the development of new therapies and device technology to improve glycemic control are rapidly evolving.

CGM devices and AID systems have improved glycemic control, reduced hypoglycemia, and enhanced quality of life for persons with T1D. Expansion of new therapies, including those involving immunomodulation and replacement of β-cell mass, is transpiring. However, the burden of daily glycemic management remains, and the ultimate desired endpoint is a permanent cure.

CLINICS CARE POINTS

- Screening of high-risk individuals for T1D can result in early identification of the presence of autoantibodies that herald the autoimmune process involved in the pathogenesis of T1D. Children identified by screening can then receive appropriate monitoring for disease progression.
- Up to 60% of children with T1D present in DKA at the time of diagnosis. Children who have been screened present in DKA less than 5% of the time.
- Children treated with teplizumab, an anti-CD3 monoclonal antibody, in stage 2 T1D (presence of at least 2 pancreatic autoantibodies and dysglycemia) have experienced at least a median delay of 2 years until progression to stage 3 (clinical diagnosis of T1D). This drug is in on-label clinical use.
- Implementation of the use of CGM systems and AID systems has resulted in improved glycemic control in patients with T1D compared to traditional insulin injection therapy.

Disclosures

The author has nothing to disclose.

References

[1] Eisenbarth GS. Type I diabetes mellitus. A chronic autoimmune disease. N Engl J Med 1986;314(21):1360–8.
[2] Atkinson MA, Eisenbarth GS. Type 1 diabetes: new perspectives on disease pathogenesis and treatment. Lancet 2001;358(9277):221–9.
[3] Atkinson MA, Eisenbarth GS, Michels AW. Type 1 diabetes. Lancet 2014;383(9911): 69–82. Available at: https://www.thelancet.com/journals/lancet/article/PIIS0140-6736(13)60591-7/fulltext.
[4] Insel RA, Dunne JL, Atkinson MA, et al. Staging presymptomatic type 1 diabetes: a scientific statement of JDRF, the endocrine Society, and the American diabetes Association. Diabetes Care 2015;38(10):1964–74.

[5] American Diabetes Association. Diagnosis and classification of diabetes: standards of care in diabetes—2025. Diabetes Care 2024;48(Supplement_1):S27–49; https://doi.org/10.2337/dc25-S002.
[6] Michels AW, Brusko TM, Evans-Molina C, et al. Challenges and opportunities for understanding the pathogenesis of type 1 diabetes: an endocrine Society scientific statement. J Clin Endocrinol Metab 2025;110(9):2496–508.
[7] Sims EK, Carr ALJ, Oram RA, et al. 100 years of insulin: celebrating the past, present and future of diabetes therapy. Nat Med 2021;27(7):1154–64.
[8] Walker JT, Saunders DC, Brissova M, et al. The human islet: mini-organ with mega-impact. Endocr Rev 2021;42(5):605–57.
[9] Besser REJ, Bell KJ, Couper JJ, et al. ISPAD clinical practice consensus guidelines 2022: stages of type 1 diabetes in children and adolescents. Pediatr Diabetes 2022;23(8): 1175–87.
[10] Citron-Zafrin K, Gandica R, Leibel N. Latest updates in prevention and screening of type 1 diabetes mellitus. Curr Pediatr Rep 2025;13(1); https://doi.org/10.1007/s40124-025-00351-z.
[11] Leichter SB, Felton JL, Rasmussen CG, et al. Establishing screening programs for presymptomatic type 1 diabetes: practical guidance for diabetes care providers. J Clin Endocrinol Metab 2025;110(8):2371–82.
[12] Phillip M, Achenbach P, Addala A, et al. Consensus guidance for monitoring individuals with islet autoantibody–positive pre-stage 3 type 1 diabetes. Diabetes Care 2024;47(8); https://doi.org/10.2337/dci24-0042.
[13] Moore DJ, Leibel NI, Polonsky W, et al. Recommendations for screening and monitoring the stages of type 1 diabetes in the immune therapy era. Int J Gen Med 2024;17:3003–14.
[14] Simmons KM, Sims EK. Screening and prevention of type 1 diabetes: where are we? J Clin Endocrinol Metab 2023;108(12):3067–79; https://doi.org/10.1210/clinem/dgad328.
[15] Sims EK, Besser REJ, Dayan C, et al. Screening for type 1 diabetes in the general population: a status report and perspective. Diabetes 2022;71(4):610–23.
[16] Mathieu C, Sims EK, Chatenoud L, et al. Toward Disease- modifying therapies in type 1 diabetes: focus on Teplizumab. Diabetes Care 2025;dci250066; https://doi.org/10.2337/dci25-0066.
[17] Ebrahimpour Y, Khatami S, Saffar M, et al. A comprehensive review of novel advances in type 1 diabetes mellitus. J Diabetes 2025;17(8); https://doi.org/10.1111/1753-0407.70120.
[18] Herold KC, Gitelman SE, Gottlieb P, et al. Teplizumab: a Disease- modifying therapy for type 1 diabetes that preserves β-Cell function. Diabetes Care 2023;46(10):1848–56.
[19] Zaitoon D, Zaitoon H. Teplizumab for stage 2 type 1 diabetes: a new era in pediatric diabetes prevention. Eur J Pediatr 2025;184(11); https://doi.org/10.1007/s00431-025-06520-y.
[20] Tzield (Teplizumab-mzwv) injection. Prescribing information. Sanofi. 2022. Available at: https://www.accessdata.fda.gov/drugsatfda_docs/label/2022/761183s000lbl.pdf. Accessed November 2, 2025.
[21] TZIELD (Teplizumab-mzwv) HCP injection 2mg/2mL I Delay stage 3 type 1 diabetes (T1D). TZIELD HCP. Available at: https://www.tzieldhcp.com/. Accessed November 2, 2025.
[22] Herold KC, Bundy BN, Long SA, et al. An Anti-CD3 antibody, Teplizumab, in relatives at risk for type 1 diabetes. N Engl J Med 2019;381(7):603–13.
[23] Ramos EL, Dayan C, Chatenoud L, et al. Teplizumab and β-Cell function in newly diagnosed type 1 diabetes. N Engl J Med 2023;389(23); https://doi.org/10.1056/nejmoa2308743.
[24] Available at: https://www.sanofi.com/en/media-room/press-releases/2025/2025-10-20-11-30-00-3169262. Accessed November 2, 2025.
[25] Holt RIG, DeVries JH, Hess-Fischl A, et al. The management of type 1 diabetes in adults. A consensus report by the American Diabetes Association (ADA) and the European Association for the Study of diabetes (EASD). Diabetes Care 2021;44(11):2589–625.

[26] Choudhary P, Rickels MR, Senior PA, et al. Evidence-informed clinical practice recommendations for treatment of type 1 diabetes complicated by problematic hypoglycemia. Diabetes Care 2015;38(6):1016–29.
[27] Vantyghem MC, Chetboun M, Gmyr V, et al. Ten-year outcome of islet alone or islet after kidney transplantation in type 1 diabetes: a prospective parallel-arm cohort study. Diabetes Care 2019;42(11):2042–9.
[28] Gamble A, Pepper AR, Bruni A, et al. The journey of islet cell transplantation and future development. Islets 2018;10(2):80–94.
[29] Bellin MD, Barton FB, Heitman A, et al. Potent induction immunotherapy promotes long-term insulin independence after islet transplantation in type 1 diabetes. Am J Transplant 2012;12 (6):1576–83.
[30] Shapiro AM. State of the art of clinical islet transplantation and novel protocols of immunosuppression. Curr Diab Rep 2011;11(5):345–54.
[31] Pagliuca FW, Millman JR, Gürtler M, et al. Generation of functional human pancreatic β cells in vitro. Cell 2014;159(2):428–39.
[32] Veres A, Faust AL, Bushnell HL, et al. Charting cellular identity during human in vitro β-cell differentiation. Nature 2019;569(7756):368–73.
[33] Rickels MR, Liu C, Shlansky-Goldberg RD, et al. Improvement in β-cell secretory capacity after human islet transplantation according to the CIT07 protocol. Diabetes 2013;62(8): 2890–7.
[34] Hering BJ, Clarke WR, Bridges ND, et al. Phase 3 trial of transplantation of human islets in type 1 diabetes complicated by severe hypoglycemia. Diabetes Care 2016;39(7): 1230–40.
[35] Reichman TW, Markmann JF, Odorico J, et al. Stem cell-derived, fully differentiated islets for type 1 diabetes. N Engl J Med 2025;393(9):858–68.
[36] Vertex. Vertex announces positive results from ongoing phase 1/2 study of VX-880 for the treatment of type 1 diabetes presented at the American Diabetes Association 84th scientific sessions. Vertex [Press Release]; 2024. Available at: https://news.vrtx.com/news-releases/news-release-details/vertex-presents-positive-data-zimislecel-type-1-diabetes. Accessed November 2, 2025.
[37] Vertex. Vertex announces positive results for Zimislecel in type 1 diabetes at the American Diabetes Associations 85th scientific sessions. Vertex [Press Release]; 2025. Available at: https://news.vrtx.com/news-releases/news-release-details/vertex-presents-positive-data-zimislecel-type-1-diabetes. Accessed November 2, 2025.
[38] Rickels MR. Innovation and progress in stem cell-derived islet-cell replacement therapy: durable glycemic control and elimination of exogenous insulin use with VX-880 in patients with type 1 diabetes (T1D) – VX-880-101 (FORWARD). In: Presented at: American Diabetes Association. 2025 Chicago, IL.
[39] Lemos JRN, Skyler JS. Challenges in beta cell replacement for type 1 diabetes. In: Hormone research in paediatrics. 2024. 2024. p. 1–34; https://doi.org/10.1159/000542206.
[40] Addissouky TA. Beyond insulin: advancing frontiers in cell-based and genetic therapies for type 1 diabetes management. Egypt J Intern Med 2025;37(1); https://doi.org/10.1186/s43162-025-00477-y.
[41] Ludwig B, Heller C, Sarangova V, et al. Islet macroencapsulation: strategies to boost islet graft oxygenation. In: Piemonti L, Odorico J, Kieffer TJ, et al, editors. Pluripotent stem cell therapy for diabetes. Cham: Springer; 2023; https://doi.org/10.1007/978-3-031-41943-0_12.
[42] Ghasemi A, Akbari E, Imani R. An overview of engineered hydrogel-based biomaterials for improved β-Cell survival and insulin secretion. Front Bioeng Biotechnol 2021;9; https://doi.org/10.3389/fbioe.2021.662084.
[43] Kaur Badwal A, Singh S. A comprehensive review on the current status of CRISPR based clinical trials for rare diseases. Int J Biol Macromol 2024;134097; https://doi.org/10.1016/j.ijbiomac.2024.134097.

[44] Banda A, Impomeni O, Singh A, et al. Precision in action: the role of clustered regularly interspaced short palindromic repeats/Cas in gene therapies. Vaccines 2024;12(6):636.
[45] Khatibi S, Sahebkar A, Bakhtiari SHA. CRISPR genome editing technology and its application in genetic diseases: a review. Curr Pharm Biotechnol 2020;21; https://doi.org/10.2174/1389201021666200621161610.
[46] Casgevy (exagamglogene autotemcel) suspension for intravenous infusion. Prescribing information. Vertex pharmaceuticals. 2023. Available at: https://pi.vrtx.com/files/uspi_exagamglogene_autotemcel.pdf. Accessed November 2, 2025.
[47] Khan S, Mahmood MS, Rahman SU, et al. CRISPR/Cas9: the Jedi against the dark empire of diseases. J Biomed Sci 2018;25(29); https://doi.org/10.1186/s12929-018-0425-5.
[48] Wahid B, Usman S, Ali A, et al. Therapeutic strategies of clustered regularly interspaced palindromic repeats-Cas systems for different viral infections. Viral Immunol 2017;30(8):552–9.
[49] Sun JY, Hu HB, Cheng YX, et al. CRISPR in medicine: applications and challenges. Brief Funct Genomics 2020;19(3):151–3.
[50] Lu XJ, Sun HM, Xu Y, et al. The applications and advances of CRISPR-Cas9 in medical research. Brief Funct Genomics 2017;16(1):1–3.
[51] Cheng X, Fan S, Wen C, et al. CRISPR/Cas9 for cancer treatment: technology, clinical applications and challenges. Brief Funct Genomics 2020;19(3):209–14.
[52] Kotagama OW, Jayasinghe CD, Abeysinghe T. Era of genomic medicine: a narrative review on CRISPR technology as a potential therapeutic tool for human diseases. BioMed Res Int 2019;2019:1369682; https://doi.org/10.1155/2019/1369682:Published 2019 Oct 7.
[53] Li T, Yang Y, Qi H, et al. CRISPR/Cas9 therapeutics: progress and prospects. Signal Transduct Targeted Ther 2023;8(1):1–23.
[54] Li R, Wang Q, She K, et al. CRISPR/Cas systems usher in a new era of disease treatment and diagnosis. Mol Biomed 2022;3(1):31.
[55] Carlsson PO, Hu X, Scholz H, et al. Survival of transplanted allogeneic beta cells with no immunosuppression. N Engl J Med 2025;393(9):887–94.
[56] Hirsch IB. Introduction: history of glucose monitoring. In: Role of continuous glucose monitoring in diabetes treatment. Arlington (VA): American Diabetes Association; 2018. p. 1.
[57] Fan W, Deng C, Zhou Z, et al. Efficacy and safety of automated insulin delivery systems in patients with type 1 diabetes mellitus: a systematic review and meta-analysis. Diabetes Metab J 2025;49:235–51.
[58] Musolino G, Dovc K, Boughton CK, et al. Reduced burden of diabetes and improved quality of life: experiences from unrestricted day-and-night hybrid closed-loop use in very young children with type 1 diabetes. Pediatr Diabetes 2019;20(6):794–9.
[59] Monaghan M, Bryant BL, Inverso H, et al. Young children with type 1 diabetes: recent advances in behavioral research. Curr Diabetes Rep 2022;22(6); https://doi.org/10.1007/s11892-022-01465-0.
[60] CGM Device Comparison. American Association of Clinical Endocrinology. Available at: https://pro.aace.com/cgm/toolkit/cgm-device-comparison. Accessed November 30, 2025.
[61] Carlson AL, Sherr JL, Shulman DI, et al. Safety and glycemic outcomes during the MiniMed™ advanced hybrid closed-loop system pivotal trial in adolescents and adults with type 1 diabetes. Diabetes Technol Ther 2022;24(3):178–89.
[62] MiniMed™ 780G Insulin Pump. Medtronic.com. Available at: https://www.medtronic.com/en-us/healthcare-professionals/products/diabetes/insulin-pumps/minimed-780g-insulin-pump.html. Accessed November 30, 2025.
[63] Choudhary P, Arrieta A, van den Heuvel T, et al. Celebrating the data from 100,000 real-world users of the MiniMed™ 780G system in Europe, Middle East, and Africa collected over 3 years: from data to clinical evidence. Diabetes Technol Ther 2024;26(S3):32–7.

[64] Healthcare Providers I omnipod® HCP Site. Available at: www.omnipod.com. Accessed November 25, 2025 https://www.omnipod.com/hcp.
[65] Brown SA, Forlenza GP, Bode BW, et al. Multicenter trial of a tubeless, On-Body automated insulin delivery system with customizable glycemic targets in pediatric and adult participants with type 1 diabetes. Diabetes Care 2021;44(7):1630–40.
[66] Forlenza GP, DeSalvo DJ, Aleppo G, et al. Real-world evidence of omnipod® 5 automated insulin delivery system use in 69,902 people with type 1 diabetes. Diabetes Technol Ther 2024;26(8):514–25.
[67] T:slim X2 Insulin Pump I Type 1 Diabetes Insulin Pump I Tandem Diabetes Care. Tandem Diabetes. Available at: https://www.tandemdiabetes.com/products/insulin-pumps/t-slim-x2-insulin-pump. Accessed November 25, 2025.
[68] Tandem mobi I Tandem diabetes care. Tandem Diabetes. Available at: https://www.tandemdiabetes.com/products/insulin-pumps/tandem-mobi. Accessed November 25, 2025.
[69] Brown SA, Kovatchev BP, Raghinaru D, et al. Six-month randomized, multicenter trial of Closed- loop control in type 1 diabetes. N Engl J Med 2019;381(18):1707–17.
[70] Kovatchev BP, Singh H, Mueller L, et al. Biobehavioral changes following transition to automated insulin delivery: a large real-life database analysis. Diabetes Care 2022;45(11): 2636–43.
[71] twiist Healthcare Professionals. Twiist.com. Available at: https://www.twiist.com/hcp-home. Accessed October 30, 2025.
[72] Lum JW, Bailey RJ, Barnes-Lomen V, et al. A real-world prospective study of the safety and effectiveness of the loop open source automated insulin delivery system. Diabetes Technol Ther 2021;23(5):367–75.
[73] Mitri J. First impressions of the twiist AID system. In: Presented at: American Diabetes Association 85th scientific sessions; Chicago, IL. 2025.
[74] iLet Bionic Pancreas. Beta bionics. Available at: https://www.betabionics.com/ilet-bionic-pancreas. Accessed November 4, 2025.
[75] Bionic Pancreas Research Group, Russell SJ, Beck RW, et al. Multicenter, randomized trial of a bionic pancreas in type 1 diabetes. N Engl J Med 2022;387(13):1161–72.

Advances in Pediatrics 73 (2026) 145–159
ADVANCES IN PEDIATRICS

Advances in Down Syndrome

Kinsa Thi Oo, MD[a,b], Najibe Abou-Antoun, MS[a,b], Soula Danopoulos, PhD[a,b], Denise Al Alam, PhD[a,b,*]

[a]Department of Pediatrics, David Geffen School of Medicine UCLA, Harbor UCLA Medical Center, 1000 W Carson Street, Torrance, CA 90509, USA; [b]Lundquist Institute for Biomedical Innovation at Harbor UCLA Medical Center, 1124 W Carson Street, Torrance, CA 90502, USA

Keywords

• Down syndrome • Trisomy 21 • Pediatric disease • Co-morbidities

Key points

- Advances in cardiac surgery, endocrine, and metabolic surveillance, respiratory medicine, neurodevelopmental care, and adult transition services have led to dramatic improvements in both survival and quality of life.
- There has been recent progress in genomic studies, particularly using gene editing technology (CRISPR/Cas9 technology) to investigate the feasibility of silencing or correcting genes on the extra chromosome 21.
- Other novel technologies, such as single-cell RNA sequencing and the use of induced pluripotent stem cells to model disease, are used to further elucidate cellular defects across multiple organ systems including the heart.

INTRODUCTION

Trisomy 21 (T21), also known as Down syndrome (DS), is the most common genetic anomaly worldwide affecting approximately 1 in 700 live births [1]. It is characterized by the presence of an extra complete or partial copy of chromosome 21. This results in intellectual disability and various physical and health-related challenges. Currently, the standard for prenatal T21 detection established by the American College of Medical Genetics and Genomics includes first-trimester biochemistry, nuchal translucency, and cell-free DNA testing. It is highly sensitive with very low false-positive rates (<0.1%) [2]. The condition presents with unique facial features, low muscle tone, and developmental

*Corresponding author. Department of Pediatrics, David Geffen School of Medicine UCLA, Harbor UCLA Medical Center, Torrance, CA. *E-mail address:* denise.alalam@lundquist.org

https://doi.org/10.1016/j.yapd.2025.12.004

Abbreviations

AD	Alzheimer's disease
ALL	acute lymphoblastic leukemia
APP	amyloid precursor protein
CHD	congenital heart defect
DS	Down syndrome
DSRD	Down Syndrome Regression Disorder
GI	gastrointestinal
IVIG	intravenous immunoglobulin
PNDM	permanent neonatal diabetes mellitus
RG	Radial Glia
T21	Trisomy 21

delays. However, the challenges associated with T21 are not limited to these early signs; patients with T21 also experience a range of complications across their lifespan, particularly in the cardiovascular, respiratory, endocrine, gastrointestinal, immunologic, and neurologic systems [3–5]. These newly occurring comorbidities vary across the life span and include higher prevalence of congenital heart malformation, ear diseases, eye disorders, autism, hypothyroidism, diabetes, and obesity in childhood [6]. Over recent decades, early prenatal diagnosis, improvements in neonatal intensive care, and structured multidisciplinary follow-up have greatly enhanced both life expectancy and functional outcomes for people with T21 [4,7]. Because of the increase in life expectancy into the 60s and beyond, neurologic decline in the form of Alzheimer's disease (AD), neurodevelopmental delays, and regression have become prominent issues for adults with T21 [3,8].

Beyond structural differences, T21 involves fundamental molecular and cellular alterations in multiple organ systems. For example, overexpression of genes encoded on chromosome 21 such as *RUNX1, SOD1, DYRK1A,* and *IFNAR1/2* affects oxidative stress regulation, neuronal development, and immune activity [5,8]. These mechanisms may help explain the broad clinical spectrum of T21, from congenital heart disease to endocrine, neurologic, and immune abnormalities. This review summarizes current evidence and new discoveries across major organ systems, focusing on practical updates for clinicians and researchers. The ongoing challenge is to translate these molecular insights into individualized care, improving outcomes across the lifespan for individuals with T21.

CARDIOVASCULAR SYSTEM

Congenital heart defects (CHDs) are the most frequent comorbidities associated with DS and are present in nearly half of all newborns [7] with DS. The most common types are atrioventricular septal defect, ventricular septal defect, and patent ductus arteriosus [7,9]. Advances in prenatal screening, cardiac surgery, and postoperative management have led to survival rates approaching those of the general population [9,10]. This has been reviewed in detail by Petrikas and colleagues [11] and Peterson and colleagues [7]. However, residual issues such as pulmonary hypertension, arrhythmia, and reduced exercise capacity remain more common in individuals with DS [10,12,13].

Adults with repaired heart defects often experience persistent right ventricular dysfunction and reduced exercise tolerance, emphasizing the need for long-term follow-up and rehabilitation [10]. Pulmonary hypertension remains a major cause of morbidity and mortality. Its persistence after surgical correction is thought to result from exaggerated hypoxic vasoconstriction and impaired vascular adaptation [12]. Early recognition and targeted use of pulmonary vasodilators have improved outcomes, but preventive strategies are still evolving [12,13].

Emerging studies have attempted to pinpoint the molecular and cellular defects underlying cardiovascular disease in individuals with DS. Whole genome sequencing revealed the association of rare variants (KIF rs138354681, GJA1 rs778110855, and PDE1C PP785745) with CHD in DS [14]. In addition, molecular studies have shown that overexpression of chromosome 21 genes influences endothelial function, vascular tone, and inflammatory signaling [8,12,13]. Altered collagen structure and increased oxidative stress contribute to vascular remodeling and chronic pulmonary hypertension, even after cardiac repair [12]. These features define a distinct cardiovascular profile in T21, marked by heightened vascular reactivity and autonomic imbalance [13]. In rodent models, studies have shown that the increase in DYRK1A gene dosage results in CHDs and is associated with mitochondrial impairment [15]. Furthermore, using human induced pluripotent stem cells and mouse models, it has been shown that the dosage of *HMGN1*, a nucleosome binding epigenetic regulator encoded on chromosome 21, can be a key contributor to the valvuloseptal defects observed in DS. Specifically, this dosage in *HMGN1* causes a shift in cell fate of human atrioventricular canal cardiomyocytes toward ventricular cardiomyocytes [16]. These studies reveal new potential biomarkers and gene target for heart disease in individuals with DS that warrant further in-depth investigations.

Overall, outcomes for congenital heart disease in DS have improved substantially, yet lifelong cardiovascular surveillance remains essential. Future research will focus on understanding vascular biology and developing therapies that address oxidative and inflammatory mechanisms underlying pulmonary hypertension and heart failure [7,9,12].

PULMONARY AND RESPIRATORY SYSTEM

Respiratory illness remains a leading cause of hospitalization and mortality in both the pediatric and adult population with DS. Contributing factors include upper airway obstruction, tracheomalacia, hypotonia, and impaired immune function. Recurrent lower respiratory tract infections, aspiration, and sleep-disordered breathing are also major concerns throughout childhood [17].

Recent studies show that airway malacia and narrowing are more common than previously thought, explaining high prevalence of obstructive sleep apnea, which is reported to affect 80% to 90% of pediatric patients with DS [18]. Early identification and treatment with adenotonsillectomy, continuous positive airway pressure, and weight control can improve neurocognitive and growth outcomes [19]. The use of atomoxetine and oxybutynin (ato-oxy) is being tested in children with T21 and obstructive sleep apnea diagnosed with polysomnography to improve cognition. The standard treatment is adenotonsillectomy, which is not as effective in general pediatric population as in children with T21. With the use of drug-induced sleep endoscopy to directly visualize the sites, children with T21 tend to have more tongue base and supraglottic obstruction, which can benefit from personalized surgery to correct the obstruction areas. These surgical approaches are currently under investigation.

Pulmonary hypertension is a hallmark complication in T21, often developing due to combined effects of congenital heart disease, chronic hypoxia, and altered vascular reactivity. Individuals with DS display unique hemodynamic responses, including exaggerated hypoxic vasoconstriction and delayed vascular remodeling. Treatment with endothelin receptor antagonists has shown significant improvement in patients with T21 [20].

However, these pulmonary complications have been demonstrated to initiate in utero. Recent studies have shown that developmental lung defects start as early as 16 weeks of gestation in approximately 75% of fetuses studied [21]. This new knowledge has significantly changed the way neonatologists consider respiratory complications in neonates with DS. Defects have been observed at all levels: in different cell types (ie, immune, epithelium, etc.) as well as different compartments (distal, proximal) of the developing T21 lung. Anomalies in the T21 pulmonary endothelium, encompassing both vascular and lymphatic components, have been characterized by defects such as congested capillaries, muscularized arteries, and dilated lymphatics [21]. In rare cases, interstitial lung disease and diffuse alveolar hemorrhage have been observed in children with DS, reflecting endothelial inflammation [22]. Within the epithelium, individuals with T21 exhibit altered cellular composition early in lung development, affecting both airway and distal regions. These changes are associated with increased secretory activity [23] and may contribute to heightened susceptibility to viral infections.

Increased susceptibility to viral infections could also be attributed to immune dysregulation. An alteration in resident immune cells within the developing lung was shown recently, with a significant decrease in B cells (paper in press). In addition, elevated senescence and inflammatory markers are observed in the T21 developing human lung [24]. Altogether, the combination of compromised epithelial architecture and a defective immune system likely contributes to altered cytokine signaling and impaired mucociliary clearance, predisposing children with DS to recurrent pneumonia and bronchiolitis. However, the cause of the reduction in mucociliary clearance is unclear and worth understanding. Some studies described a decrease in ciliary beat frequency in T21 airway that was attributed to recurrent infections. Detailed analyses of the development of early airway composition and airway cell differentiation in

T21 are lacking and would better inform the cause of the defective mucociliary clearance. Preventive vaccination, early infection control, and coordinated pulmonary care remain critical for maintaining respiratory health.

GASTROINTESTINAL SYSTEM

Gastrointestinal (GI) abnormalities are common in T21, ranging from congenital malformations to functional and autoimmune disorders [25]. The most frequent GI associated congenital defects in babies with DS are Hirschsprung disease, duodenal atresia, and imperforate anus [25,26]. Less frequent congenital disorders of the GI tract in individuals with DS include congenital megacolon, esophageal atresia, annular pancreas, and esophageal compression [27]. Whereas recent studies have found that individuals with DS do not have higher medical or surgical complications than the general population [28], postoperative recovery is often prolonged due to feeding difficulties, delayed healing, and increased risk of infection [29].

In older infants and children, other GI problems include motility problems such as gastroesophageal reflux, constipation [30] and autoimmune conditions. Hypotonia, delayed gastric emptying, and oropharyngeal incoordination contribute to feeding difficulties that may persist into adulthood [30,31]. Nutritional therapy and noninvasive feeding interventions are usually effective, while surgery is reserved for refractory cases. Both nutrient deficiencies and obesity are prevalent in this population, underscoring the need for continuous nutritional monitoring and counseling throughout life [32]. A review study confirmed that different exercise modalities for adults with DS are prone to improve muscle strength, redox balance, and inflammatory profile. A tailored training is needed to be prescribed for better results [33].

Celiac disease affects approximately 5% to 12% of individuals with T21, and regular serologic screening is now standard. A gluten-free diet has been shown to improve growth and GI symptoms once the diagnosis is confirmed. Individuals with DS are 18 times more likely to get celiac disease than the general population [31]. Villus atrophy, commonly described in T21 intestine, is often attributed to the presence of celiac disease. However, a recent study showed that 50% of patients who underwent esophagogastroduodenoscopy presented with abnormal duodenal histology, half of whom had villus atrophy in the absence of celiac disease diagnosis [34]. The GI tract is one of the least studied organs in DS. There is a dire need for a better understanding of GI complications in this patient population.

ENDOCRINE SYSTEM

Endocrine disorders are also very common in people with T21. In particular, thyroid dysfunction commonly presents in childhood with subclinical hypothyroidism that can be caused by autoimmune thyroiditis, thyroid hypoplasia, or even dysgenesis [35,36]. This highlights the importance of routine screening as early as the first year of life to avoid growth and neurologic delays in patients. Early thyroxine therapy has been shown to improve cognitive and physical outcomes, although some may argue that therapy should only be started after 1 year of age [36,37]. Furthermore, the treatment should be avoided when the defect is not attributable to transient hypothyroidism, which may resolve without thyroxine therapy in the follow-up thyroid function tests [36,37].

In addition to thyroid disorders, type 1 and type 2 diabetes are also commonly associated with T21. Hyperinsulinism is more prevalent in individuals with DS than the general population [38]. While type 1 diabetes is usually associated with other autoimmune diseases, type 2 diabetes is mostly due to obesity and insulin resistance, which are also common in adolescents and adults with T21. For example, type 1 diabetes is commonly associated with conditions such as celiac disease, with the likelihood of developing celiac disease in individuals with DS who have type 1 diabetes being 4.7 times higher compared with type 1 diabetic patients without DS [39]. Glycemic control is also better in individuals with T21 compared with those with type 1 diabetes likely due to the less resistance to routine diet and exercise with less complicated lifestyles [39]. In addition, permanent neonatal diabetes mellitus (PNDM) was found at higher rates in individuals with T21, in the absence of any pathogenic variants in the 24 known PNDM genes, suggesting that T21 is causative of PNDM. The etiology of DS-PNDM is believed to be autoimmune, suggestive of a prenatal onset of B-cell dysfunction [40]. These observations are corroborated by a new study in a DS mouse model that confirms impaired glucose metabolism and defective insulin production with no change in beta cell mass in vivo [41].

Another proposed mechanism for obesity and type 2 diabetes in T21 involves thermogenic adipose tissue dysfunction. In this model, the conversion of brown adipose tissue–which supports insulin sensitivity and metabolic regulation–into white adipose tissue leads to increased oxidative stress. This shift is marked by elevated oxidative stress markers such as 4-HNE, SOD1, and SOD2 ultimately impairing glucose metabolism and insulin signaling in DS mouse models [42].

Obesity is another major problem in the DS population that is associated with type 2 diabetes, thyroid dysfunction, obstructive sleep apnea, and diminished exercise. Contributing factors include low muscle tone, reduced energy expenditure, and hyperphagia or preoccupation with food in the context of intellectual disability [43]. Growth retardation is another common problem in the T21 population which might be due to insulin like growth factor 1 deficiency with normal or mildly elevated growth hormone resulting in growth hormone resistant disorders [44]. This may be caused by increased inflammatory pathways such as tumor necrosis factor- alpha (TNFa) [44]. Therefore, growth monitoring with specific growth charts from the Down Syndrome Growing Up study for people with T21 is very important. Monitoring body mass index (BMI) and following up on growth and body weight are recommended from birth until 20 years of age so that early recognition of obesity and suboptimal growth, as well as timely interventions like healthy eating habits, tailored exercise programs, and avoidance of sedentary lifestyles can be done with better outcomes [45].

NEUROLOGY AND NEURODEVELOPMENTAL SYSTEM

Neurologic and neurodevelopmental disorders define much of the T21 phenotype. Intellectual disability is present in all individuals with T21, typically ranging from mild to moderate. Delays in speech, motor skills, and social development are common in childhood. The neurologic defects in T21 start in utero through reduced Radial Glia (RG) neural stem cell proliferation, reduced cortical volume, and imbalanced neural cell types [46,47]. A recent study showed an early emergence of cortical inhibitory neurons, an accelerated maturation of RG and an elevated interferon response in T21 human developing brains [48] which could explain the early onset of neurodegenerative diseases in individuals with T21. New research on early white matter microstructure in infants with DS found reduced structural integrity, disrupted myelination, and increased neurite dispersion in fibers critical for cognitive functions [49]. Gene overexpression, particularly of *DYRK1A, RCAN1,* and *APP,* disrupts synaptic development and neuronal signaling, contributing to learning and memory challenges [50,51]. Autism spectrum disorder is also more prevalent in T21, affecting about 15% to 20% of children.

After early childhood, neurodegenerative diseases, especially early-onset AD, become major concerns. The overexpression of the *APP* gene (amyloid precursor protein) on chromosome 21 leads to early amyloid plaque formation in the brain, which accelerates neurodegeneration. Studies have shown that by age 50%, 50% to 70% of adults with T21 will exhibit symptoms of AD [52,53]. Because of the early-onset AD, there are more significant challenges in managing cognitive decline, as many individuals may show signs of memory loss, confusion, and personality changes decades earlier than the general population. Anti-amyloid antibodies like aducanumab, which were developed for sporadic AD, are being tested in the T21 population. Additionally, small molecule inhibitors, like Leucettinib-21, targeting overexpressed genes like *DYRK1A* are currently in phase 1 clinical trial after showing efficacy in animal models [54]. These emerging therapies, including cholinesterase inhibitors and anti-amyloid antibodies, have shown limited but encouraging results [55,56].

In addition to AD, a rare but significant issue in T21 is regression in adolescence or early adulthood, known as Down Syndrome Regression Disorder (DSRD). DSRD involves a sudden loss of previously acquired skills, often accompanied by behavioral changes, insomnia, and sometimes catatonia. While the cause is not fully understood, it may be linked to autoimmune or inflammatory processes, and some cases have shown improvement with immunotherapy or psychiatric interventions [57,58]. This regression further complicates the care of older individuals with T21 and makes the transition from childhood to adulthood very challenging. New research into DSRD has revealed that some individuals improve with treatments such as intravenous immunoglobulin (IVIG), corticosteroids, or immunomodulators. Protocols are now being developed to better diagnose and treat DSRD based on suspected autoimmune or neuroinflammatory mechanisms [59]. A phase IIb clinical trial is aiming at comparing the safety and efficacy of 3 medications: lorazepam, IVIG, and tofacitinib, a JAK inhibitor in the treatment of DSRD.

Furthermore, epilepsy, especially infantile spasms (West syndrome), is more common in T21 than in the general population [60]. Early diagnosis and treatment of infantile spasms can improve long-term developmental outcomes. Sleep disturbances and behavioral conditions such as anxiety, depression, and autism spectrum traits are also common. A multidisciplinary approach that integrates neurology, psychiatry, and developmental care provides the best outcomes.

Together, ongoing research in neurobiology and early intervention (speech therapy, physical therapy, and occupational therapy) is transforming the management of neurodevelopmental challenges in T21. Early developmental therapy and structured educational programs significantly improve communication and adaptive functioning. Advances in early intervention have underscored the importance of stimulation during infancy when neuroplasticity is highest.

HEMATOLOGY, IMMUNOLOGY DYSREGULATION, AND INFLAMMATION

Hematologic and immune abnormalities are characteristic of T21. Compared with the general population, individuals with T21 are at a higher risk of developing acute leukemia before the age of 5 years [61,62]. In myeloid leukemia, newborns with T21 commonly present with transient myeloproliferative disorder which can be self-limiting in the first 3 months of life or can progress to acute myeloid leukemia linked to *GATA1* gene mutations and *CTCF, RAS, or JAK/STAT* pathway genes [63]. Acute lymphoblastic leukemia (ALL) associated with T21 differs from non-T21 ALL in that it exhibits a higher frequency of mutations in CRLF2, JAK2, and genes within the RAS signaling pathway [63,64]. There are several ongoing clinical trials, including one evaluating the effectiveness of blinatumomab alone versus blinatumomab combined with nivolumab in patients experiencing a first relapse of B-cell ALL, including those with T21. Blinatumomab is a bispecific antibody that targets and destroys cancer cells, whereas nivolumab is an immune checkpoint inhibitor that enhances immune response. The rationale is that combining these agents may inhibit or delay cancer progression.

Another characteristic of T21 is chronic inflammation and immune dysregulation which could be due to the consistent activation of interferon pathway as 4 of the 16 interferon receptors are encoded on chromosome 21, thus causing activation of the pathway and downstream targets [8]. This hyperactivation of interferon pathway can result in a condition called interferonopathy with complications of many systems with the neurologic and immune systems being the most affected. New therapies targeting the interferon-activated kinase like JAK are now being studied to treat the various complications from this interferon-related chronic inflammation in T21. A recent study focusing on the JAK inhibitor tofacitinib reported promising results where although tofacitinib does not completely suppress the interferon pathways in people with T21, it reduces the inflammatory markers by lowering the interferon (IFN) scores and cytokine scores to the general population's level. This can significantly benefit individuals with T21 in terms of controlling the autoimmune-related conditions [65]. The use of tofacitinib is also being tested in the treatment of autoimmune skin conditions in DS.

OTHER AND MULTISYSTEM FINDINGS

Beyond the major organ systems, children with T21 also have an increased risk of musculoskeletal problems like pes planus, inflammatory arthritis, delayed ambulation, hip problems, and scoliosis. Scoliosis, hip dysplasia, and low bone mineral density occur more often in adolescence and adulthood [66]. A delay in diagnosing these conditions can result in many adverse events like developmental delay, obesity due to low level of movements, and injuries due to instability. The annual musculoskeletal assessment helps with early diagnoses of these complications, for a timely referral, early intervention, and multidisciplinary management for overall improvement. Optimized calcium and vitamin D intake, and weight-bearing exercise are key preventive strategies [67].

Furthermore, people with T21 have more ligamentous laxity and joint hypermobility, which makes them at a higher risk for atlantoaxial dislocation. Currently, surgical corrections are recommended only for symptomatic patients. However, recent studies recommend prophylactic surgical interventions in those with atlanto-dens interval greater than 5 in radiographic screenings given their high chance of eventual development to progressive myelopathy and other complications [68].

Dedicated multidisciplinary clinics now coordinate care across specialties, improving adherence to screening, vaccination, and preventive guidelines. These programs address adult health issues, reproductive counseling, and caregiver support–ensuring comprehensive care throughout life [69].

BIOMARKERS FOR EARLY DETECTION

More biomarkers have been found for early detection of AD in T21. The development of blood-based biomarkers such as plasma amyloid-beta, tau, or neurofilament light chain levels holds promise for noninvasive screening [70]. The magnetic resonance spectroscopy could also be a good noninvasive alternative for the detection of AD-stage biomarkers; it was recently used for the analysis of AD metabolite markers (myo-inositol and N-acetyl-aspartate) [71]. Biomarker studies for CHD revealed significantly higher levels of plasma bone morphogenetic protein receptor type II (BMPR-II) and VE-cadherin in individuals with DS and pulmonary hypertension but without CHD than those with CHD; while the opposite was observed for hypoxia-inducible factor (HIF)-1 alpha [72]. These could allow for earlier diagnosis and intervention before significant complication occurs.

SUMMARY

The past decade has transformed our understanding and clinical care of individuals with T21. Advances in cardiac surgery, endocrine and metabolic surveillance, respiratory medicine, neurodevelopmental care, and adult transition services have led to dramatic improvements in both survival and quality of life. Importantly, recognition of immune dysregulation and neurodegeneration has opened new avenues for research and therapy.

There has been recent progress in genomic studies, particularly using CRISPR/Cas9 technology to investigate the feasibility of silencing or correcting genes on the extra chromosome 21 [73]. While still in preclinical stages, these approaches could represent a major step toward personalized and potentially curative therapies for T21-related complications. Other novel technologies, such as single-cell RNA sequencing and the use of induced pluripotent stem cells to model disease, are used to further elucidate cellular defects across multiple organ systems including the heart. Applications of these to DS research are rapidly improving our understanding of comorbidities.

Despite progress, challenges persist. These include disparities in access to multidisciplinary care, late diagnoses of comorbid conditions, and under-recognition of adult-onset diseases. Future priorities should focus on long-term surveillance strategies, integration of genomic and proteomic biomarkers, and development of targeted therapies to modulate inflammation, neurodegeneration, and metabolic complications.

With continued research, collaboration, and advocacy, individuals with T21 can look forward to longer, healthier, and more meaningful lives–supported by systems that meet their medical, developmental, and psychosocial needs throughout the lifespan.

CLINICS CARE POINTS

- Nearly half of newborns with Down Syndrome have congenital heart defects (CHD); early detection and intervention are critical for survival and quality of life.
- Respiratory illness is a leading cause of hospitalization and mortality; early recognition of abnormalities and sleep-disordered breathing is vital.
- Screen for congenital GI anomalies (eg, Hirschsprung disease, duodenal atresia) and celiac disease that affects 5–12% of patients with DS.
- Routine screening for thyroid dysfunction should begin in the first year of life; early thyroxine therapy can improve outcomes in case of confirmed hypothyroidism.
- Early intervention for neurodevelopmental disorders (speech, physical, occupational therapy) is crucial for developmental progress.
- Children with Down Syndrome are at higher risk for acute leukemia, especially before age 5; monitor for hematologic abnormalities.
- Annual musculoskeletal assessments help detect and manage conditions like scoliosis, hip dysplasia, and low bone density.
- Pearls: Advances in prenatal screening, cardiac surgery, and multidisciplinary care have significantly improved survival and functional outcomes.

- Early recognition and management of obstructive sleep apnea, pulmonary hypertension, and feeding difficulties can prevent long-term complications.
- Routine screening for thyroid dysfunction, diabetes, and celiac disease is essential, with tailored nutritional and exercise interventions improving growth and metabolic health.
- Early developmental therapies and structured educational programs enhance neurocognitive and adaptive functioning, and improve the overall quality of life.
- New biomarkers and therapies are emerging for Alzheimer's disease, regression disorders, and autoimmune complications.
- Annual musculoskeletal assessments and preventive strategies (eg, vitamin D, weight-bearing exercise) reduce risk of orthopedic complications.
- Multidisciplinary clinics and coordinated care improve adherence to preventive guidelines and address evolving needs across the lifespan.
- Pitfalls: Delaying or omitting surveillance for cardiac, respiratory, endocrine, or hematologic complications can result in missed opportunities for early intervention and increased morbidity.
- Attributing all gastrointestinal symptoms to celiac disease or all neuropsychiatric changes to behavioral issues may overlook treatable conditions.
- Over- or under-treating thyroid dysfunction without confirming persistence can lead to unnecessary therapy or missed benefits.
- Failing to recognize regression disorders or subtle signs of instability, delayed ambulation, or growth failure may delay critical interventions.
- Neglecting the need for lifelong, coordinated, and multidisciplinary follow-up risks under-recognition of adult-onset diseases and disparities in care.

Disclosures

The authors have nothing to disclose.

Funding

Dr Danopoulos acknowledges funding support from NIH, Office of the director (R01HL155104); Dr Al Alam acknowledges funding support from NIH/NHLBI (R01HL171915-01A1) and California Institute for Regenerative Medicine (CIRM/DISC0-15654).

References

[1] Parker SE, Mai CT, Canfield MA, et al, National Birth Defects Prevention Network. Updated National Birth Prevalence estimates for selected birth defects in the United States, 2004-2006. Birth Defects Res A Clin Mol Teratol 2010;88(12):1008–16.

[2] Palomaki GE, Smith WE, Bajaj K, et al. Prenatal screening for trisomy 21 (Down syndrome) using first- and second-trimester biochemistry and nuchal translucency: a technical standard of the American College of Medical Genetics and Genomics (ACMG). Genet Med 2025;27(9):101505; https://doi.org/10.1016/j.gim.2025.101505:PubMed PMID: 40778613.

[3] Bull MJ. Down Syndrome. N Engl J Med 2020;382(24):2344–52.

[4] de Graaf G, Skladzien E, Buckley F, et al. Estimation of the number of people with Down syndrome in Australia and New Zealand. Genet Med 2022;24(12):2568–77.

[5] Sullivan KD, Evans D, Pandey A, et al. Trisomy 21 causes changes in the circulating proteome indicative of chronic autoinflammation. Sci Rep 2017;7(1):14818; https://doi.org/10.1038/s41598-017-13858-3:PubMed PMID: 29093484; PMCID: PMC5665944.
[6] Alexander M, Petri H, Ding Y, et al. Morbidity and medication in a large population of individuals with Down syndrome compared to the general population. Dev Med Child Neurol 2016;58(3):246–54.
[7] Peterson JK, Clarke S, Gelb BD, et al. Council on cardiovascular R, intervention. Trisomy 21 and congenital heart disease: impact on health and functional outcomes from birth through adolescence: a scientific statement from the American Heart Association. J Am Heart Assoc 2024;13(19):e036214; https://doi.org/10.1161/JAHA.124.036214:PubMed PMID: 39263820; PMCID: PMC11681493.
[8] Sullivan KD, Lewis HC, Hill AA, et al. Trisomy 21 consistently activates the interferon response. eLife 2016;5:20160729; https://doi.org/10.7554/eLife.16220:PubMed PMID: 27472900; PMCID: PMC5012864.
[9] Dimopoulos K, Constantine A, Clift P, et al. Cardiovascular complications of Down syndrome: scoping review and expert consensus. Circulation 2023;147(5):425–41, PubMed PMID: 36716257; PMCID: PMC9977420.
[10] Engsner S, Giang KW, Dellborg M, et al. Impact of Down syndrome on survival among patients with congenital heart disease. J Am Heart Assoc 2024;13(2):e031392; https://doi.org/10.1161/JAHA.123.031392:PubMed PMID: 38214262; PMCID: PMC10926807.
[11] Petrikas M, Choi S, Cavanaugh K, et al. A change of heart: the evolution of care for children with Trisomy 21 and CHD. Cardiol Young 2025;35(9):1759–65.
[12] Bush DS, Ivy DD. Pulmonary hypertension in the population with Down syndrome. Cardiol Ther 2022;11(1):33–47, PubMed PMID: 35037192; PMCID: PMC8933583.
[13] Cilhoroz BT, Receno CN, Heffernan KS, et al. Cardiovascular physiology and pathophysiology in Down syndrome. Physiol Res 2022;71(1):1–16, PubMed PMID: 35043643; PMCID: PMC8997681.
[14] Ganguly A, Pal S, Chatterjee S, et al. Rare and novel variant load threshold for KIF7, GJA1 and PDE1C genes elevates the risk of severity of congenital heart defects in Down syndrome. PLoS One 2025;20(6):e0326566; https://doi.org/10.1371/journal.pone.0326566:PubMed PMID: 40569905; PMCID: PMC12200707.
[15] Lana-Elola E, Aoidi R, Llorian M, et al. Increased dosage of DYRK1A leads to congenital heart defects in a mouse model of Down syndrome. Sci Transl Med 2024;16(731):eadd6883; https://doi.org/10.1126/scitranslmed.add6883:PubMed PMID: 38266108; PMCID: PMC7615651.
[16] Ranade SS, Li F, Whalen S, et al. Myocardial reprogramming by HMGN1 underlies heart defects in trisomy 21. Nature 2025;647(8091):979–87.
[17] DeBoer E, Wolter-Warmerdam K, Hickey F, et al. Large airway and lung findings in symptomatic children and young adults with Down syndrome. Pediatr Pulmonol 2025;60(10):e71339; https://doi.org/10.1002/ppul.71339:PubMed PMID: 41090283.
[18] Nerfeldt P, Sundelin A. Obstructive sleep apnea in children with Down syndrome - prevalence and evaluation of surgical treatment. Int J Pediatr Otorhinolaryngol 2020;133:109968; https://doi.org/10.1016/j.ijporl.2020.109968:PubMed PMID: 32126418.
[19] Shan S, Wang S, Yang X, et al. Effect of adenotonsillectomy on the growth, development, and comprehensive cognitive abilities of children with obstructive sleep apnea: a prospective single-arm study. BMC Pediatr 2022;22(1):41, PubMed PMID: 35033050; PMCID: PMC8760659.
[20] Kermeen FD, Franks C, O'Brien K, et al. Endothelin receptor antagonists are an effective long term treatment option in pulmonary arterial hypertension associated with congenital heart disease with or without trisomy 21. Heart Lung Circ 2010;19(10):595–600.

[21] Danopoulos S, Bhattacharya S, Deutsch G, et al. Prenatal histological, cellular, and molecular anomalies in trisomy 21 lung. J Pathol 2021;255(1):41–51, PubMed PMID: 34050678; PMCID: PMC9109699.
[22] Bloom JL, Frank B, Weinman JP, et al. Diffuse alveolar hemorrhage in children with trisomy 21. Pediatr Rheumatol Online J 2021;19(1):114, PubMed PMID: 34273981; PMCID: PMC8285855.
[23] Bhattacharya S, Frauenpreis A, Cherry C, et al. The transcriptional landscape of developing human trisomy 21 lungs. Am J Respir Cell Mol Biol 2025; https://doi.org/10.1165/rcmb.2025-0217OC.
[24] Belgacemi R, Cherry C, Thompson M, et al. Elevated senescence markers in developing trisomy 21 human lungs. Am J Respir Cell Mol Biol 2025;73(2):251–63, PubMed PMID: 40019852; PMCID: PMC12334841.
[25] Zrinyi A, Lum Min SA, Bello EA, et al. Effect of trisomy 21 on long-term gastrointestinal outcomes in duodenal atresia. Pediatr Surg Int 2023;39(1):84.
[26] Elgendy MM, Cortez J, Saker F, et al. Prevalence and outcomes of gastrointestinal anomalies in Down syndrome. Am J Perinatol 2024;41(15):2047–52.
[27] Bermudez B, de Oliveira CM, de Lima Cat MN, et al. Gastrointestinal disorders in Down syndrome. Am J Med Genet 2019;179(8):1426–31.
[28] Cairo SB, Zeinali LI, Berkelhamer SK, et al. Down syndrome and postoperative complications in children undergoing intestinal operations. J Pediatr Surg 2019;54(9):1832–7.
[29] Gely Y, Moreci R, Roberts H, et al. Trisomy 21 children with duodenal atresia or anorectal malformation: NSQIP-P surgical outcomes study. J Surg Res 2025;310:194–202.
[30] Ravel A, Mircher C, Rebillat AS, et al. Feeding problems and gastrointestinal diseases in Down syndrome. Arch Pediatr 2020;27(1):53–60.
[31] Ostermaier KK, Weaver AL, Myers SM, et al. Incidence of celiac disease in Down syndrome: a longitudinal, population-based birth cohort study. Clin Pediatr 2020;59(12):1086–91, PubMed PMID: 32664755; PMCID: PMC8108108.
[32] Nordstrom M, Retterstol K, Hope S, et al. Nutritional challenges in children and adolescents with Down syndrome. Lancet Child Adolesc Health 2020;4(6):455–64.
[33] DE Luca Corrêa H, Dos Santos Rosa T, Marques RS, et al. Exercise therapy in Down syndrome: a systematic review and meta-analysis focused on muscle strength, redox balance, and inflammatory profile. Med Sci Sports Exerc 2025;57(9):2073–82.
[34] Alexander E, Stahl M, Weaver A, et al. The spectrum of duodenal histologic findings in patients with trisomy 21: a multicenter study. J Pediatr Gastroenterol Nutr 2023;77(2):184–90.
[35] Cebeci AN, Guven A, Yildiz M. Profile of hypothyroidism in Down's syndrome. J Clin Res Pediatr Endocrinol 2013;5(2):116–20, PubMed PMID: 23748065; PMCID: PMC3701917.
[36] Mulu B, Fantahun B. Thyroid abnormalities in children with Down syndrome at St. Paul's hospital millennium medical college, Ethiopia. Endocrinol Diabetes Metab 2022;5(3):e00337; https://doi.org/10.1002/edm2.337:PubMed PMID: 35426257; PMCID: PMC9094469.
[37] Karlsson B, Gustafsson J, Hedov G, et al. Thyroid dysfunction in Down's syndrome: relation to age and thyroid autoimmunity. Arch Dis Child 1998;79(3):242–5, PubMed PMID: 9875020; PMCID: PMC1717691.
[38] Hewat TI, Laver TW, Houghton JAL, et al. Increased referrals for congenital hyperinsulinism genetic testing in children with trisomy 21 reflects the high burden of non-genetic risk factors in this group. Pediatr Diabetes 2022;23(4):457–61, PubMed PMID: 35294086; PMCID: PMC9310623.
[39] Rohrer TR, Hennes P, Thon A, et al. Down's syndrome in diabetic patients aged <20 years: an analysis of metabolic status, glycaemic control and autoimmunity in comparison with type 1 diabetes. Diabetologia 2010;53(6):1070–5.
[40] Johnson MB, De Franco E, Greeley SAW, et al. Trisomy 21 is a cause of permanent neonatal diabetes that is autoimmune but not HLA associated. Diabetes 2019;68(7):1528–35, PubMed PMID: 30962220; PMCID: PMC6609990.

[41] Tolu S, Hamze R, Moreau M, et al. Beta cell function and global glucose metabolism are impaired in Dp(16)1Yey mouse model of Down syndrome. Diabetes Obes Metab 2025;27 (3):1477–87.
[42] Castelli S, Tramutola A, Perluigi M, et al. Oxidative stress characterizes the dysfunction of thermogenic adipose tissue in a mouse model of Down syndrome. Free Radic Biol Med 2025;237:101–9.
[43] Foerste T, Sabin M, Reid S, et al. Understanding the causes of obesity in children with trisomy 21: hyperphagia vs physical inactivity. J Intellect Disabil Res 2016;60(9):856–64.
[44] Araya P, Kinning KT, Coughlan C, et al. IGF1 deficiency integrates stunted growth and neurodegeneration in Down syndrome. Cell Rep 2022;41(13):111883; https://doi.org/10.1016/j.celrep.2022.111883:PubMed PMID: 36577365; PMCID: PMC9876612.
[45] Zemel BS, Pipan M, Stallings VA, et al. Growth charts for children with Down syndrome in the United States. Pediatrics 2015;136(5):e1204–11, PubMed PMID: 26504127; PMCID: PMC5451269.
[46] Stagni F, Giacomini A, Emili M, et al. Neurogenesis impairment: an early developmental defect in Down syndrome. Free Radic Biol Med 2018;114:15–32.
[47] Zorrilla de San Martin J, Delabar JM, Bacci A, et al. GABAergic over-inhibition, a promising hypothesis for cognitive deficits in Down syndrome. Free Radic Biol Med 2018;114:33–9.
[48] Ding JW, Kim CN, Steyert MR, et al. Accelerated tempo of cortical neurogenesis in Down syndrome. bioRxiv 2025; https://doi.org/10.1101/2025.09.29.679346.
[49] Azrak O, Garic D, Nasir A, et al. Early white matter microstructure alterations in infants with Down syndrome. Neuroimage 2025;321:121489; https://doi.org/10.1016/j.neuroimage.2025.121489:PubMed PMID: 41038591; PMCID: PMC12629210.
[50] Dang T, Duan WY, Yu B, et al. Autism-associated Dyrk1a truncation mutants impair neuronal dendritic and spine growth and interfere with postnatal cortical development. Mol Psychiatry 2018;23(3):747–58, PubMed PMID: 28167836; PMCID: PMC5822466.
[51] Martin KR, Corlett A, Dubach D, et al. Over-expression of RCAN1 causes Down syndrome-like hippocampal deficits that alter learning and memory. Hum Mol Genet 2012;21(13): 3025–41.
[52] Mann DM, Esiri MM. The pattern of acquisition of plaques and tangles in the brains of patients under 50 years of age with Down's syndrome. J Neurol Sci 1989;89(2–3):169–79.
[53] Mann DM. The pathological association between Down syndrome and Alzheimer disease. Mech Ageing Dev 1988;43(2):99–136.
[54] Laham AJ, El-Awady R, Saber-Ayad M, et al. Targeting the DYRK1A kinase prevents cancer progression and metastasis and promotes cancer cells response to G1/S targeting chemotherapy drugs. npj Precis Oncol 2024;8(1):128, PubMed PMID: 38839871; PMCID: PMC11153725.
[55] Qizilbash N, Whitehead A, Higgins J, et al. Cholinesterase inhibition for Alzheimer disease: a meta-analysis of the tacrine trials. Dementia Trialists' Collaboration. JAMA 1998;280 (20):1777–82.
[56] Waite LM. New and emerging drug therapies for Alzheimer disease. Aust Prescr 2024;47 (3):75–9, PubMed PMID: 38962384; PMCID: PMC11216914.
[57] Connors MH, Sachdev PS, Colebatch JG, et al. Case report: down syndrome regression disorder, catatonia, and psychiatric and immunomodulatory interventions. Front Psychiatry 2024;15:1416736; https://doi.org/10.3389/fpsyt.2024.1416736:PubMed PMID: 39132313; PMCID: PMC11316268.
[58] Santoro JD, Spinazzi NA, Filipink RA, et al. Immunotherapy responsiveness and risk of relapse in Down syndrome regression disorder. Transl Psychiatry 2023;13(1):276, PubMed PMID: 37553347; PMCID: PMC10409776.
[59] Santoro JD, Partridge R, Tanna R, et al. Evidence of neuroinflammation and immunotherapy responsiveness in individuals with Down syndrome regression disorder. J Neurodev Disord 2022;14(1):35, PubMed PMID: 35659536; PMCID: PMC9164321.

[60] Kumada T, Ito M, Miyajima T, et al. Multi-institutional study on the correlation between chromosomal abnormalities and epilepsy. Brain Dev 2005;27(2):127–34.
[61] Hasle H, Clemmensen IH, Mikkelsen M. Risks of leukaemia and solid tumours in individuals with Down's syndrome. Lancet 2000;355(9199):165–9.
[62] Marlow EC, Ducore J, Kwan ML, et al. Leukemia risk in a cohort of 3.9 million children with and without Down syndrome. J Pediatr 2021;234:172–80.e3, PubMed PMID: 33684394; PMCID: PMC8238875.
[63] Labuhn M, Perkins K, Matzk S, et al. Mechanisms of progression of myeloid preleukemia to transformed myeloid leukemia in children with Down syndrome. Cancer Cell 2019;36(2); https://doi.org/10.1016/j.ccell.2019.06.007:123-38.e10.
[64] Peroni E, Gottardi M, D'Antona L, et al. Hematologic neoplasms associated with Down syndrome: cellular and molecular heterogeneity of the diseases. Int J Mol Sci 2023;24 (20):20231018; https://doi.org/10.3390/ijms242015325:PubMed PMID: 37895004; PMCID: PMC10607483.
[65] Rachubinski AL, Wallace E, Gurnee E, et al. JAK inhibition decreases the autoimmune burden in Down syndrome. eLife 2024;13:20241231; https://doi.org/10.7554/eLife.99323:PubMed PMID: 39737640; PMCID: PMC11687933.
[66] Foley C, Killeen OG. Musculoskeletal anomalies in children with Down syndrome: an observational study. Arch Dis Child 2019;104(5):482–7, PubMed PMID: 30472668; PMCID: PMC6557226.
[67] Baksh RA, Pape SE, Chan LF, et al. Multiple morbidity across the lifespan in people with Down syndrome or intellectual disabilities: a population-based cohort study using electronic health records. Lancet Public Health 2023;8(6):e453–62.
[68] Gao Y, Xu N, Tian Y, et al. Surgical management strategies for atlantoaxial instability/dislocation in Down syndrome. J Orthop Surg Res 2025;20(1):723, PubMed PMID: 40745318; PMCID: PMC12315429.
[69] VanZant JS, McCormick AA. Health care transition for individuals with Down syndrome: a needs assessment. Am J Med Genet 2021;185(10):3019–27.
[70] Kubota M, Bun S, Takahata K, et al. Plasma biomarkers for early detection of Alzheimer'S disease: a cross-sectional study in a Japanese cohort. Alzheimers Res Ther 2025;17(1): 131, PubMed PMID: 40483474; PMCID: PMC12144780.
[71] Voevodskaya O, Poulakis K, Sundgren P, et al. Brain myoinositol as a potential marker of amyloid-related pathology: a longitudinal study. Neurology 2019;92(5):e395–405, PubMed PMID: 30610093; PMCID: PMC6369900.
[72] Widjaja SL, Anniazi ML, Artiko B, et al. BMPR-II, caspase-3, HIF-1alpha, and VE-cadherin profile in Down syndrome children with and without congenital heart disease and pulmonary hypertension. Narra J 2025;5(1):e1244; https://doi.org/10.52225/narra.v5i1.1244:PubMed PMID: 40352250; PMCID: PMC12059882.
[73] Hashizume R, Wakita S, Sawada H, et al. Trisomic rescue via allele-specific multiple chromosome cleavage using CRISPR-Cas9 in trisomy 21 cells. PNAS Nexus 2025;4(2): pgaf022; https://doi.org/10.1093/pnasnexus/pgaf022:PubMed PMID: 39967679; PMCID: PMC11832276.

Advances in Pediatrics 73 (2026) 161–178
ADVANCES IN PEDIATRICS

Paradigm Shifts in Cystic Fibrosis Newborn Screening and Care in Infancy

MacKenzie L. Wyatt, MD[a,*], Jessica Clarion, MD[b], Meghan McGarry, MD, MAS[a]

[a]Division of Pulmonary and Sleep Medicine, Seattle Children's Hospital, Center for Respiratory Biology and Therapeutics, University of Washington, Seattle, WA, USA; [b]Division of Pulmonary and Sleep Medicine, Seattle Children's Hospital, University of Washington, Seattle, WA, USA

Keywords

• Cystic fibrosis (CF) • Newborn screening (NBS) • Cystic fibrosis transmembrane conductance regulator (CFTR)-Related metabolic syndrome (CRMS)
• Cystic fibrosis screen positive • Inconclusive diagnosis (CFSPID) • Modulators
• Highly effective modulator therapy (HEMT) • Health equity

Key points

- There have been advances in pediatric cystic fibrosis (CF) care including cystic fibrosis conductance regulator and universal newborn screening (NBS).
- NBS improves early detection of CF but children from minoritized backgrounds are more likely to be missed on NBS.
- Some children screen positive on CF NBS but do not meet full diagnostic criteria for CF, called CFTR-related metabolic syndrome.

INTRODUCTION

Cystic fibrosis (CF) is an autosomal recessive genetic disease with multisystem involvement; its disease manifestations are most prominent in the lungs, sinuses, pancreas, and reproductive system, although no organ system is entirely spared [1]. CF is also rare, affecting an estimated 105,000 individuals worldwide and approximately 40,000 children and adults in the United States [2].

*Corresponding author. Division of Pulmonary and Sleep Medicine, Seattle Children's Hospital, 4800 Sand Point Way NE, Seattle, WA 98115. *E-mail address:* mackenzielanwyatt@gmail.com

https://doi.org/10.1016/j.yapd.2026.02.002

Abbreviations

ACMG	American College of Medical Genetics and Genomics
ACOG	American College of Obstetrics and Gynecology
ACT	action
ADA	adenosine deaminase
ALT	alanine aminotransferase
AST	aspartate aminotransferase
CF	cystic fibrosis
CFF	Cystic Fibrosis Foundation
CFSPID	cystic fibrosis screen positive, inconclusive diagnosis
CFTR	cystic fibrosis transmembrane conductance regulator
CFTR-RD	cystic fibrosis transmembrane conductance regulator–related disorder
CRMS	cystic fibrosis transmembrane conductance regulator–related metabolic syndrome
ETI	elexacaftor/tezacaftor/ivacaftor
GGT	gamma-glutamyltransferase
HEMT	highly effective modulator therapy
ICP	intracranial pressure
IRT	immunoreactive trypsinogen
MFM	maternal fetal medicine
NBS	newborn screening
NGS	next-generation sequencing
PwCF	people with cystic fibrosis
TMA	targeted variant analysis
VUS	variants of unknown significance
VVCCs	variants of varying clinical consequences

In people with CF (PwCF), variants in the CFTR gene lead to an absent or dysfunctional cystic fibrosis transmembrane conductance regulator (CFTR) chloride channel. Gene variants are typically classified into one of several categories depending on their downstream impact on CFTR production, processing, function, or quantity. The most common genetic variant identified is F508del (c.1521_1523delCTT), a protein processing variant, which occurs in around 85% of PwCF in the US Cystic Fibrosis Foundation (CFF) patient registry [3]. CFTR variants produce a nonfunctional ion channel at the cell membrane; this change disrupts salt transport, leading to higher intracellular chloride levels and ultimately thick mucus that obstructs the exocrine glands of multiple organs [1]. This results in chronic sinus and obstructive lung disease in the respiratory tract. In the gastrointestinal system, clinical manifestations include pancreatic insufficiency, meconium ileus, weight loss, constipation, and distal intestinal obstruction syndrome.

CF is an autosomal recessive disease. In order to have CF, a child must have 2 CF-causing gene variants to develop the disease and/or an elevated sweat chloride test $\geq$ 60 mmol/L [4]. CFTR2 is an international database that classifies *CFTR* genetic variants as CF-causing, non-CF–causing, or variants of varying clinical consequences (VVCCs). VVCCs only lead to the phenotype of CF sometimes. We increasingly know more about the genetics for CF, but these unknown VVCCs can lead to indeterminate diagnoses.

There have been many vital advances in the care of PwCF that allow for disease identification and management very early in childhood; 2 of particular importance are: (1) the rise of CFTR modulator therapy (pharmacologic treatment intended to correct the malfunctioning CFTR protein) and (2) refinement of CF newborn screening (NBS) processes. Newborn screening for CF, has transformed the health of infants with CF because it has allowed for earlier diagnosis and treatment prior to onset of serious CF-related complications. However, there remain shortcomings in current CF NBS strategies as well as uncertainty surrounding interpretation of newborn screening test results, specifically, clinical phenotypes that are indeterminate for the diagnosis of CF. General pediatricians, obstetricians, family practitioners, and advanced practice providers in these fields are the first-line medical personnel faced with interpreting CF newborn screening results including indeterminate diagnose. Additionally, there have been advancements in prenatal diagnosis of CF, and current studies are examining modulator therapy prenatally to prevent CF complications. This review is intended to provide an overview for first-line clinicians on the rapidly changing landscape of CF diagnosis and care in infancy.

EPIDEMIOLOGY

CF occurs in about one in every 3000 to 4000 live births [5]. It has traditionally, though mistakenly, been taught that CF was a disease found exclusively in people of northern European descent [6]. In fact, CF affects people of all races, ethnicities, and ancestries [7]. Moreover, the CF community is becoming increasingly diverse: 23.3% of people newly diagnosed with CF in 2024 within the CF Foundation Registry (a registry that tracks PwCF in the United States) identified as Asian, Black, Hispanic, multiracial, or another race or ethnicity other than white [8]. Within the US CF population, 10.1% identified as Hispanic and 3.3% identified as Black [8], with an important caveat that only 84% of individuals consent to having their data included in the CF Foundation Registry, possibly leading to an underestimation of prevalence in some groups [9]. Fortunately, there is an increasing awareness of CF outside of the United States, including countries previously believed to have exceedingly low prevalence of CF. For example, in India, where CF was once thought to be nearly nonexistent, the incidence is now estimated at one in every 7000 to 12,000 live births based on immigrant data from the United States and the United Kingdom [10]. As we learn more about CF, we anticipate revised prevalence estimates in other parts of the world outside of the United States and Europe.

CYSTIC FIBROSIS IN THE ERA BEFORE CYSTIC FIBROSIS TRANSMEMBRANE CONDUCTANCE REGULATOR MODULATORS

In 1970, an individual with a diagnosis of CF had an average life expectancy of only 17 years [11]. In short, a diagnosis of CF often meant significant morbidity followed by death in childhood or adolescence. Development of and attention to aggressive preventive management strategies improved survival to an average of 36 years of life by 2011 [12]. These strategies included early and intense focus on nutrition, specifically, initiation of pancreatic enzyme replacement therapy to combat pancreatic insufficiency as well as high-calorie, high-fat diets to optimize nutritional status early in life [13]. The other major element of preventive management strategies is pulmonary therapies directed at improving lung function. Airway clearance with mucolytics (like dornase alpha), inhaled hypertonic saline, and chest physiotherapy lead to decreased mucous burden and a reduced risk of pulmonary infections and exacerbations [14]. Inhaled antibiotics such as tobramycin and anti-inflammatory agents like azithromycin similarly lead to improved outcomes [14]. While these therapies continue to be beneficial in the management of CF, they each address signs and symptoms rather than the disease pathogenesis.

ADVANCES IN CYSTIC FIBROSIS: CYSTIC FIBROSIS TRANSMEMBRANE CONDUCTANCE REGULATOR MODULATORS

CFTR modulators are gene-specific medications that treat the underlying pathology of CF by directly targeting the dysfunctional protein that ultimately becomes the CFTR chloride channel (Table 1). In most cases, to benefit from CFTR modulators, an individual must have specific CFTR variants [7]. Modulators were first introduced in 2011 and multiple are now approved for clinical use, including for the pediatric population. Broad categories of these medications include: (1) correctors like lumacaftor or tezacaftor, which promote correct 3-dimensional folding of the CFTR protein and its trafficking to the cell surface, and (2) potentiators such as ivacaftor and elexacaftor, which work to keep the ion channel open to allow appropriate chloride efflux from the cell [15,16]. Ivacaftor (Kalydeco) remains available as a monotherapy however other CFTR modulators are now available as a combination of a corrector and potentiator; examples of these combination medications include lumacaftor/ivacaftor (Orkambi), tezacaftor/ivacaftor (Symdeko), elexacaftor/tezacaftor/ivacaftor (ETI) (Trikafta), and most recently vanzacaftor/tezacaftor/deutivacaftor (Alyftrek).

The combination of ETI is noteworthy because it has been classified as a highly effective modulator therapy (HEMT) [17]. HEMT are distinguished from other modulators by their superior positive impact on lung function, pulmonary exacerbations, nutritional status, and quality of life. HEMT are also associated with improvement in fertility for women and a reduction in hospitalization days and lung transplantation. However, ivacaftor monotherapy was initially found to be effective solely for patients with gating mutations like G551D (c.1652G>A), which affects only about 5% of the CF population [16]. In contrast, ETI could be used in people with the much more common F508del mutation. Consequently, with the release of ETI in 2020, the vast majority of PwCF (around 90%) in the United States became eligible for a therapy

Table 1
Modulators in cystic fibrosis approved for infants with cystic fibrosis

CF modulator	Brand name	Age approved	Mechanism of action	Effects	Side effects
Ivacaftor	Kalydeco	1 mo	CFTR potentiator—increases probability CFTR channel opens	Improves lung function, nutrition, and symptoms	Elevated liver enzymes, cataracts, GI symptoms, and headaches
Lumacaftor/Ivacaftor	Orkambi	1 y	Lumacaftor—CFTR corrector—improves protein folding and trafficking	Modest improvement in lung function, nutrition, and symptoms	Dyspnea, chest tightness, increased blood pressure, and elevated liver enzymes
ETI	Trikafta	2 y	Elexacaftor/Tezacaftor—CFTR corrector	Substantial improvement in lung function, nutrition, and symptoms	Mental health, rash, elevated liver enzymes, headaches, and gastroenterology (GI) symptoms

that radically improves both day-to-day symptoms and overall life expectancy [18]. In fact, life expectancy for PwCF in the United States who are homozygous for the F508del mutation and eligible for HEMT in childhood is now projected to be 82.5 years of age [19] which is comparable to the US population as a whole.

Despite the staggering range of clinical benefits, CFTR modulators are not widely available for infants with CF. Only ivacaftor is approved for children as young as 1 month of age and who have one of 97 specific CFTR variants, which comprises between 5% to 10% of the US population of PwCF [20]. Lumacaftor/ivacaftor is approved for children 1 year of age and more who are homozygous F508del [21]. ETI is approved for children aged 2 years and older who have at least one copy of the F508del variant or one of another 271 specific variants–approximately 90% of children with CF in the United States meet these criteria and are therefore eligible for ETI therapy [22][(p3)].

MODULATORS: SIDE EFFECTS AND MONITORING

For modulators including ivacaftor, the most common side effects include abdominal pain, rash, and elevation of transaminases (aspartate aminotransferase [AST] and alanine aminotransferase [ALT]) [23]. Ivacaftor was also shown to have a risk of noncongenital cataracts in animal studies, but not in humans [22]. However, congenital cataracts have been described in infants exposed to ETI in utero or during breastfeeding [24]. Lumacaftor/ivacaftor can cause blood pressure changes and dyspnea [25]. ETI is typically well-tolerated, but postdrug monitoring has shown increased risk for psychiatric disorders [26]. In children, mental health side effects of ETI can manifest as anxiety and depression, sleep disturbances, aggression, and attention deficit disorders [27,28]. A rare but particularly severe side effect of ETI is increased intracranial pressure (ICP) [29].

With regard to drug monitoring for patients on modulator therapy, it is recommended that children on ETI undergo annual ophthalmologic examinations due to the risk of cataracts [30]. Liver function testing including AST, ALT, gamma-glutamyltransferase (GGT), bilirubin, and alkaline phosphatase is recommended before drug initiation, followed by quarterly lab monitoring in the first year and then annual labs thereafter [31]. There is also the potential for drug-drug interactions since CFTR modulators are metabolized by the CYP3A family of enzymes. Routine mental health screening is advised for school-aged children and adolescents due to the side effects in ETI [28]. Behavioral concerns and symptoms of elevated ICP such as headaches should be queried in the patient history and review of systems [29].

HEALTH EQUITY: MODULATORS

Although the advent of modulators has revolutionized CF care, not all PwCF benefit from these medications on the basis of their CF genotype [32]. Moreover, CFTR genetic variant distribution differs between racial and ethnic groups [7]. It is believed that F508del and other more common CFTR genetic variants originated more than 50,000 years ago in a population that is distinct from any European group currently present [33]. These variants spread throughout the European continent, where the F508del now has a frequency of about 70%. The most common CFTR variant in sub-Saharan Africa is 3120 + 1G → A, identified in 46% of PwCF in that region [34]. This variant is also the second most common in PwCF who identify as Black [35]. Thus, CFTR variants differ by ancestral backgrounds.

A cross-sectional study of patients in the 2018 CFF Patient Registry showed that PwCF who are Black, Indigenous, Hispanic, Asian or other people of color were less likely to have a genetic variant amenable to CFTR modulators compared to PwCF who were non-Hispanic white [32]. Additionally, few modulator clinical trials to date included PwCF who are racial and ethnic minorities [36,37]. Of all CF clinical pharmacology trials from 1999 to 2015, 80% did not report the race and/or ethnicity of their subjects [7]. Of the trials that did report race and ethnicity, PwCF from non-white backgrounds were included at disproportionately lower rates than what is reported in the US CFF patient registry [37]. This lack of diversity inclusion in drug studies creates the misleading impression that these medications are effective for most PwCF, ignoring that non-white PwCF are more likely to have a variant not amenable to currently available CFTR modulators.

For most children with CF living in high-income nations such as the United States, Canada, Australia, and most countries in Western and Northern Europe, there is ready access to CFTR modulator therapies. However, access remains limited in low-income and middle-income regions of the world due to high cost and regulations [38]. In addition to available CFTR modulators being less likely to effectively treat PwCF with certain variants, there are other barriers to CFTR medication. In high-income countries lacking universal health care such as the United States, financial barriers–in those who are uninsured or underinsured–may interfere with CFTR modulator affordability and access. Another growing barrier to optimal medication use, deserving further attention, is an inability to tolerate the side effects associated with CFTR modulators [39,40].

NEWBORN SCREENING: HISTORY

Diagnosis of CF earlier in life allows for prompt intervention and leads to improved pulmonary and nutritional outcomes over time [9]. This understanding has led to development of NBS-based testing for CF, first developed in Colorado and Wisconsin in 1982 [41,42]. With continued demonstration of improved outcomes attributable to earlier diagnosis, CF was added to the Recommended Uniform Screening Panel for NBS in 2006 [43].

As of 2010, all 50 states screen for CF. However, despite implementation of universal NBS testing for CF, there is variability in the screening process across states because each state's NBS program determines its own CF algorithm. Common features across all states include: reliance on blood spot screening, measurement of immunoreactive trypsinogen (IRT), which will be elevated when there is pancreatic duct blockage (Fig. 1) [44,45], and assessment for CFTR genetic variants when IRT levels are elevated. Where states differ is in the IRT cutoff level indicating a positive result and how they screen for genetic variants, specifically, whether they use targeted variant analysis (TMA) with a specific gene panel, (which can screen for anywhere between 23 to >300 CFTR genetic variants), or by whole gene sequencing.

Depending on the state, a child's NBS is considered positive if one or 2 CFTR genetic variants are identified, or if a patient has a very high IRT despite lack of identified CFTR genetic variants. In all states, infants with a positive CF NBS should undergo diagnostic CF testing. The gold standard diagnostic test for CF is measurement of sweat chloride concentrations, which will be elevated (≥60 mmol/L) in children with CF. Sweat chloride testing should be completed as soon as possible after a positive CF NBS result, ideally by 4 weeks of age. With all of this in mind, general pediatricians and other primary care providers play a critical role in the NBS process, as they typically receive and review NBS results, communicate these to patients' families, and direct timely specialty follow-up for confirmatory diagnostic testing and disease management. The American College of Medical Genetics and Genomics (ACMG) created action (ACT) sheets to educate pediatricians and primary care physicians on how to communicate CF newborn screening findings to families [46].

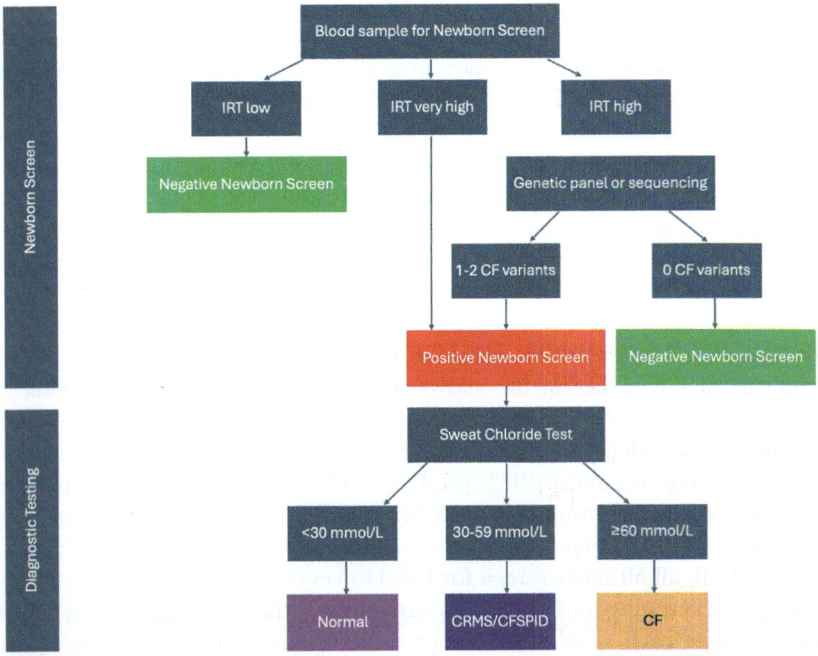

Fig. 1. General NBS and CF diagnosis schema.

NEWBORN SCREENING: NEW GUIDELINES AND ADVANCES

The 2024 CF NBS consensus guidelines recommend implementing a *floating* IRT cutoff rather than a fixed IRT level [47] to trigger testing for CFTR genetic variants and/or sweat chloride testing. The floating cutoff refers to IRT levels more than an established statistical benchmark, typically the 95th-98th percentile for all NBS samples analyzed over a discrete time period (typically 1 day or 1 week). This flexible threshold strategy is used to account for seasonal changes in IRT and different testing conditions, such as reagent lot changes, ensuring that samples with elevated IRT levels relative to the population undergo testing for CFTR variants. Minimizing false negative results is an important tenet of NBS and the floating IRT cut-off approach improves sensitivity, although using a floating cut-off typically results in more samples being tested for CFTR variants and higher costs. Most states also consider an IRT level at or greater than the 99th percentile to be positive regardless of whether CFTR variants were detected.

For identification of genetic variants, the new guidelines also recommend testing all CF-causing variants in the CFTR2 database to maximize detection across all ancestral groups [48]. Genetic sequencing of CFTR is encouraged when a panel cannot test all known variants. Next-generation sequencing (NGS) is a relatively new DNA analysis technology that can rapidly examine the CFTR gene in even more granular detail, identifying rare or even previously unknown gene variants. NGS can evaluate the entire CFTR gene, including noncoding areas like introns or regulatory elements that are not routinely analyzed through TMA but host several increasingly recognized CF-causing variants [49]. Additionally, some countries are conducting pilot studies of infant whole genome sequencing as a form of newborn screening, such as France's Perigenomed Project.

HEALTH EQUITY CONSIDERATIONS IN NEWBORN SCREENING

Although CF NBS has improved pulmonary and nutritional outcomes through earlier CF diagnosis, there are still persistent health care disparities within this system. CFTR genetic variant panels were developed based on non-Hispanic, white populations; as such, the genes tested for in the common variant panels represent the variants more commonly found in individuals of Northern and Western European ancestry [50]. Thus, children from other backgrounds that have rare or de novo genetic CFTR variants are less likely to screen positive on currently available CF NBS panels. The outcome of these false negative results is ultimately that children with CFTR variants that are more common in non-white populations are more likely to have delayed CF diagnoses potentially resulting in more severe disease at presentation and compromising nutritional and pulmonary outcomes, which has life-long health implications [51].

Pediatricians in the United States should be aware of what their state's CF NBS algorithm entails and its potential gaps. Some states such as Washington only screen for 43 genes, whereas others like California and New York test for more than 300 genes. Studies have shown that larger variant panels and genetic sequencing can detect more children from non-white, non-Hispanic backgrounds and improve test sensitivity. Moreover, NBS is not a definitive diagnostic test; as such, clinical suspicion for CF should remain high if an infant or child is showing signs of CF such as failure to thrive, chronic cough, chronic sinusitis, or recurrent pancreatitis, regardless of NBS results and the child's racial or ethnic background.

SPECIAL CASES OF NEWBORN SCREENING

In addition to state-to-state variability in NBS practices within the United States, providers should recognize that NBS programs throughout the world differ in terms of diseases tested for, if NBS is available at all. For example, Japan does not include CF in its NBS disease panel due to the historically low prevalence of CF in their population; however, if the child of an active-duty US service member stationed in Japan were to be born in a host nation hospital, that child may not undergo US-based NBS, risking delayed CF diagnosis as a result [52]. Currently, the US Department of Defense does not have a uniform policy for NBS testing in active-duty dependents born overseas nor means to systematically assess the impact of delayed diagnoses Similar concerns are relevant to other American families working and living abroad. Furthermore, in the face of concerning symptoms, consideration for undiagnosed CF should be heightened in highly mobile and immigrant populations whose children may not have undergone NBS and/or completed confirmatory testing. Finally, the rise of elective births at home in the United States has also played a negative role in the uptake of NBS and presents another potential challenge to advancing timely CF diagnosis [53].

In the same vein, while countries in Latin America continue to expand their public NBS programs, population coverage of NBS can be highly variable and the inclusion of CF on these testing panels is not universal, and this produces implications for the timely diagnosis of children of US immigrant families from this region, among others [54]. It is important to note that access to confirmatory testing may also be limited abroad.

UNIQUE DIAGNOSES: CYSTIC FIBROSIS TRANSMEMBRANE CONDUCTANCE REGULATOR–RELATED METABOLIC SYNDROME /CYSTIC FIBROSIS SCREEN POSITIVE, INCONCLUSIVE DIAGNOSIS

Most US primary care providers who care for infants have received NBS results with an indeterminate result for CF, prompting questions about significance and next steps. The identification of infants who have an indeterminate diagnosis of CF is an unintended consequence of universal CF NBS. CF is an autosomal recessive disease, which means an individual must have two CF-causing gene variants to develop the disease and/or an elevated sweat chloride test $\geq$ 60 mmol/L [4]. Some children have CFTR variants whose phenotypes are not well-defined as disease-causing or have symptoms of CF but an intermediate sweat chloride level (30–59 mmol/L). The combination of an abnormal NBS for CF and an abnormal but not clearly elevated sweat chloride test may lead to a diagnosis of CFTR-related metabolic syndrome (CRMS), or, as it is referred to in Europe, CF screen positive, inconclusive diagnosis (CFSPID); it is now common to refer to these collectively as CRMS/CFSPID. For a diagnosis of CRMS/CFSPID, a child must have a positive NBS and either (1) an intermediate sweat chloride test (30–59 mmol/L) and one or no CF-causing variants or (2) any sweat test ≤60 mmol/L and 2 CFTR variants with at least 1 that has unclear consequences (Table 2).

Knowledge of CFTR variants continues to expand, for example, through genetic sequencing as a component of NBS. As of the most recent update of CFTR2 in 2024, there are 1085 known CF-causing variants and 27 non-CF causing variants that have phenotypic consequences [48]. Variants not found in CFTR2 are referred to as variants of unknown significance (VUS). However, CFTR2 includes 55 variants of VVCCs that can sometimes cause CF but have incompletely understood clinical manifestations. These VVCCs can also be reported per ACMG with terminology such *likely pathogenic, uncertain* significance, or likely benign, which can lead to additional confusion for clinical interpretation.

Some genetic panels used in NBS test for some VVCCs and others do not. With the rise of genetic sequencing in CF NBS programs, there will likely

Table 2
Diagnostic criteria for cystic fibrosis and cystic fibrosis transmembrane conductance regulator–related metabolic syndrome/cystic fibrosis screen positive, inconclusive diagnosis

Genetic CFTR Variants		Sweat Chloride Concentration		
Variant 1	Variant 2	Normal (<30 mmol/L)	Intermediate (30-60 mmol/L)	Elevated (>60 mmol/L)
CF-causing	CF-causing	CF	CF	CF
CF-causing, VVCC, or VUS	VVCC or VUS	CRMS/CFSPID	CRMS/CFSPID	CF
CF-causing, VVCC, or VUS	Non CF-causing	Normal (Carrier)	CRMS/CFSPID	CF
Non CF-causing	Non CF-causing	Normal	CRMS/CFSPID	CF

Wyatt, M et al., Refining CFTR-Related Metabolic Syndrome (CRMS)/Cystic Fibrosis Screen Positive, Inconclusive Diagnosis (CFSPID) Diagnosis: Impact of CFTR2 Variant Classifications. Int. J. Neonatal Screen. 2025, 11, 60. https://doi.org/10.3390/ijns11030060.

continue to be increased detection of VVCCs and subsequently more CRMS/CFSPID diagnoses [55]. Additionally, children with CRMS/CFSPID are more likely to be racial or ethnic minorities due to a lack of understanding of genetic variants from different ancestry. Fortunately, the majority of children with CRMS/CFSPID are healthy; however, it is estimated that 5% to 11% of children with CRMS/CFSPID develop clinical features of CF and are then given a diagnosis CF [56]. This diagnostic uncertainty is a new challenge for CF care teams and is immensely stressful for affected families [57]. To date, there is no reliable way to predict which individuals will have their diagnosis converted from CRMS/CFSPID to CF. However, conversion has been associated with presence of one CF-causing CFTR variant and an increase in sweat chloride concentration [58].

MANAGEMENT OF UNIQUE DIAGNOSES: CYSTIC FIBROSIS-RELATED METABOLIC SYNDROME/CYSTIC FIBROSIS SCREEN POSITIVE, INCONCLUSIVE DIAGNOSIS

Because children with CRMS/CFSPID can still go on to be reclassified to the diagnosis of CF, they should be followed by a CFF-accredited care center. Before 2024, there were no guidelines on CRMS/CFSPID management, and so the approach differed heavily between individual providers and centers. However, published recommendations now advise children with CRMS/CFSPID be evaluated by a CF clinician at time of diagnosis, then attend annual visits until at least 8 years of age [59]. Due to the risk of conversion to CF, it is recommended to repeat sweat chloride testing at 6 months old and then annually until age 8. Genetic sequencing and genetic counseling are offered as well. There are no current guidelines on how to determine conversion to CF. However, typical considerations that would prompt a diagnosis of CF after previous CRMS/CFSPID classification include a repeat sweat chloride level results as ≥ 60 mmol/L, if a person's variants reclassify on CFTR2 as CF-causing, or they develop clinical features of CF.

It is important that providers of pediatric care understand CRMS/CFSPID, as a portion of these children may not be followed in CF clinics until awareness of new guidelines builds. It is suspected that there is a high loss to follow-up when the diagnosis is indeterminate. Primary care providers also play a key role in screening for further symptoms that might point to a conversion to CF and knowing when to refer patients back to a CF care center.

UNIQUE DIAGNOSES: CYSTIC FIBROSIS TRANSMEMBRANE CONDUCTANCE REGULATOR-RELATED DISORDER

Children who have CRMS/CFSPID screen positive for CF but do not meet the full diagnostic criteria for the disease. In addition to CRMS/CFSPID, other individuals do not meet full diagnostic criteria for CF or screen negative for CF on NBS but go on to develop signs of the disease later in life (Table 3). The latter is known as CFTR-related disorder (CFTR-RD). Individuals with CFTR-RD have evidence of decreased CFTR function such as congenital

Table 3
Cystic fibrosis transmembrane conductance regulator-related metabolic syndrome/cystic fibrosis screen positive, inconclusive diagnosis versus cystic fibrosis transmembrane conductance regulator–related disorder

	Cystic fibrosis transmembrane conductance regulator–related metabolic syndrome/cystic fibrosis screen positive, inconclusive diagnosis	Cystic fibrosis transmembrane conductance regulator–related disorder
Definition	Inconclusive CF diagnosis after NBS	CFTR dysfunction that doesn't meet CF criteria; typically monosymptomatic
Typical presentation	Asymptomatic infants	Isolated organ involvement - Bronchiectasis, recurrent pancreatitis, congenital bilateral absence of vas deferens
Newborn screen	+	Typically – but can be +
Sweat chloride test	≤60 mmol/L	≤60 mmol/L
Symptoms	+/−	<2 systems typically
Risk of CF progression	Variable 5%–11% estimated Can also progress to CFTR-RD	Rare progression
Management	Annual follow-up	Organ specific management

bilateral absence of vas deferens, recurrent pancreatitis, or bronchiectasis, but do not meet other clinical criteria for CF [60]. They have a sweat chloride level lesser than 60 mmol/L and have less than 2 CF-causing variants. Children with CRMS/CFSPID can convert to CFTR-RD.

ON THE HORIZON IN CYSTIC FIBROSIS: MODULATOR USE IN UTERO

In addition to the initiation of CFTR modulator therapy in infancy or early childhood, new case reports and animal studies have demonstrated that HEMT can benefit the fetus with CF in utero as well. A fetus might be exposed to ETI or other modulators in 2 ways: if the pregnant mother has CF or is a CF carrier, or if the child is diagnosed with CF or as a CF carrier through prenatal testing [61].

Prenatal diagnosis of CF is becoming more widely available. The American College of Obstetrics and Gynecology (ACOG) recommends prenatal carrier screening for certain genetic disorders, including CF, be offered to all women considering pregnancy. This is typically performed through a gene panel, with partner testing to follow in the event of a positive result. If a fetus with CF is not diagnosed through genetic methods beforehand, the prenatal ultrasound is the next possible method of diagnosis. Up to 20% of fetuses with CF can have meconium ileus, manifesting on ultrasound as echogenic bowel with or without dilation. Genetic confirmation of CF, either before or after ultrasound, can occur through invasive testing via chorionic villus sampling (placental cell sample at 10–13 weeks) or amniocentesis (amniotic fluid sample at 15–20 weeks) or noninvasive testing via cell free DNA test (blood test at 12–14 weeks) [62]. Maternal fetal medicine (MFM) physicians typically lead the prenatal diagnosis and treatment of fetuses with CF in collaboration with CF centers.

In animal models of CF, prenatal modulator use in utero has been shown to reverse meconium ileus, restore pancreatic function, and preserve vas deferens development [63]. Once modulator therapy is removed, pancreatic function again declines but vas deferens protection can be sustained and allow for fertility preservation. Similar findings have been seen in case reports in humans [64]. The ongoing study Maternal and Fetal Outcomes in the Era of Modulators (MAYFLOWERS) has enrolled 300 women with CF and their infants to examine the natural effect of continuing modulator therapy during pregnancy and lactation [65]. Retrospective data has shown safety in continuing HEMT and ETI during pregnancy, with no difference in miscarriage rates from the general population. Due to promising findings, in utero modulator use has been initiated off-label for pregnant people whose fetus has been prenatally diagnosed fetus with CF. HEMT may also be continued in pregnant females with CF. However, more research is needed. It is currently recommended that infants exposed to ETI in utero undergo regular ophthalmologic screening as there is a risk of cataracts found from case studies [24]. There is a risk of ETI withdrawal after discontinuation of the exposure, for example, at the time of birth or with breastfeeding. Like children and adults on ETI therapy, infants in the United States with prenatal exposure are typically monitored for evidence of hepatotoxicity but there are no official guidelines.

SPECIAL CASES OF NEWBORN SCREENING: MODULATOR USE IN UTERO

As more women with CF on HEMT become pregnant, it is important for primary care providers who care for their infants to understand the implications of HEMT on NBS results, specifically that in utero use of modulators can lead to false negative NBS in CF and false negative diagnostic sweat chloride testing. Due to restoration of pancreatic function with HEMT in utero, the IRT level can be falsely low and lead to a false negative result for children with CF with 2 CF-causing variants [66]. Additionally, sweat chloride results can also be lower (<60 mmol/L) than anticipated in this group. MFMs must be in communication with the newborn's primary care provider and CF centers to ensure accurate CF testing in children who have been exposed to CFTR modulators in utero. In some states, these newborns bypass the NBS as their IRT level can be low and go directly to CFTR genetic sequencing and monitoring by a CF center [61].

SUMMARY

Cystic fibrosis has fundamentally evolved from a life-limiting childhood illness to a manageable chronic condition with continued hope for ongoing improved care on the horizon. Beyond nutritional and pulmonary management, this transformation is best attributed to implementation and refinement of newborn screening programs as well as the development of CFTR modulator therapies. However, these advancements have revealed new diagnostic challenges, particularly the entities of CRMS/CFSPID or CFTR-RD, as well as health inequities that primarily impact individuals from non-white, non-Hispanic backgrounds. Frontline providers, particularly those caring for infants and pregnant patients, are integral to addressing these concerns. We encourage every person involved in the care of PwCF to appreciate the diversity of the CF population, maintain awareness of advances in diagnosis and treatment as well as the specific practices of their institution, and continue fostering multidisciplinary collaboration to sustain this progress.

CLINICS CARE POINTS

- CF care has advanced due to therapies with CFTR modulators.
- NBS is a good tool for early diagnosis of CF, but children from minoritized backgrounds might be missed. There must be a high clinical suspicion for diagnosis and workup.
- Some children do not meet full criteria for CF diagnosis but have some features known as CRMS if screened positive on NBS or CFTR-RD if diagnosed later.
- Prenatal modulator use is an evolving field as a a potential target for CF therapy.

Disclosure

The research of Dr M.L. Wyatt is funded by the Cystic Fibrosis Foundation, United States (CFF) Clinical Fellowship Award, grant number WYATT24B0 and WYATT25D0, the Rosenfeld Funds, and the Corkery Endowment. The work of Dr M. McGarry is funded by the National Institutes of Health, United States (NIH), grant number 5K23HL133437-05, and the Cystic Fibrosis Foundation (CFF), grant number MCGARR16A0.

References

[1] Ong T, Ramsey BW. Cystic fibrosis: a review. JAMA 2023;329(21):1859.

[2] Guo J, Garratt A, Hill A. Worldwide rates of diagnosis and effective treatment for cystic fibrosis. J Cyst Fibros 2022;21(3):456–62.

[3] Grasemann H, Ratjen F. Cystic fibrosis. N Engl J Med 2023;389(18):1693–707.

[4] Farrell PM, White TB, Ren CL, et al. Diagnosis of cystic fibrosis: Consensus guidelines from the cystic fibrosis foundation. J Pediatr 2017;181:S4–15.e1.

[5] Knapp EA, Fink AK, Goss CH, et al. The cystic fibrosis foundation patient registry. Design and methods of a national observational disease registry. Ann Am Thorac Soc 2016;13(7):1173–9.

[6] Khoury MJ, McCabe LL, McCabe ERB. Population screening in the age of genomic medicine. N Engl J Med 2003;348(1):50–8.

[7] McGarry ME, Gibb ER, Oates GR, et al. Left behind: the potential impact of CFTR modulators on racial and ethnic disparities in cystic fibrosis. Paediatr Respir Rev 2022;42:35–42.
[8] 2024 Patient registry highlights I cystic fibrosis foundation. Available at: https://www.cff.org/medical-professionals/2024-patient-registry-highlights. Accessed October 15, 2025.
[9] Rosenfeld M, Ostrenga J, Cromwell EA, et al. Real-world associations of US cystic fibrosis newborn screening programs with nutritional and pulmonary outcomes. JAMA Pediatr 2022;176(10):990–9.
[10] Farrell PM, Paul GR, Varkki SD. India: the last and best frontier for cystic fibrosis newborn screening with perspectives on special challenges. Int J Neonatal Screen 2025;11(2):27.
[11] Burgener EB, Cornfield DN. Delivering a new future for people with cystic fibrosis. Pediatrics 2023;152(4):e2023062985.
[12] Stephenson AL, Sykes J, Stanojevic S, et al. Survival comparison of patients with cystic fibrosis in Canada and the United States: a population-based cohort study. Ann Intern Med 2017;166(8):537–46.
[13] McDonald CM, Alvarez JA, Bailey J, et al. Academy of nutrition and dietetics: 2020 cystic fibrosis evidence analysis center evidence-based nutrition practice guideline. J Acad Nutr Diet 2021;121(8):1591–636.e3.
[14] Mogayzel PJ, Naureckas ET, Robinson KA, et al. Cystic fibrosis pulmonary guidelines. Am J Respir Crit Care Med 2013;187(7):680–9.
[15] Dwight M, Marshall B. CFTR modulators: transformative therapies for cystic fibrosis. J Manag Care Spec Pharm 2021;27(2); https://doi.org/10.18553/jmcp.2021.27.2.281.
[16] Ramsey BW, Davies J, McElvaney NG, et al. A CFTR potentiator in patients with cystic fibrosis and the G551D mutation. N Engl J Med 2011;365(18):1663–72.
[17] Elexacaftor–tezacaftor–ivacaftor for cystic fibrosis with a single Phe508del allele I new England journal of medicine. Available at: https://www.nejm.org/doi/full/10.1056/NEJMoa1908639. Accessed October 15, 2025.
[18] Graeber SY, Mall MA. The future of cystic fibrosis treatment: from disease mechanisms to novel therapeutic approaches. Lancet 2023;402(10408):1185–98.
[19] Lopez A, Daly C, Vega-Hernandez G, et al. Elexacaftor/tezacaftor/ivacaftor projected survival and long-term health outcomes in people with cystic fibrosis homozygous for F508del. J Cyst Fibros 2023;22(4):607–14.
[20] Who is KALYDECO® (ivacaftor) for?. Available at: https://www.kalydeco.com/who-kalydeco. Accessed October 15, 2025.
[21] ORKAMBI® (lumacaftor/ivacaftor) I patient information. Available at: https://www.orkambi.com/. Accessed October 15, 2025.
[22] Zhu Y, Li D, Reyes-Ortega F, et al. Ocular development after highly effective modulator treatment early in life. Front Pharmacol 2023;14:1265138.
[23] Terlizzi V, Fevola C, Cecchetti M, et al. Effect of elexacaftor-tezacaftor-ivacaftor on liver transient elastography, fibrosis indices and blood tests in children with cystic fibrosis. J Cyst Fibros 2025;24(3):574–80.
[24] Jain R, Wolf A, Molad M, et al. Congenital bilateral cataracts in newborns exposed to elexacaftor-tezacaftor-ivacaftor in utero and while breast feeding. J Cyst Fibros 2022;21(6):1074–6.
[25] Heneghan M, Southern KW, Murphy J, et al. Corrector therapies (with or without potentiators) for people with cystic fibrosis with class II CFTR gene variants (most commonly F508del). Cochrane Database Syst Rev 2023;11(11):CD010966.
[26] Piehler L, Thalemann R, Lehmann C, et al. Effects of elexacaftor/tezacaftor/ivacaftor therapy on mental health of patients with cystic fibrosis. Front Pharmacol 2023;14:1179208.
[27] Pasley K, Dell ML, May A. Diagnosis and treatment of ADHD in pediatric patients during the first year of elexacaftor/tezacaftor/ivacaftor. Pediatr Pulmonol 2024;59(12):3524–9.
[28] Pham H, Vandeleur M, Mainzer RM, et al. Mental health, sleep, and respiratory health after initiating elexacaftor/tezacaftor/ivacaftor treatment in children with cystic fibrosis. Pediatr Pulmonol 2024;59(10):2606–13.

[29] Southern KW, Barben J, Goldring S, et al. Raised intracranial pressure in three children with cystic fibrosis receiving Elexacaftor-Tezacaftor-Ivacaftor modulator therapy. Am J Respir Crit Care Med 2023;208(1):103–5.
[30] Elexacaftor, Tezacaftor and Ivacaftor. In: Drugs and lactation database (LactMed®). National Institute of Child Health and Human Development; 2006. Available at: http://www.ncbi.nlm.nih.gov/books/NBK556372/. Accessed October 15, 2025.
[31] Southern KW, Castellani C, Lammertyn E, et al. Standards of care for *CFTR* variant-specific therapy (including modulators) for people with cystic fibrosis. J Cyst Fibros 2023;22(1):17–30.
[32] McGarry ME, McColley SA. Cystic fibrosis patients of minority race and ethnicity less likely eligible for CFTR modulators based on CFTR genotype. Pediatr Pulmonol 2021;56(6):1496–503.
[33] Morral N, Bertranpetit J, Estivill X, et al. The origin of the major cystic fibrosis mutation (delta F508) in European populations. Nat Genet 1994;7(2):169–75.
[34] Masekela R, Zampoli M, Westwood AT, et al. Phenotypic expression of the 3120+1G>A mutation in Non-Caucasian children with cystic fibrosis in South Africa. J Cyst Fibros 2013;12(4):363–6.
[35] Macek M, Mackova A, Hamosh A, et al. Identification of common cystic fibrosis mutations in African-Americans with cystic fibrosis increases the detection rate to 75%. Am J Hum Genet 1997;60(5):1122–7.
[36] Milinic T, Burdis N, Gill E, et al. Research coordinators' perspectives on recruitment of minoritized people with cystic fibrosis into clinical trials. BMC Pulm Med 2025;25:325.
[37] McGarry ME, McColley SA. Minorities are underrepresented in clinical trials of pharmaceutical agents for cystic fibrosis. Ann Am Thorac Soc 2016;13(10):1721–5.
[38] Kerem E. Expanding the impact of new cystic fibrosis therapies in low- and middle-income countries. Pediatr Pulmonol 2025;60(Suppl 1):S90–1.
[39] Ramos KJ, Pilewski JM, Taylor-Cousar JL. Challenges in the use of highly effective modulator treatment for cystic fibrosis. J Cyst Fibros 2021;20(3):381–7.
[40] Kramer-Golinkoff E, Camacho A, Kramer L, et al. A survey: understanding the health and perspectives of people with CF not benefiting from CFTR modulators. Pediatr Pulmonol 2022;57(5):1253–61.
[41] Gregg RG, Simantel A, Farrell PM, et al. Newborn screening for cystic fibrosis in Wisconsin: comparison of biochemical and molecular methods. Pediatrics 1997;99(6):819–24.
[42] Sontag MK, Lee R, Wright D, et al. Improving the sensitivity and positive predictive value in a cystic fibrosis newborn screening program using a repeat immunoreactive trypsinogen and genetic analysis. J Pediatr 2016;175:150–8.e1.
[43] Ross LF. Newborn screening for cystic fibrosis: a lesson in public health disparities. J Pediatr 2008;153(3):308–13.
[44] Rehani MR, Marcus MS, Harris AB, et al. Variation in cystic fibrosis newborn screening algorithms in the United States. Pediatr Pulmonol 2023;58(3):927–33.
[45] Raraigh KS, Aksit MA, Hetrick K, et al. Complete CFTR gene sequencing in 5,058 individuals with cystic fibrosis informs variant-specific treatment. J Cyst Fibros 2022;21(3):463–70.
[46] ACT sheets and algorithms. Available at: https://www.acmg.net/ACMG/Medical-Genetics-Practice-Resources/ACT_Sheets_and_Algorithms.aspx. Accessed October 15, 2025.
[47] McGarry ME, Raraigh KS, Farrell P, et al. Cystic fibrosis newborn screening: a systematic review-driven consensus guideline from the United States cystic fibrosis foundation. International Journal of Neonatal Screening 2025;11(2):24.
[48] Welcome to CFTR2 | CFTR2. Available at: https://cftr2.org/. Accessed October 15, 2025.
[49] Cambraia A, Junior MC, Zembrzuski VM, et al. Next-generation sequencing for molecular diagnosis of cystic fibrosis in a Brazilian cohort. Dis Markers 2021;2021:9812074.
[50] McGarry ME, Ren CL, Wu R, et al. Detection of disease-causing CFTR variants in state newborn screening programs. Pediatr Pulmonol 2023;58(2):465–74.

[51] McColley SA, Martiniano SL, Ren CL, et al. Disparities in first evaluation of infants with cystic fibrosis since implementation of newborn screening. J Cyst Fibros 2023;22(1):89–97.
[52] Scotet V, Gutierrez H, Farrell PM. Newborn screening for CF across the globe-where is it worthwhile? Int J Neonatal Screen 2020;6(1):18.
[53] Stein-Zamir C, Shoob H, Katan S, et al. Non-uptake of newborn screening in planned home-birth is associated with preventive health practices for infants: a retrospective case-control study. Int J Neonatal Screen 2025;11(1):15.
[54] Gonzaga-Jauregui C, Moreno-Salgado R, Tovar-Casas J, et al. Newborn screening in Mexico and Latin America: present and future. RDODJ 2024;3(3); https://doi.org/10.20517/rdodj.2024.02.
[55] Wyatt M, Quinn A, Shade L, et al. Refining CFTR-related metabolic syndrome (CRMS)/cystic fibrosis screen positive, inconclusive diagnosis (CFSPID) diagnosis: impact of CFTR2 variant classifications. International Journal of Neonatal Screening 2025;11(3):60.
[56] Sciortino S, Graham S, Bishop T. Diagnostic transitions of cystic fibrosis and CRMS compared after 12 years of newborn screening in California. J Pediatr 2025;276:114287.
[57] Ginsburg DK, Salinas DB, Cosanella TM, et al. High rates of anxiety detected in mothers of children with inconclusive cystic fibrosis screening results. J Cyst Fibros 2023;22(3):420–6.
[58] Terlizzi V, Manti S, D'Amico F, et al. Biochemical and genetic tools to predict the progression to cystic fibrosis in CRMS/CFSPID subjects: a systematic review. Paediatr Respir Rev 2024;51:46–55.
[59] Green DM, Lahiri T, Raraigh KS, et al. Cystic fibrosis foundation evidence-based guideline for the management of CRMS/CFSPID. Pediatrics 2024;153(5):e2023064657.
[60] Castellani C, De Boeck K, De Wachter E, et al, ECFS Diagnostic Network Working Group. ECFS standards of care on CFTR-related disorders: updated diagnostic criteria. J Cyst Fibros 2022;21(6):908–21.
[61] Szentpetery S, Riva D, Blumenfeld YJ, et al. PRenatal mOdulator treatment to PrEvent CF complicaTions (PROTECT) workshop report. J Cyst Fibros 2025;24(6); https://doi.org/10.1016/j.jcf.2025.07.015.
[62] Wynn J, Rego S, Chandler-Brown D, et al. Routine cell-free DNA prenatal screening identifies pregnancies at high risk for cystic fibrosis that may benefit from fetal therapy. J Cyst Fibros 2025 S1569-1993(25)01563-2.
[63] Evans IA, Sun X, Liang B, et al. In utero and postnatal ivacaftor/lumacaftor therapy rescues multiorgan disease in CFTR-F508del ferrets. JCI Insight 2024;9(8):e157229.
[64] Metcalf A, Martiniano SL, Sagel SD, et al. Outcomes of prenatal use of elexacaftor/tezacaftor/ivacaftor in carrier mothers to treat meconium ileus in fetuses with cystic fibrosis. J Cyst Fibros 2025;24(3):466–8.
[65] Jain R, Magaret A, Vu PT, et al. Prospectively evaluating maternal and fetal outcomes in the era of CFTR modulators: the MAYFLOWERS observational clinical trial study design. BMJ Open Respir Res 2022;9(1):e001289.
[66] Fortner CN, Seguin JM, Kay DM. Normal pancreatic function and false-negative CF newborn screen in a child born to a mother taking CFTR modulator therapy during pregnancy. J Cyst Fibros 2021;20(5):835–6.

Advances in Pediatrics 73 (2026) 179–190

ELSEVIER

ADVANCES IN PEDIATRICS

Gastrointestinal and Pancreatic Manifestations of Cystic Fibrosis in the Era of Highly Effective Modulators

Sasha-Jane Abi-Aad, MD, MSc[a], Sridevi Narayanan, DO[b], Racha T. Khalaf, MD, MSCS[a,*]

[a]Department of Pediatrics, Division of Gastroenterology, Hepatology and Nutrition, University of South Florida Morsani College of Medicine, 13101 Bruce B. Downs Boulevard, Tampa, FL 33612, USA; [b]Department of Pediatrics, University of South Florida Morsani College of Medicine, 13101 Bruce B. Downs Boulevard, Tampa, FL 33612, USA

Keywords

• CFTR modulators • Digestive diseases • Pancreatic insufficiency
• Motility disorders • Cystic fibrosis
• Cystic fibrosis transmembrane conductance regulator

Key points

- Early data on the use of triple cystic fibrosis transmembrane conductance regulator (CFTR) modulators have shown mild improvements in gastrointestinal manifestations of cystic fibrosis.
- Triple CFTR modulators improve nutrition and growth; however, the majority of individuals with cystic fibrosis remain pancreatic insufficient with some data showing a reduction in the dose of pancreatic enzyme replacement therapy.
- While symptoms of gastrointestinal diseases remain burdensome, data suggest improvements in microbiome dysbiosis and intestinal inflammation with the use of highly effective modulators.
- Long-term data on the effects of triple CFTR modulators on gastrointestinal manifestations of cystic fibrosis are scarce and highly needed.

INTRODUCTION

Cystic fibrosis (CF) is an inherited disorder caused by mutations in the *cystic fibrosis transmembrane conductance regulator* (CFTR) gene. The defective CFTR

*Corresponding author. *E-mail address:* khalafr@usf.edu

https://doi.org/10.1016/j.yapd.2025.11.001

Abbreviations

AP	acute pancreatitis
CF	cystic fibrosis
CFTR	cystic fibrosis transmembrane conductance regulator
CI	confidence interval
CRC	colorectal cancer
CwCF	children with CF
DIOS	distal intestinal obstruction syndrome
EPI	exocrine pancreatic insufficiency
ETI	elexacaftor–tezacaftor–ivacaftor
FDA	US Food and Drug Administration
FE-1	fecal elastase-1
GERD	gastroesophageal reflux disease
GI	gastrointestinal
HEMT	highly effective modulator therapy
M2-PK	M2-pyruvate kinase
PERT	pancreatic enzyme replacement therapy
PI-CF	pancreatic-insufficient CF
PPI	proton pump inhibitor
pwCF	people with CF
QoL	quality of life
VTD	vanzacaftor–tezacaftor–deutivacaftor

protein disrupts chloride ion transport across epithelial cells, resulting in thickened mucus and impaired secretions that primarily affect the respiratory and gastrointestinal (GI) systems. CF affects more than 105,000 individuals worldwide, including about 40,000 in the United States [1].

Over the past decade, the advent of modulator therapy, which is a therapeutic that corrects or improves the function of the defective CFTR protein, has evolved from monotherapy to triple combination therapy. With an increase in efficacy, these medications have transformed the clinical landscape of CF, yielding marked improvements in pulmonary, survival, and quality of life (QoL) outcomes [2]. Elexacaftor–tezacaftor–ivacaftor (ETI), a highly effective modulator therapy (HEMT), is currently approved for people with CF (pwCF) aged 2 years or older with at least one *F508del* or other responsive *CFTR* mutations [3–5]. According to the 2024 CF Patient Registry, median predicted survival in CF now approaches 65 years, up from 40 years a decade ago, with approximately 76% of pwCF receiving ETI and 5% receiving other modulators [6].

In late 2024, vanzacaftor–tezacaftor–deutivacaftor (VTD) was approved by the US Food and Drug Administration (FDA) for use in individuals aged 6 years or older with at least one *F508del* or other responsive mutations. Similar to ETI, this new combination modulator therapy has demonstrated significant improvements in lung function, sweat chloride concentration, and QoL [7,8]. Fig. 1 illustrates the progression of CFTR care and modulator therapies.

As individuals with CF live longer, GI complications have become increasingly prominent contributors to morbidity. Defective CFTR function promotes intestinal inflammation, mucus inspissation, and dysbiosis, which together drive

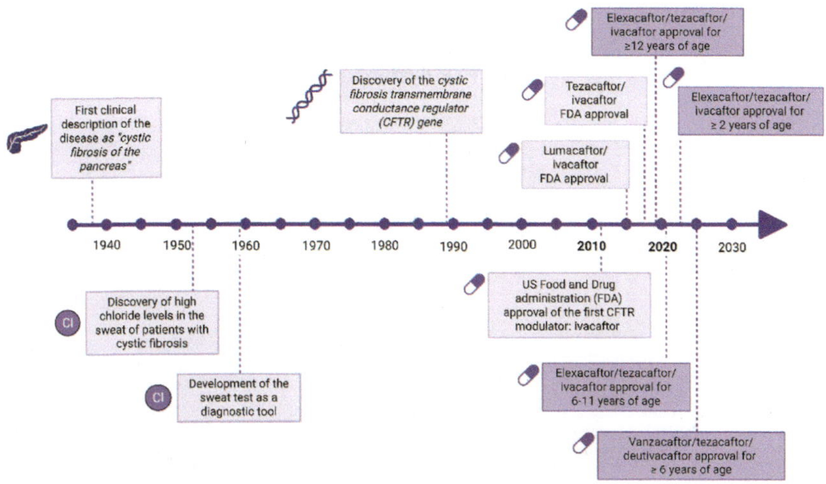

Fig. 1. Milestones in cystic fibrosis care. This timeline illustrates the major evolution in cystic fibrosis knowledge and management over the years as it relates to gastrointestinal care [3–5,7,8,41,42]. (Created in BioRender. Abi-Aad, S. (2025) https://BioRender.com/jzx38ky.)

a broad spectrum of GI manifestations. These include pancreatic insufficiency and fat malabsorption; gastroesophageal reflux disease (GERD); and motility disorders such as gastroparesis, meconium ileus, constipation, distal intestinal obstruction syndrome (DIOS), and small intestinal bacterial overgrowth. Fig. 2 presents the pathophysiology of GI manifestations of CF [9]. In a cohort of 7649 pwCF aged under 21 years in the United States (between 2010 and 2020), 73% had at least one GI disorder compared with less than 1% in the general population. The prevalence of pancreatobiliary disorders was approximately 43%, diseases of the esophagus to duodenum 34%, and intestinal diseases 43%, all markedly higher than in unaffected individuals. These manifestations are associated with a high burden of GI-directed pharmacotherapy [10].

The introduction of HEMT has led to modest improvements in GI symptoms, yet the full impact of ETI and of newer HEMT on these manifestations remains incompletely characterized. This review provides an update on the latest advancements in GI manifestations of CF in the era of triple CFTR modulator therapy, with a primary focus on luminal and pancreatic disorders. Although hepatobiliary involvement is common, it is beyond the scope of this review.

Gastroesophageal reflux disease

GERD is among the most prevalent luminal manifestations of CF and is associated with declining lung function, as microaspirations and GERD-related bronchospasms can exacerbate chronic bronchopulmonary disease [11]. Despite limited evidence of long-term clinical benefit, many pwCF remain on long-term acid suppression therapy. A matched cohort study reported that chronic proton pump inhibitor (PPI) use increased the risk of respiratory

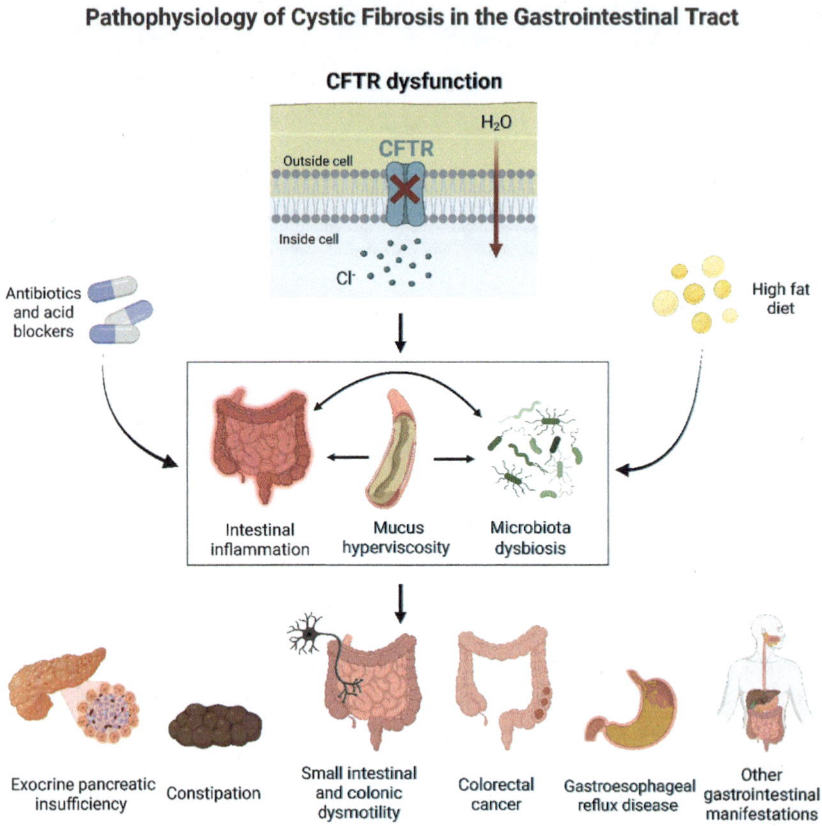

Fig. 2. Factors contributing to the pathophysiology of gastrointestinal manifestations of cystic fibrosis. (Created in BioRender. Abi-Aad, S. (2025) https://BioRender.com/5h18ta4.)

colonization with *Pseudomonas aeruginosa,* with an adjusted mean difference in percentage of positive culture of 23.1% ($P = .0002$) over a mean follow-up of 23 ± 17 months [12]. A recent survey data indicated that 63% of pwCF are on chronic PPIs, 16% on antihistamines, and 16% on other antiacid medications. Among CF practitioners, 93% prescribed acid blockers to treat GERD and 80% to enhance the efficacy of pancreatic enzyme replacement therapy (PERT), highlighting the widespread use of acid suppression in this population [13].

Since the introduction of highly effective CFTR modulators, there has been very limited data on GERD prevalence and changes in symptoms. In a study comparing children with CF (CwCF) and pancreatic insufficiency, on versus off ETI, authors used International Classification of Diseases 10th Revision (ICD-10) codes to assess disease prevalence. ETI therapy was associated with a decrease in GERD prevalence from 54% to 48%, and GERD without esophagitis from 53% to 48%; however, these changes were not statistically significant after Bonferroni correction [14]. In pwCF with advanced lung disease, ETI led to a significant reduction in the reflux symptom index, with median scores decreasing from 15 (11–23) at baseline to 5 (2.8–7.3) after 6 months ($P < .0001$). According to survey data, 42% of pwCF successfully discontinued PPI therapy with ETI, indicating a meaningful reduction in GERD therapy burden with HEMT [15]. While early data are promising, further studies are needed to define the long-term impact of CFTR modulators on GERD prevalence, symptom burden, related pulmonary complications, and outcomes secondary to de-escalation of acid suppression.

Exocrine pancreatic insufficiency and nutritional outcomes

Exocrine pancreatic insufficiency (EPI) affects more than 85% of pwCF and is defined by the need for PERT. In contrast, acute pancreatitis (AP) has been traditionally considered rare in pancreatic-insufficient CF (PI-CF) due to early life parenchymal destruction [16]. Since the advent of ETI, case series have suggested a potential increase in AP incidence in PI-CF, potentially related to partial restoration of pancreatic ducts [16–18]. However, large cohort studies indicate no overall increase, and some report a reduction in AP among pwCF receiving CFTR modulators. In a population-wide database study, there was no significant difference in the prevalence of AP in PI-CF before and after treatment with ETI [14]. Similarly, a metanalysis reported an overall incidence of AP of 0.11 per patient-year with CFTR modulator use, compared with 0.73 per patient-year prior to modulator therapy (rate ratio 0.15, 95% confidence interval [CI] 0.04, 0.52). Among pancreatic-sufficient subjects, AP incidence decreased from 0.76 to 0.1 per patient-year, but there was no significant change in AP incidence among PI-CF subjects [19].

Despite these findings, ETI is associated with only partial restoration of pancreatic function. In a prospective cohort of 29 adults with CF treated with ETI, the mean (±SD) PERT dose significantly decreased over 24 weeks from 7471.1 (±4108.5) to 6,002.8 (±3,926.9) units of lipase/kg/day, with a mean change of -1968.56 ± 2443.55 units/kg/day ($P < .001$). However, of 22 individuals with fecal elastase-1 (FE-1) measurements, only 1 achieved pancreatic sufficiency while the others remained insufficient [20]. Similarly, in a study of 30 children with PI-CF on PERT and ETI, only 7 showed an increase in FE-1 of at least 100 μg/g from the baseline, considered responders, whereas 23 children were nonresponders [21].

Early initiation of triple CFTR modulators may be associated with improved outcomes and normalization of pancreatic function in infants and young children. Case reports describe newborns with homozygous *F508del* mutations who maintained normal pancreatic function and elevated FE-1 levels when mothers received ETI during pregnancy; however, continued ETI therapy after breastfeeding was required to maintain function [22,23]. These cases suggest that in utero ETI exposure may prevent or delay the development of EPI, but ongoing therapy is necessary to maintain normal function. Furthermore, 48 children with PI-CF aged 2 to 6 years showed that 28% converted to pancreatic sufficiency after 6 months of ETI ($P = .0005$) [24]. While promising, multicenter long-term studies are needed to better understand the impact of ETI on pancreatic function and to determine the optimal timing for treatment initiation.

Beyond pancreas function, ETI has also been associated with improved nutritional outcomes including increases in body mass index, weight, and fat-soluble vitamin levels [25–27]. Among 169 pwCF aged over 12 years on ETI, median vitamin A levels increased from 422.0 to 471.0 mcg/L ($P < .001$) and vitamin D from 28.5 to 30.8 ng/mL ($P = .003$) over 2 years after ETI initiation, with no significant change in vitamin E or international normalized ratio (INR; a surrogate for vitamin K) [28]. In another cohort of 80 pwCF on CFTR modulators (29 on ETI), vitamin D level increased from 23.5 ± 7.6 to 29.2 ± 9.5 ng/mL ($P = .015$), vitamin A from 37.4 ± 13.0 to 47.4 ± 15.8 mcg/dL ($P = .011$), and vitamin E from 1054.3 ± 208.0 mcg/dL to 1213.4 ± 219.3 ($P = .006$), reflecting improved fat absorption with HEMT [29]; however, the effect of ETI on vitamin E levels varies across studies. Despite improved pancreatic and nutritional outcomes, dysregulated intestinal immunity and microbiome imbalance continue to characterize the GI tract in CF.

Intestinal inflammation in cystic fibrosis

CFTR dysfunction can also alter the gut microbiome and induce intestinal dysbiosis, which are key contributors to intestinal inflammation and GI manifestations of CF. PwCF often exhibit reduced microbial diversity, depletion of anti-inflammatory microbes, and enrichment of proinflammatory pathogens [30]. Intestinal dysbiosis in CF is multifactorial resulting from defective CFTR function, viscous mucus secretions, frequent antibiotic exposure, and a high fat diet [31]. A common clinical manifestation of this imbalance is small intestinal bacterial overgrowth characterized by excessive bacterial proliferation in the small intestine, leading to symptoms such as bloating, nausea, diarrhea, excessive gas, or abdominal pain.

ETI use has been associated with partial restoration of microbial diversity. In a matched case–control cohort study, stool microbiota diversity initially decreased after 6 months of ETI but significantly increased with prolonged therapy, shifting toward a composition more similar to healthy controls, though still distinct [32]. Similarly, a longitudinal study on 39 CwCF demonstrated a significant increase in fecal alpha diversity which measures the variety of species within individual samples (Shannon index, $P = .021$) and a significant increase in species richness (median 83–109 species, $P = .026$) after 6 to 12 months of ETI. Fecal calprotectin, a marker of intestinal inflammation, decreased from 109 to 44.8 μg/g after ETI, with a mean reduction of 64.2 μg/g (95% CI −16.1, −112.3), and a 30% decrease in the abundance of microbiome-encoded antibiotic resistance genes from 1180 to 829 reads per kilobase of reference sequence per million sample reads ($P = .0097$), likely reflecting reduced antibiotic use during the study period [33].

In contrast, the "PROMISE" study analyzing 345 fecal samples from 124 participants showed statistically significant reductions in the relative abundances of 7 species including *Escherichia coli*, *Staphylococcus aureus*, and *Clostridium scindens* after 6 months of ETI initiation. These microbial shifts correlated with reductions in calprotectin levels, suggesting that ETI may mitigate intestinal inflammation by improving dysbiosis [34].

Relationship between inflammation, dysbiosis, and quality of life

ETI use has also been linked to improvements in GI symptoms and QoL. Caley and colleagues [35] conducted a prospective study on 68 adults pwCF, and used validated CF-specific patients' reported outcome measures to determine the total CF abdominal scores (CFAbd-Scores), which are composed of 28 questions grouped in 5 domains (pain, GERD, disorder of bowel movement, disorders of appetite, and QoL). The scores significantly decreased from 20.4 ± 1.6 points pre-ETI to 15.3 ± 1.9 points at a median of 25 weeks after ETI ($P = .005$) and 16.8 ± 1.6 points ($P = .014$) at a median of 148 weeks of ETI. These findings indicate that prolonged ETI use might improve GI symptoms and disease burden. Likewise, the domains of QoL significantly improved after 1.5 years or less of ETI therapy ($P = .013$).

Similarly, the "RECOVER" study also demonstrated a significant reduction in the total CF abdominal scores among 108 pwCF over 12 years of age from 15.0 ± 1.4 at baseline to 10.2 ± 1.1 at 1 month, and 9.8 ± 1.2 at 12 months of ETI therapy ($P < .001$). Additionally, among 93 participants who provided stool samples, mean (±SD) fecal calprotectin concentrations decreased significantly from 70 ± 8.9 to 27.4 ± 3.4 μg/g, $P < .0001$ at 1 month of therapy, and median [interquartile range] M2-pyruvate kinase (M2-PK) concentrations declined from 12.0 [4.4–20.0] to 2.9 [1.0–8.0] U/mL, $P < .0001$. M2-PK concentrations correlated with CFAbd-scores at 6 months (Spearman's rho=0.31, P=.02), while fecal calprotectin did not, suggesting that improvements in abdominal symptoms may reflect broader reductions in intestinal inflammation rather than direct biomarker correlations [36].

Colon cancer risk in cystic fibrosis

Addressing intestinal inflammation in pwCF should remain critical, as intestinal dysbiosis and inflammation have been linked to increased colorectal cancer (CRC) risk. PwCF are known to have a higher lifetime CRC risk, and current screening recommendations are based on premodulator data. In a prospective study comparing stool samples from pwCF, individuals with CRC, and healthy controls, alpha diversity was significantly lower in pwCF than in both CRC and controls, and beta diversity profiles, which assess the difference in microbial composition between samples, differed between pwCF and both comparator groups. Among 20 taxa enriched in CRC, 6 (*Peptostreptococcus*, *Blautia*, *Lachnoclostridium*, *Streptococcus*, *Hungatella*, and *Veillonella*) were also enriched in pwCF compared to controls, and among 6 depleted taxa in the CRC group, 2 (*Faecalibacterium* and *Anaerostipes*) were also depleted in CF [37]. These findings suggest shared microbial signatures that may underlie the increased CRC risk in CF, highlighting the importance of optimizing gut dysbiosis management in pwCF. However, the long-term impact of ETI on CRC incidence remains unknown, emphasizing the need for future registry-based studies to define modulator-related cancer risk [38].

Dysmotility and slower transit

While ETI has revolutionized CF care, important gaps persist in understanding its impact on dysmotility-related disorders. Fig. 3A–D shows thickened mucus in the proximal and distal intestinal tracts, which contributes to increased incidence of constipation and dysmotility in CF.

Beyond its effects on microbiota, ETI appears to modulate intestinal physiology, promoting intestinal motility. In a longitudinal study of 24 children and adults with CF aged 12 years or greater, ETI use led to increased small bowel water content after 6 months, reduced oro-fecal transit time after 18 months, and decreased total colonic volume, consistent with enhanced small bowel transit and improved bowel dynamics based on MRI findings. The imaging biomarkers obtained throughout the study aligned with symptomatic relief reported by pwCF on ETI [39]. In addition, a large database

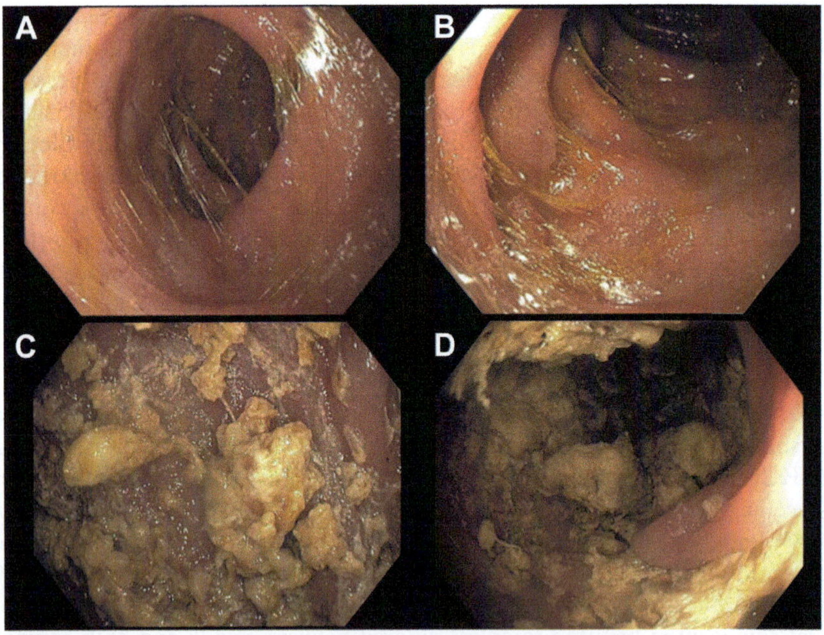

Fig. 3. Endoscopic images from a patient with cystic fibrosis seen at the University of South Florida, Department of Pediatric Gastroenterology. Images captured when patient was actively on elexacaftor-tezacaftor-ivacaftor (ETI), but compliance was not assessed. (*A*) and (*B*) show thick mucus tinged with bile in the duodenum, and (*C*) and (*D*) show thick adherent stool in the cecum and ascending colon, even after a 3 day cleanout.

study of 6 and 21 year old individuals with PI-CF also demonstrated a significant reduction in the prevalence of constipation from 65% to 58% ($P < .0001$) and a nonsignificant reduction in laxative prescriptions from 76% to 70% with ETI use [14]. Despite this, only modest improvement has been described with ETI use. The "PROMISE-GI" study followed 438 pwCF ≥12 year old receiving ETI and reported significant reductions in patients' reported GI outcomes across all domains except rectal symptoms, using validated questionnaires: the patient assessment of constipation-quality of life (PAC-QOL) and the patient assessment of constipation-symptom severity index (PAC-SYM). However, these improvements in QOL indices were considered mild by the authors and remained lower than those of healthy controls, with clinically significant changes mostly observed in pwCF who had severe baseline symptoms [27]. In addition, current evidence suggests that there are no changes in DIOS rates, despite mild improvements observed in intestinal motility. A retrospective single-center study of pwCF aged 18 years or older found no significant reduction in the incidence of DIOS-related hospital admissions and emergency visits during the 3 years following the initiation of CFTR modulators, compared with the 3 years prior [40]. Therefore, multicenter longitudinal studies are needed to clarify the long-term effects of triple CFTR modulators on GI motility disorders, especially with younger individuals who are on these therapies.

FUTURE PERSPECTIVE

With the introduction of HEMT, some measurable improvements in GI manifestations and disease burden have been documented in both children and adults with CF. However, these benefits are often modest and may not reach clinical significance for all individuals. Given the absence of long-term outcome data and the potential for persistent GI inflammation to contribute to complications such as malignancy or irreversible pancreatic damage, there is an urgent need for multicenter longitudinal studies and clinical trials to evaluate the long-term impact of triple CFTR modulator therapy on GI health.

Future investigations should also focus on the mechanisms linking CFTR modulation to microbiome restoration, intestinal inflammation, and medication burden, as these factors may critically influence QoL and long-term nutritional outcomes. As next-generation modulators, such as VTD, advance into clinical use, dedicated studies are warranted to assess their efficacy in ameliorating GI pathology in CF.

SUMMARY

Triple CFTR modulator therapy with ETI has led to modest and variable improvements across GI manifestations of CF, including GERD, intestinal dysmotility, dysbiosis, and inflammation. Nevertheless, persistent intestinal inflammation, ongoing microbiome alterations, and residual symptoms burden remain common, indicating that complete GI restoration has not yet been achieved. Given that current data are limited to short-term and medium-term observations, longitudinal studies are essential to define the durability and clinical significance of these effects and to guide strategies for comprehensive GI care in the era of CFTR modulation.

CLINICS CARE POINTS

- CFTR modulator therapy is associated with modest improvements in patients' reported GI outcomes.
- Clinicians should continue to monitor symptoms longitudinally and manage them using a symptom-directed approach.
- Despite new advances in therapuetics, GI medication burden remains high, including the use of PERT, acid blockers, and laxatives.

Funding sources

Dr R.T. Khalaf receives funding from the Cystic Fibrosis Foundation, United States (#005206Q123, 005583Q123, and 009319Y125).

Disclosure

None.

References

[1] Cystic Fibrosis Foundation. Secondary cystic fibrosis foundation. Available at: https://www.cff.org/intro-cf/about-cystic-fibrosis. Accessed October 19, 2025.

[2] Bacalhau M, Camargo M, Magalhães-Ghiotto GAV, et al. Elexacaftor-tezacaftor-ivacaftor: a life-changing triple combination of CFTR modulator drugs for cystic fibrosis. Pharmaceuticals 2023;16(3); https://doi.org/10.3390/ph16030410.

[3] Middleton PG, Mall MA, Dřevínek P, et al. Elexacaftor-tezacaftor-ivacaftor for cystic fibrosis with a single Phe508del allele. N Engl J Med 2019;381(19):1809–19 [published Online First: 20191031].

[4] Zemanick ET, Taylor-Cousar JL, Davies J, et al. A phase 3 open-label study of elexacaftor/tezacaftor/ivacaftor in children 6 through 11 years of age with cystic fibrosis and at least one F508del allele. Am J Respir Crit Care Med 2021;203(12):1522–32.

[5] Goralski JL, Hoppe JE, Mall MA, et al. Phase 3 open-label clinical trial of elexacaftor/tezacaftor/ivacaftor in children aged 2-5 years with cystic fibrosis and at least one F508del allele. Am J Respir Crit Care Med 2023;208(1):59–67.

[6] 2024 Cystic Fibrosis Foundation Patient Registry Highlights Report. Secondary 2024 cystic fibrosis foundation patient registry highlights report. Available at: https://www.cff.org/sites/default/files/2025-05/2024-Patient-Registry-Highlights-Report.pdf. Accessed October 19, 2025.

[7] Hoppe JE, Kasi AS, Pittman JE, et al. Vanzacaftor–tezacaftor–deutivacaftor for children aged 6–11 years with cystic fibrosis (RIDGELINE trial VX21-121-105): an analysis from a single-arm, phase 3 trial. Lancet Respir Med 2025;13(3):244–55.

[8] Keating C, Yonker LM, Vermeulen F, et al. Vanzacaftor–tezacaftor–deutivacaftor versus elexacaftor–tezacaftor–ivacaftor in individuals with cystic fibrosis aged 12 years and older (SKYLINE trials VX20-121-102 and VX20-121-103): results from two randomised, active-controlled, phase 3 trials. Lancet Respir Med 2025;13(3):256–71.

[9] Sabharwal S. Gastrointestinal manifestations of cystic fibrosis. Gastroenterol Hepatol 2016;12(1):43–7.

[10] Trocchia C, Mosha M, Hamner B, et al. Prevalence and characteristics of gastrointestinal disorders, medication use, and diagnostic interventions in pediatric patients with cystic fibrosis: a nested case–control analysis from the TriNetX EMR-derived global research network real-world dataset. Front Gastroenterol 2025;3; https://doi.org/10.3389/fgstr.2024.1489876.
[11] Bongiovanni A, Manti S, Parisi GF, et al. Focus on gastroesophageal reflux disease in patients with cystic fibrosis. World J Gastroenterol 2020;26(41):6322–34.
[12] Zazzeron L, Alicandro G, Daccò V, et al. Effects of prolonged proton pump inhibitor treatment on nutritional status and respiratory infection risk in cystic fibrosis: a matched cohort study. Dig Liver Dis 2023;55(3):360–5.
[13] Sathe M, Moshiree B, Aliaj E, et al. Need to study simplification of gastrointestinal medication regimen in cystic fibrosis in the era of highly effective modulators. Pediatr Pulmonol 2023;58(3):811–8.
[14] Abi-Aad S-J, Trocchia C, Mosha M, et al. Gastrointestinal burden in patients with pancreatic insufficient cystic fibrosis before and after Elexacaftor/Tezacaftor/Ivacaftor use. Pancreas 2025; https://doi.org/10.1097/mpa.0000000000002522.
[15] Shakir S, Echevarria C, Doe S, et al. Elexacaftor-tezacaftor-ivacaftor improve gastro-oesophageal reflux and sinonasal symptoms in advanced cystic fibrosis. J Cyst Fibros 2022;21(5):807–10.
[16] Sellers ZM. Pancreatic complications in children with cystic fibrosis. Curr Opin Pediatr 2020;32(5):661–7.
[17] Sadras I, Cohen-Cymberknoh M, Kerem E, et al. Acute pancreatitis in pancreatic-insufficient cystic fibrosis patients treated with CFTR modulators. J Cyst Fibros 2023;22(4):777–9.
[18] Gould MJ, Smith H, Rayment JH, et al. CFTR modulators increase risk of acute pancreatitis in pancreatic insufficient patients with cystic fibrosis. J Cyst Fibros 2022;21(4):600–2.
[19] Ramsey ML, Li SS, Lara LF, et al. Cystic fibrosis transmembrane conductance regulator modulators and the exocrine pancreas: a scoping review. J Cyst Fibros 2023;22(2):193–200.
[20] Stastna N, Kunovsky L, Svoboda M, et al. Improved nutritional outcomes and gastrointestinal symptoms in adult cystic fibrosis patients treated with elexacaftor/tezacaftor/ivacaftor. Dig Dis 2024;42(4):361–8 [published Online First: 20240403].
[21] Sankararaman S, Prunty L, Pamer C, et al. Impact of elexacaftor/tezacaftor/ivacaftor on fecal Elastase-1 in children with cystic fibrosis. Pediatr Pulmonol 2025;60(6); https://doi.org/10.1002/ppul.71156.
[22] Fortner CN, Seguin JM, Kay DM. Normal pancreatic function and false-negative CF newborn screen in a child born to a mother taking CFTR modulator therapy during pregnancy. J Cyst Fibros 2021;20(5):835–6 [published Online First: 20210409].
[23] Kowalik A, Roberts E, Harris AH, et al. Clinical outcomes of two infants with cystic fibrosis, including presence of the vas deferens, born to a woman with cystic fibrosis taking CFTR modulators during both pregnancies. J Cyst Fibros 2024;23(5):1027–30.
[24] Schembri L, Jones D, Bentley S, et al. Real-world pancreatic function recovery and fluctuation in young children with cystic fibrosis on elexacaftor/tezacaftor/ivacaftor. J Cyst Fibros 2025; https://doi.org/10.1016/j.jcf.2025.09.004.
[25] Stewart KL, Szczesniak R, Liou TG. Predicting weight gain in patients with cystic fibrosis on triple combination modulator. Pediatr Pulmonol 2024;59(6):1724–30 [published Online First: 20240412].
[26] Enaud R, Languepin J, Lagarrigue M, et al. Dietary intake remains unchanged while nutritional status improves in children and adults with cystic fibrosis on elexacaftor/tezacaftor/ivacaftor. Clin Nutr 2025;50:76–82.
[27] Schwarzenberg SJ, Vu PT, Skalland M, et al. Elexacaftor/Tezacaftor/ivacaftor and gastrointestinal outcomes in cystic fibrosis: report of promise-GI. J Cyst Fibros 2023;22(2):282–9 [published Online First: 20221021].

[28] Hergenroeder GE, Faino A, Bridges G, et al. The impact of elexacaftor/tezacaftor/ivacaftor on fat-soluble vitamin levels in people with cystic fibrosis. J Cyst Fibros 2023;22(6): 1048–53 [published Online First: 20230808].
[29] Francalanci M, Terlizzi V, Fevola C, et al. Nutritional status and circulating levels of fat-soluble vitamins in cystic fibrosis patients: a cohort study and evaluation of the effect of CFTR modulators. Children 2023;10(2); https://doi.org/10.3390/children10020252 [published Online First: 20230130].
[30] Green N, Chan C, Ooi CY. The gastrointestinal microbiome, small bowel bacterial overgrowth, and microbiome modulators in cystic fibrosis. Pediatr Pulmonol 2024;59(Suppl 1):S70–80.
[31] Wrigley-Carr HE, Van Dorst JM, Ooi CY. Intestinal dysbiosis and inflammation in cystic fibrosis impacts gut and multi-organ axes. Med Microecol 2022;13:100057; https://doi.org/10.1016/j.medmic.2022.100057.
[32] Marsh R, Santos CD, Yule A, et al. Impact of extended elexacaftor/tezacaftor/ivacaftor therapy on the gut microbiome in cystic fibrosis. J Cyst Fibros 2024;23(5):967–76.
[33] Reasoner SA, Bernard R, Waalkes A, et al. Longitudinal profiling of the intestinal microbiome in children with cystic fibrosis treated with elexacaftor-tezacaftor-ivacaftor. mBio 2024;15(2); https://doi.org/10.1128/mbio.01935-23.
[34] Duong JT, Hayden HS, Verster AJ, et al. Fecal microbiota changes in people with cystic fibrosis after 6 months of elexacaftor/tezacaftor/ivacaftor: findings from the promise study. J Cyst Fibros 2025;24(4):792–800.
[35] Caley LR, Gillgrass L, Zagoya C, et al. Longer term follow-up of abdominal symptoms (CFAbd-Score) after initiation of elexacaftor/tezacaftor/ivacaftor in adults with cystic fibrosis. J Cyst Fibros 2025; https://doi.org/10.1016/j.jcf.2025.01.010.
[36] Mainz JG, Lester K, Elnazir B, et al. Reduction in abdominal symptoms (CFAbd-Score), faecal M2-pyruvate-kinase and calprotectin over one year of treatment with Elexacaftor-Tezacaftor-Ivacaftor in people with CF aged ≥12 years - the RECOVER study. J Cyst Fibros 2024;23(3):474–80 [published Online First: 20231007].
[37] Caley LR, Wood HM, Bottomley D, et al. The gut microbiota in adults with cystic fibrosis compared to colorectal cancer. J Cyst Fibros 2024;23(2):262–8.
[38] Taichman DB, Grasemann H, Ratjen F. Cystic fibrosis. N Engl J Med 2023;389(18): 1693–707.
[39] Yule A, Ng C, Recto A, et al. A longitudinal study assessing the impact of elexacaftor/tezacaftor/ivacaftor on gut transit and function in people with cystic fibrosis using magnetic resonance imaging (MRI). J Cyst Fibros 2024;23(5):984–90 [published Online First: 20240905].
[40] Wongjarupong N, Delbrune MF, Alp J, et al. Effect of cystic fibrosis transmembrane conductance regulator modulators and dedicated cystic fibrosis gastrointestinal clinic visits on the incidence of distal intestinal obstructive syndrome in persons with cystic fibrosis. PLoS One 2025;20; https://doi.org/10.1371/journal.pone.0328015.
[41] Davis PB. Cystic fibrosis since 1938. Am J Respir Crit Care Med 2006;173(5):475–82.
[42] Administration UFaD. Secondary. Available at: https://www.accessdata.fda.gov/scripts/cder/daf/index.cfm. Accessed October 19, 2025.

Advances in Pediatrics 73 (2026) 191–211

ADVANCES IN PEDIATRICS

The Hidden Burden

Endocrinopathies in Adolescents after Hematopoietic Stem Cell Transplantation

Harinder Dosanjh Raipuria, DNP[a,b,*], Catherine M. Gordon, MD, MS[a,b]

[a]Pediatric Endocrinology, *Eunice Kennedy Shriver* National Institute of Child Health and Human Development, National Institutes of Health, Bethesda, MD, USA; [b]Section on Adolescent Bone Health & Body Composition, *Eunice Kennedy Shriver* National Institute of Child Health and Human Development, National Institutes of Health, Bethesda, MD, USA

Keywords

• Adrenal insufficiency • Bone mineral density • Glucocorticoids
• Gonadotoxic therapies • Hematopoietic stem cell transplantation
• Hyperglycemia • Immunosuppression • Premature ovarian insufficiency

Key points

- Hematopoietic stem cell transplantation (HSCT) is an established curative therapy for adolescent patients with malignancy, hemoglobinopathies, bone marrow failure, inborn errors of metabolism, and immunodeficiency.
- Endocrine sequalae can occur secondary to the use of immunosuppressants, glucocorticoids, and gonadotoxic agents required for the transplant process.
- Glucocorticoid use alone, essential for management, can lead to iatrogenic adrenal insufficiency, reduced bone mineral density, and medication-induced hyperglycemia.
- Premature ovarian insufficiency can occur in females secondary to the gonadotoxic preparatory conditioning regimen.
- Assessment, monitoring, and management of endocrinopathies after HSCT require consideration in clinical practice.

*Corresponding author. Eunice Kennedy Shriver National Institute of Child Health and Human Development, National Institutes of Health, Building 10 CRC - Room 5-2583, 10 Center Drive, Bethesda, MD 20892. *E-mail address:* harinder.raipuria@nih.gov

https://doi.org/10.1016/j.yapd.2025.12.011

Abbreviations

ACTH	adrenocorticotropic hormone
AI	adrenal insufficiency
AMH	antimullerian hormone
BMD	bone mineral density
DXA	dual-energy X-ray absorptiometry
FSH	follicle stimulating hormone
GVHD	graft versus host disease
HPA	hypothalamic-pituitary-adrenal
HRT	hormone replacement therapy
HSCT	hematopoietic stem cell transplant
LH	luteinizing hormone
OTC	ovarian tissue cryopreservation
POI	premature ovarian insufficiency
PTH	parathyroid hormone

INTRODUCTION

Around 4000 cases of leukemia and 2300 cases of lymphoma are newly diagnosed annually in adolescents aged 10 to 19 in the United States (US) [1–3]. Hematopoietic stem cell transplant (HSCT) is a curative treatment that replaces dysfunctional bone marrow with healthy hematopoietic stem cells, taken from either peripheral blood mononuclear cells, umbilical cord blood, or bone marrow [4]. Indications for HSCT have broadened, with 2500 transplants performed each year in the US, reflecting a rise of 5% to 10% [5]. A chemotherapeutic conditioning regimen is administered to eliminate existing bone marrow and create space for donor cell engraftment, in the initial preparatory phase. Recipient T cells are eliminated to reduce the risk of rejection and if indicated, treat the primary malignancy [4]. Stem cells are then infused intravenously with delivery to the bone marrow to stimulate hematopoiesis. Donor stem cells are termed allogenic and autologous cells derive from the recipient.

Malignancies, hemoglobinopathies, bone marrow failure, inborn errors of metabolism, and immunodeficiency are indications for HSCT in adolescents [6]. Essential agents used pre-transplant and post-transplant include gonadotoxic agents for conditioning, immunosuppressants to promote graft acceptance, and glucocorticoids to suppress inflammation. Secondary endocrine sequalae can occur, including adrenal insufficiency (AI), altered bone turnover and reduced bone mineral density (BMD), medication-induced hyperglycemia, and premature ovarian insufficiency (POI). With increasing indications, treatment-related morbidity merits consideration. Adolescents are in a critical period for growth and bone mineral acquisition, with endocrine factors affecting accrual [7]. Adolescent patients will have an extended inpatient hospital stay, up to 100 days following transplant, during which time endocrinopathies can develop. This requires assessment and further medical management, leading to health care burden.

The focus of this review is upon the endocrine sequalae seen among adolescents after HSCT. With increased rates of survivorship post-transplant at

100 days (93%) and at 3 years (74%), long-term health is at risk [8]. The primary aim is to raise awareness for clinicians caring for adolescents, for early detection and evaluation of endocrinopathies and immediate initiation of treatment. This ensures health outcomes are preserved and long-term sequelae are minimized.

CLINICAL SIGNIFICANCE

Adolescents undergo a process of physical maturation to reach sexual maturity and attain reproductive capabilities, termed puberty. Hormone production from the hypothalamus, pituitary gland, adrenal glands, and gonads trigger the process [9]. This is a crucial time for development, which can be compromised due to hormonal and endocrine disarrangement in adolescents following HSCT.

Up to 70% of patients after HSCT develop graft versus host disease (GVHD) within the first 100 days, where transplanted graft cells attack host cells, causing an array of complications [3]. The gastrointestinal tract is most affected due to antigen-presenting cells, translocating microbial products [10]. Consequent symptoms of nausea, vomiting, abdominal pain, and diarrhea occur, resulting in poor appetite. Inadequate nutritional intake is associated with pubertal delay and compromised bone accrual. First-line treatment of GVHD includes high-dose glucocorticoids, often associated with pubertal delay [11]. Long-term use of supraphysiologic glucocorticoids can impair bone health, with increased bone resorbing osteoclastogenesis and decreased bone-forming osteoblastogenesis, coupled with altered calcium homeostasis in the kidney and intestines, which heightens the risk of fractures [12]. Adolescence is a critical period for the acquisition of peak bone mass and negative effects on bone health have implications for osteoporosis later in life [13]. Adolescent girls with POI are in a hypoestrogenic state, which impairs BMD via activation of resorbing osteoclasts, decreased gut calcium absorption, and increased renal calcium excretion [14]. AI has implications for puberty, with inadequate production of androgens, required for pubarche [15]. Prolonged medication-induced hyperglycemia can lead to long-term microvascular and macrovascular complications [16].

Multiple factors impair pubertal progression, potential for attaining full height velocity, growth patterns, and the attainment of peak bone mass. Underlying chronic disease, impaired nutritional status, glucocorticoid use, and impaired androgen and gonadotropin production are contributors. With the potential for extensive negative impact on a patient's health, evaluation for endocrinopathies is essential, to minimize long-term complications.

ENDOCRINOPATHIES

As long-term survivorship increases, consideration of multiple coexisting endocrinopathies in adolescents after HSCT requires consideration, along with the associated high burden of chronic disease [17]. Our focus is on four prevalent endocrine conditions–iatrogenic AI, reduced BMD, medication-induced hyperglycemia, and POI.

ADRENAL INSUFFICIENCY

Pathogenesis

AI encompasses inadequate production and secretion of glucocorticoids or mineralocorticoids from the adrenal cortex [18]. Damage to the adrenal glands causes loss of steroid secretion in primary AI [19]. Suppression of the hypothalamic-pituitary-adrenal (HPA) axis results in suppressed adrenocorticotropic hormone (ACTH) secretion from the anterior pituitary, causing adrenal cortex atrophy, termed secondary AI [19,20]. This is also a form of central AI. Prolonged use of supraphysiologic glucocorticoids is the leading cause of secondary AI, also termed iatrogenic or glucocorticoid-induced [21]. Physiologic release of hypothalamic corticotropin-releasing hormone stimulates ACTH secretion from the anterior pituitary, which in turn stimulates adrenal steroidogenesis.

HSCT recipients require glucocorticoids for their primary disease and post-transplant sequelae. Synthetic glucocorticoid use triggers the negative feedback loop, causing downregulation of ACTH from the anterior pituitary in response to exogenous exposure, which mimics the presence of endogenous cortisol [19]. Mineralocorticoid secretion is preserved in secondary AI, as this is stimulated via the renin-angiotensin-aldosterone system [22]. Prednisolone doses $\geq$ 5 mg/day for over 4 weeks or a hydrocortisone equivalent of $\geq$15 mg per day heighten risk of secondary AI [19]. Higher glucocorticoids doses are often required for optimal disease and symptom control. Physiologic stress requires further supraphysiologic dosing, as absent adrenal function results in suboptimal cortisol secretion, crucial in the face of an acute stressor [18].

Clinical presentation

The clinical presentation is variable and a patient may be asymptomatic or have nonspecific symptoms including myalgia, weakness, and fatigue [19]. Even vague symptoms in high-risk patients after HSCT should prompt evaluation [18]. The goal is to avoid adrenal crisis, an acute life-threatening process [18,21]. Malaise, fatigue, generalized weakness, weight loss, anorexia, nausea, dizziness, and abdominal pain can indicate AI [23]. Symptoms can be acute or insidious. Physical examination may reveal pallor, dehydration (decreased skin turgor and dry mucous membranes), and hypotension [18,19]. Prompt identification of AI in the differential diagnosis is crucial to reduce the risk of cardiovascular shock, metabolic encephalopathy, and coma [22]. Patient presentation can mimic a primary chronic disease flare, posing a clinical challenge [19].

Evaluation

The diagnosis is based on history, laboratory findings, and clinical suspicion (Fig. 1 and Table 1). A history of known AI, ongoing glucocorticoid use, glucocorticoid noncompliance, and recent etiology of gastrointestinal or flu-like

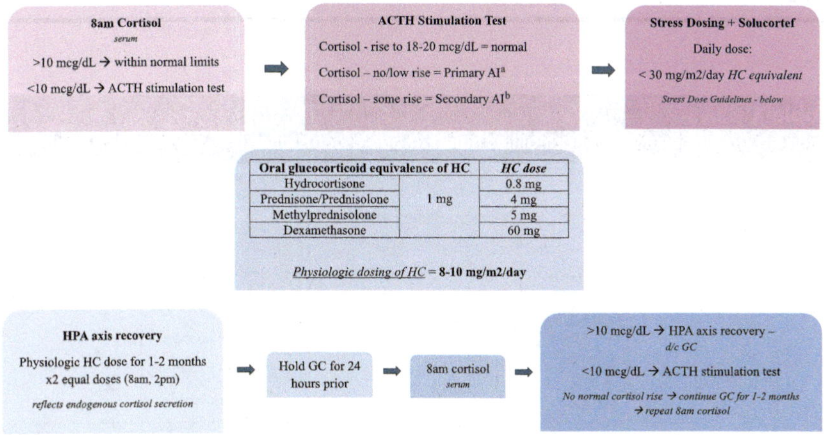

Stress Dose Guidelines

	Symptoms	Hydrocortisone Dose
Minor	• Mild cold symptoms, without fever • Routine sports/physical activity • Psychological stress (exam, interview)	*No change to usual dose*
Mild	• Mild URI or other infection with low grade fever (99.5 - 102 F) • Emesis x1 • Diarrhea x1-2	~25mg/m²/day *or* twice usual dose *Q6 – equal doses (round up)*
Moderate	• Anesthesia for diagnostic or minimally invasive procedures • Persistent diarrhea • Emesis >1 (but can keep tablets down) • URI or other infection with fever > 39°C (102°F) • GI infection • Dental surgery • Fracture • Seizure (first time or unexpected) • Concussion/head trauma • All-day sports tournament	~50mg/m²/day *or* 3x usual dose *Q6 – equal doses (round up)*
Severe	• Major trauma – e.g., MVA • Sepsis/septic shock • Repeated emesis • Signs of dehydration • Change in mental status • Unconscious • 911/ER	Solu-Cortef IM: 25 mg - (0-2 years) 50 mg - (2- 8 years) 100 mg - (>8 years)

Fig. 1. Adrenal insufficiency assessment, management, and recovery. [a]Primary AI: adrenal gland dysfunction = ↓ aldosterone ↓ cortisol [Addison's Disease, adrenal gland bleeding, infection, genetic disease, adrenalectomy]. [b]Secondary AI: hypothalamic dysfunction = ↓ ACTH ↓ cortisol [iatrogenic, pituitary tumor, irradiation, hypophysectomy, head trauma, infection]. ER, emergency room; d/c, discontinue; GC, glucorticoid, GI, gastrointestinal; HC, hydrocortisone; HPA, hypothalamic-pituitary-adrenal; MVA, motor vehicle accident; URI, upper respiratory infection. (*Data from* National Institutes of Human Health & Development Stress Dose + Weaning Glucorticoid Guidelines, 2025; Original Figure using previously published data: Data from National Institutes of Human Health & Development Stress Dose + Weaning Glucorticoid Guidelines, 2025.)

Table 1
Imaging and laboratory abnormalities noted in adolescents after HSCT with endocrinopathies

Endocrinopathy	Mechanism	Evaluation findings[a]		Follow up evaluation	
Adrenal Insufficiency	Suppression of HPA axis secondary to supraphysiologic glucocorticoid use = iatrogenic/central AI	8am ACTH 8am Cortisol ACTH stimulation test	↓ ↓ ↓ *Basal cortisol fails to rise at least 7 mcg/dL in response to stimulation*	ACTH stimulation test once on physiologic dose of glucocorticoids [*hydrocortisone equivalent 8-10 mg/m2/day*]	Cortisol > 18mcg/dL Restoration of HPA axis
Bone Mineral Density	Altered bone metabolism secondary to glucocorticoid use and/or estrogen deficiency	DXA Whole Body Composition – *total body less head* *Serum testing:* Calcium 25-hydroxyvitamin D PTH Phosphorous Alkaline phosphatase TSH FT4	BMD Z-score ≤ - 2.0 *after adjustment for height*[b] ↓ ↓ ↓/↑ ↓/↑ ↓ ↓/↑ ↓/↑	Repeat DXA Repeat serum testing *Serum values are highly variable*	As per clinician judgment following therapy – *calcium (dietary preferred) + vitamin D supplementation; consideration of bisphosphonates when skeletal fragility is documented*
Hyperglycemia	Secondary to use of diabetogenic medications including glucocorticoids and immunosuppressants	Fasting plasma glucose - *x2 on separate occasions* Fructosamine – *evaluates average glucose for prior 2-3 weeks*	≥ 126 mg/dL ↑	Fasting plasma glucose Fructosamine after diabetogenic medications are discontinued or dose reduced	≤ 126 mg/dL < 238 (μmol/L) concordant with A1c of 6.5%
Premature Ovarian Insufficiency	Acquired hypergonadotropic hypogonadism and ovarian tissue damage secondary to gonadotoxic agents used for conditioning	β-HCG FSH Estradiol Anti-Müllerian hormone Prolactin - *rule out insidious prolactinoma* TSH	(-) >25 mIU/mL ↓ ↓ <23.3 ng/mL ↑/↓	Initiate use of transdermal estradiol to reduce risk of low BMD and cardiovascular disease	Measure gonadotropins every 3-6 months when titrating estradiol dose

Abbreviations: A1c, hemoglobin A1c; β-HCG, beta-human chorionic gonadotropin; FT4, free thyroxine; TSH, thyroid stimulating hormone.

[a]Laboratory values will differ depending on the assay used.

[b]Z-scores are adjusted for height using the Children's Hospital of Philadelphia Pediatric Bone Density Calculator.

illness should raise a high index of suspicion [22]. Before confirmation of the diagnosis, clinicians need to start empiric glucocorticoid therapy [19]. With acute presentation, the priority is to assess a serum metabolic panel, complete blood count with differential, cortisol, ACTH, aldosterone, renin and thyroid stimulating hormone. Any delay in evaluation increases the risk of acute decompensation and potential adrenal crisis. Patients with secondary AI have low serum cortisol (<10 mcg/dL), low normal serum ACTH, hypoglycemia, normocytic normochromic anemia, lymphocystis, and eosinophilia [18,22,23]. The etiology of the triggering illness should be investigated, to identify precipitating factors and treat accordingly. Atypical symptoms of vision impairment, headache or polyuria and/or polydipsia suggestive of diabetes insipidus, require a full pituitary panel with MRI [19].

Once hemodynamically stable and empiric glucocorticoids have been administered, a confirmatory diagnosis can be pursued. An 8 AM serum cortisol and ACTH should be obtained simultaneously. Serum cortisol measurement less than 10 mcg/dL with low-normal ACTH level is suggestive of secondary AI and warrants an ACTH stimulation test [19]. For inconclusive results, an ACTH stimulation test is also recommended. This is the gold standard for evaluation and a measure of adrenal reserve and the HPA-axis [18]. Baseline serum cortisol is drawn, 250 mcg of cosyntropin administered intramuscularly, then cortisol drawn at 30 and 60 minutes [20]. A cortisol value of less than 18 mcg/dL at 60 minutes confirms the diagnosis of AI [23]. The abnormal response to stimulation is indicative of downregulation of ACTH receptors and consequent adrenal cortex atrophy [19].

Management

The mainstay of treatment is glucocorticoid replacement, balancing patient needs with risks of therapy. Treatment objectives are to use the lowest dose for the shortest period. The primary disease status and HSCT sequelae can make this challenging. However, glucocorticoid replacement can restore good health and is essential for recovery [21].

The management of adrenal crisis requires hemodynamic stability and correction of metabolic effects from glucocorticoid deficiency [23]. Fluid resuscitation, bolus glucocorticoid administration with hydrocortisone, and intravenous dextrose to treat hypoglycemia are required [18,23]. Precipitating causes requires treatment, such as antibiotics for an infectious disease process [22]. Long-term supraphysiologic glucocorticoid therapy causes cortisol peaks, increasing the risk of morbidity [24]. Mortality, adrenal crisis, cardiometabolic effects of diabetes mellitus, hypertension and dyslipidemia; depression, anxiety, chronic fatigue, impaired quality of life, and increased hospitalizations are known adverse outcomes of AI [19,22].

Daily hydrocortisone is recommended, as this replacement mimics physiologic cortisol secretion, when given 2 to 3 times a day. Administration upon waking, at midday and 5 PM; avoiding dosing 4 hours before bedtime due to the risk of insomnia, is the ideal regimen [18]. If using twice daily replacement, a higher dose should be given upon waking, followed by a lower dose 6 hours later [19]. Patient and caregiver education for management, stress dosing for illness and emergencies are critical. Adolescents should be empowered to take control of their medical management [18,24] Sick day rules with instructions for acute illness need to be provided, based on the severity of illness (see Fig. 1). Major trauma, sepsis, repeated emesis, change in mental status, and loss of consciousness require urgent administration of 100 mg of intramuscular hydrocortisone, followed by calling 911 [25]. The need for stress dosing, never missing a dose, and clinical follow-up require emphasis [18]. Caregivers should be able to demonstrate how to administer emergency hydrocortisone. Patients should carry a steroid emergency card, wear a medical alert bracelet, keep extra doses on hand and have 2 doses of parenteral glucocorticoids for emergencies [18,22]. For any procedures including dental, stress dosing must be discussed with the provider in advance, so that the glucorticoid replacement dose can be increased before the procedure. Families require education on signs and symptoms of AI, including abdominal pain, nausea, vomiting, weight loss, dizziness, fatigue, and anorexia, with a need for urgent hydrocortisone treatment and immediate emergency care [22].

A glucocorticoid taper can be considered with close monitoring of symptoms when clinical improvement occurs, with incremental reductions to dosing. An individualized approach is recommended, to avoid glucocorticoid withdrawal, which presents similarly to an adrenal crisis [19]. The goal is to minimize cardiometabolic morbidity and optimize HPA axis recovery [19]. All patients should be switched to hydrocortisone with twice daily dosing, upon waking and after 6 hours, to best match physiologic cortisol release [25]. Once at a physiologic dose of hydrocortisone 8 to 10 mg/m^2/day for 1 to 2 months, adrenal function recovery testing can occur [25]. Glucocorticoids should be held for 24 hours, and then an 8 AM serum cortisol obtained. If serum cortisol is greater than 10 mcg/dL the HPA axis is considered recovered, and glucocorticoids can be discontinued. If indeterminate, an ACTH stimulation test is an appropriate next step, with a peak serum cortisol of 18 mcg/dL at 60 minutes, indicative of adrenal function restoration [23]. If cortisol remains low, the physiologic dose should be continued for 1 to 2 months, then an 8 AM cortisol repeated [25]. Secondary AI is a reversible endocrinopathy and most patients will achieve recovery of the HPA axis within one year [19].

BONE MINERAL DENSITY

Pathogenesis

Bone is a living tissue, and its mineral components are evaluated with a BMD measurement, a marker of bone health [26]. Greater levels of bone mineralization reflect greater strength and capacity for weight-bearing. Calcium, phosphorus, inorganic salts, and bone collagen compose the foundation of osteocytes, osteoclasts, osteoblasts, stem cells, and the bone matrix [27]. Bone remodeling occurs with osteoclast activated bone resorption, followed by osteoblast activated bone formation [27]. This allows for maintenance of structural integrity and for the continual cycle of mineralization [27]. If the equilibrium between these cells is compromised, remodeling is under threat. Decreased osteoblast activity, irrespective of osteoclast activity, results in higher bone resorption over formation, causing bone microstructure destruction [27]. Adequate serum levels of calcium, vitamin D, and parathyroid hormone (PTH) are required for optimal bone health. Significant for adolescents after HSCT, glucocorticoids are the most common iatrogenic cause of reduced BMD due to increased bone resorption and decreased bone formation [28]. Compromised nutritional intake, chronic disease, minimized physical activity, and prolonged glucocorticoid use collectively reduce BMD. Chronic disease impairs physical activity, contributing to bone mass loss [26]. Up to 75% of patients experience loss of BMD after HSCT, concerning for the accrual of peak bone mass [17,26]. Disease-related cytokines from hematologic and inflammatory disorders have an additive negative effect and also impact bone metabolism [29].

Clinical presentation

The clinical presentation is variable, as the patient may be asymptomatic, have vague back pain suggestive of a vertebral fracture, a history of multiple low impact fractures inappropriate for the mechanism of action or pathologic fractures and found incidentally. For high-risk patients taking osteotoxic medications including glucocorticoids with chronic disease, there should be a low index of suspicion for compromised bone health [30]. To preserve bone integrity and halt disease progression, clinicians need to identify high risk patients promptly [31]. At-risk markers including glucocorticoid use, chronic disease, immobility and poor nutrition, need early identification and timely intervention. A 10% increase in peak bone mass during adolescence, delays the onset of osteoporosis by 13 years [13].

Assessment

The gold standard for the assessment of bone health is dual-energy X-ray absorptiometry (DXA) imaging; a validated method of measure with low radiation exposure (Tables 1 and 2) [32]. Patient history should include loss of linear height velocity, dose and duration of glucocorticoid use, pubertal status, fracture history, and primary disease status [29]. Vertebral height loss can be assessed from growth charts. The physical examination should include palpation of posterior spinous processes for tenderness and assessment for Cushingoid features indicating prolonged glucorticoid exposure [29]. The anteroposterior spine and total body less head are preferred assessment sites in adolescents, as there is robust normative pediatric data for analysis [30]. Spinal imaging allows for a vertebral fracture to be ruled out. Decreased BMD reflected in DXA measurements supports compromised mechanical strength and an increased fracture risk [31]. Of note, DXA does not differentiate between trabecular and cortical compartments. Glucocorticoids mostly affect trabecular bone within vertebrae and at the ends of long bones, making patients more vulnerable to vertebral fractures, with greater exposure and duration of use representing an additive effect [29]. Lateral spine radiographs or DXA vertebral fracture assessment allow for assessment of fractures at this compromised skeletal site [29]. While an initial screening tool, DXA reporting can be confounded by small adolescent bone size with short stature and/or pubertal delay. Vertebral imaging before initiating glucocorticoids is recommended

Table 2
Choice of dual-energy X-ray absorptiometry imaging site in adolescents

Site		Rationale	Adjustment for Height	Interpretation
Total Body Less Head	✓	Assess cortical bone = 80% of bone mass	Height adjusted Z-score (HAZ) using BMD Children's Hospital of Philadelphia Calculator *(number of standard deviations below the age matched mean)*	BMD (g/cm²) ≤ - 2.0 = "low bone mass/BMD for chronological age" - 2.0 → + 2.0 = "normal bone mass/BMD for chronological age"
Posterior: Anterior Spine	✓	Assess trabecular bone[a] Validated site (*pediatric/adolescent*) Robust normative data Assess for vertebral fractures		
Proximal Femur	☒	Size/shape of bone is evolving Transition from cartilage → bone Closure of growth plates pending Bone mass accrual incomplete Skull = 40% skeletal mass, minimal change Lack of normative data		
Femoral Neck	☒			
Distal Radius	☒			
Total Body	☒			

Clinical Pearls

- Discontinue calcium and vitamin D supplementation 48 hours prior to imaging.
- If patient has received contrast agent, wait 14 days to perform.
- No metal or jewelry to be worn due to potential for artifact.
- T-scores are *not appropriate* for reporting results in adolescents as bone mineral accrual is incomplete.
- Terms of 'osteopenia/osteoporosis' should *not* be used unless there is evidence of skeletal fragility; preferred terminology 'low bone mass/low bone mineral density for chronological age'.

[a]Glucorticoids have a greater impact on trabecular versus cortical bone.

with periodic follow-up. BMD is reported using Z-scores as peak bone mass and full skeletal development have not yet been attained. *Low bone mass or low bone mineral density for age* is the preferred terminology, corresponding to a BMD Z-score threshold ≤ 2.0 [30]. *Osteoporosis* should not be used unless there is evidence of skeletal fragility. Osteoporosis in an adolescent cannot be diagnosed with the absence of pathologic and/or multiple fractures. Adjustment of BMD Z-scores for height, using the Children's Hospital of Philadelphia pediatric bone density calculator, is required [33]. This allows for BMD to be compared to that of a healthy individual of the same age, sex, and ethnicity. BMD Z-scores may be falsely low due to short stature, poor linear height velocity, weight loss, and pubertal delay [29]. Biochemical evaluation of serum calcium, phosphorus, 25-hydroxyvitamin D, PTH, alkaline phosphatase, thyroid stimulating hormone, and free thyroxine is warranted.

Management

Treatment objectives are to reduce skeletal morbidity and glucocorticoid sequelae. The goal is receipt of the lowest glucocorticoid dose, for the least amount of time. As discussed, in clinical practice this may be unfeasible due to transplant rejection, treatment sequelae and primary disease. The treatment approach is multifaceted with a need to treat pubertal delay with hormone replacement therapy (HRT), supplement nutritional deficiencies, encourage weight-bearing activities albeit cautiously in patients with low BMD, and discuss fall prevention strategies. As weight-bearing activity supports bone strength and optimizes BMD accrual, moderate activity is always recommended [7]. Adequate nutritional calcium intake is important as low circulating levels lead to increased bone calcium resorption, in order to supply calcium for life-sustaining activities of muscle contractility, cardiac rhythm regulation, and nerve impulse transmission [27]. About 99% of calcium is stored within bone and a nutritional intake of 1300 mg of elemental calcium daily via dairy products, leafy green vegetables, fatty fish, and fortified cereals is recommended [34]. As insulin-like growth factor 1 is nutrition-dependent and a signaling factor for osteoblasts, adequate protein intake and healthful nutrition promotes bone formation [7]. Vitamin D3 supplementation is recommended, as its direct action on target organs bypassing any need for hepatic or renal activation, promotes homeostasis [27]. This allows for greater calcium absorption, increased bone mineralization and reduced bone resorption. A serum 25-OHD level less than 20ng/mL requires supplementation, with dosing dependent on the level of deficiency [35]. The sun provides 95% of 25-OHD through cutaneous synthesis, however deficiency is common as many adolescents have inadequate exposure [35]. Calcium supplements can have adverse gastrointestinal effects and should be reserved for use for patients with dietary restrictions. Circulating calcium is the primary driver of PTH secretion, with the 25-OHD level regulating intestinal calcium absorption. If conservative measures are not successful and skeletal fragility or osteoporosis noted, the first-line treatment is intravenous bisphosphonate infusions. Bisphosphonates inhibit bone resorption and are used along with vitamin D3 supplementation and high dietary calcium intake [27]. Zoledronic acid is the preferred agent, with its greater potency, a shorter infusion time, and lower dosing intervals. A standard pediatric dose of 0.05 mg/kg every 6 months, with a maximum dose of 4 mg is recommended [29]. Dental evaluation and treatment is recommended beforehand, due to the rare risk of jaw osteonecrosis. Bone strength is dependent on size, microarchitecture, macroarchitecture, mineralization, and the organic matrix. A 10% increase in peak bone mass leads to 50% reduced risk of a later life fragility fracture, highlighting the need for timely identification and intervention [7].

HYPERGLYCEMIA

Pathogenesis

Diabetogenic agents are required following HSCT to prevent transplant rejection. Glucocorticoids increase glucose levels by 68% from baseline but are crucial for their anti-inflammatory and immunosuppressive properties [36]. Concurrent use of antiproliferative immunosuppressants and/or calcineurin inhibitors heighten the risk of medication-induced hyperglycemia [37]. Prophylactic triazoles for immunocompromised patients further cause metabolic derangements [38]. Parenteral nutrition exacerbates hyperglycemia, with its high glucose content, yet is required if nutritional intake is compromised from gastrointestinal GVHD [39]. Medication interference of glucose homeostasis is multifaceted, occurring in a dose-dependent manner, with systemic glucocorticoids posing the greatest risk [40]. Insulin resistance via similar mechanisms to type 2 diabetes mellitus can occur. Glucocorticoids interfere with liver, muscle, and adipose tissue insulin receptors. Further, they hinder beta cell-activity with induction of cellular apoptosis, promoting hyperglycemia [36,37]. Glucocorticoids stimulate hepatic gluconeogenesis, increasing serum glucose [41]. Glucocorticoids inhibit peripheral glucose uptake creating a hyperglycemic and hyperinsulinemic state, the hallmark of insulin resistance [40]. Antiproliferative immunosuppressants required for a successful post-transplant course, exacerbate beta cell dysfunction [40]. Calcineurin inhibitors induce beta cell apoptosis, while a mammalian target of rapamycin agent decreases glycogen production, and reduces skeletal tissue glucose uptake [42]. Compensatory mechanisms that should maintain normoglycemia are disrupted [37].

Clinical presentation

The clinical presentation is variable. Typical signs of hyperglycemia include polyuria, polydipsia, polyphagia, fatigue, weight loss and blurred vision. As patients require extended hospitalization after HSCT, hyperglycemia is often identified incidentally on routine serum testing. Risk factors of glucocorticoid use, chronic disease, history of glycemic deviations, family history of diabetes mellitus, and use of concomitant diabetogenic medications, require timely evaluation [39,41]. Hyperglycemia increases with greater glucocorticoid doses and duration of use [43]. Complaints of feeling faint, trembling, diaphoresis, and confusion especially overnight or early morning, requires assessment, as the glucocorticoid's mechanism of action wears off resulting in hypoglycemia [44].

Assessment

Ideally, HbA1c is assessed before starting glucocorticoids. However, this has limited diagnostic use for patients after HSCT, as hemoglobinopathies, a common indication for transplant, alter the red blood cell lifespan (see Table 1) [37,41]. Fructosamine provides accurate glycemic representation over the preceding 2 to 3 weeks and should be used [43]. Fasting glucose is of little diagnostic use, due to the mechanism of action of glucocorticoids. Intermediate-acting agents such as methylprednisolone and prednisone, peak 4 to 6 hours after administration. When given as a single daily morning dose, post-prandial hyperglycemia occurs in the late afternoon/early evening [36]. Post-prandial glucose obtained 2 hours after lunch has the highest diagnostic value and sensitivity [40]. Glycemic variability occurs from systemic insulin resistance and impaired insulin secretion. Normoglycemia and hypoglycemia can be seen when glucocorticoids wear off overnight or in the early morning [37]. Diagnosis can be made with random blood glucose greater than 250 mg/dL+, fasting 140 mg/dL+, pre-prandial greater than 150 mg/dL + or 2 hours post-prandial greater than 200 mg/dL+ [37,39]. Point-of-care testing with capillary blood glucose is preferred for glycemia assessment. After identification of hyperglycemia, fasting, pre-prandial, post-prandial, and evening glucose levels should be assessed for 2 days [39].

Management

Treatment objectives are to reduce microvascular and macrovascular sequelae of long-term hyperglycemia and achieve normoglycemia. Principles of care apply as for any diabetic patient. Insulin is efficacious, has a strong safety profile, immediate onset of action, and is easily titratable depending on glycemic values [43]. For intermediate acting agents including prednisone, administration of Neutral Protamine Hagedorn (NPH), an intermediate acting insulin concurrently, matches the pharmacokinetics of the glucocorticoid mechanism of action, providing greater glycemic control [42,44]. For long-acting glucocorticoids including dexamethasone, longer acting glargine insulin can be used [42]. Assessing the pattern of glucocorticoid-induced hyperglycemia and matching it with the pharmacodynamics of antidiabetic agents, offers the strongest coverage [40]. A basal-bolus insulin regimen mimics pancreatic physiologic insulin release [39,40]. This regimen can be used with correction dosing and a continuous glucose monitor if hyperglycemia persists [37]. Oral antidiabetic agents are another option. Metformin, a biguanide, increases insulin sensitivity and improves insulin resistance [37]. In practice, oral agents are not always ultilized due to their side effect profile and potential for these to mimic GVHD (eg, the gastrointestinal adverse events related to metformin use). Dipeptidyl peptidase-4-inhibitors are deemed beneficial, as they enhance insulin secretion and inhibit glucagon, with cardiovascular and renal benefits [39,42]. Hyperglycemia causes acute inflammatory processes, endothelial dysfunction, longer admissions, slower wound healing, higher infection rates, increased mortality and metabolic dysfunction [36,41]. Structural and functional cardiac damage is associated with insulin resistance [45]. Up to 65% of patients have glucocorticoid induced hyperglycemia and early identification is crucial [42]. Patient education about symptoms of hyper and hypoglycemia, monitoring, methods to treat and nutritional guidance are required from a diabetes educator [37,39]. Insulin doses need adjustment when weaning glucocorticoids to avoid hypoglycemia [43].

PREMATURE OVARIAN INSUFFICIENCY

Pathogenesis

Loss of menses for at least 4 months, with elevated serum follicle stimulating hormone (FSH) and low serum estradiol, before 40 years of age, define POI across the age spectrum [14]. Gonadotoxic conditioning regimens before HSCT heighten the risk of hypergonadotropic hypogonadism, due to end organ ovarian damage [46,47]. Myeloablative conditioning with high-dose gonadotoxic alkylating agents including busulfan and cyclophosphamide, coupled with total body irradiation is considered the gold standard preparatory regimen [48]. Reduced intensity regimens using fludarabine, melphalan and cyclophosphamide lower gonadal damage risk [48]. POI risk is dose-dependent, determined in part by the cyclophosphamide equivalent dose (CED). Prepubertal females receiving greater than 12 gm/m^2 CED and pubertal females receiving >8 mg/m2 CED are at highest risk for gonadal damage [46,49]. Amenorrhea can be primary with delayed pubertal onset and no lifetime menses, or secondary with new onset cessation of previous menses [50]. POI is a heterogenous diagnosis with eventual depletion of ovarian follicles and hormonal dysregulation [49]. Iatrogenic causes are most prevalent, and the triad of amenorrhea, elevated gonadotropins, and hypoestrogenism represent gonadal dysfunction [17,51]. Females who are prepubertal or younger than 13 year old, exhibit gonadotoxicity resistance, as the hypothalamic-pituitary-ovarian axis is not yet fully established, resulting in a higher chance of spontaneous puberty and ovarian recovery [47,52].

Clinical presentation

The clinical presentation varies with delayed pubertal onset, a lack of breast development followed by menarche 2 to 3 years later; pubertal arrest, new onset menses cessation, no lifetime menses or oligomenorrhea [14,49,53]. To note, menstrual irregularities are the most common initial symptom; however, asymptomatic presentation is possible [50,54]. Anxiety, low mood, sleep disturbance, vulvar-vaginal discomfort, vasomotor symptoms, low libido, and poor concentration all reflect hypoestrogenism [53,54].

Assessment

The assessment should include obtaining a transplant, radiation, medical diagnoses, and hematological clotting disorder history (Fig. 2 and Table 1). Lifetime fractures should be noted as POI is an independent predictor of BMD due to hypoestrogenism, which causes increased bone resorption and reduced bone formation compromising bone accrual [46,49]. DXA imaging can be used for BMD assessment. Physical examination requires thelarche and pubarche Tanner staging, midparental height assessment, and examination for androgen excess, as hirsutism can indicate polycystic ovary syndrome, a cause of menstrual irregularities [14,48]. Growth chart review allows for skeletal growth assessment. Hypothyroidism and hyperprolactinemia need to be ruled out as they both can disrupt menses [14]. The hypothalamic-pituitary-gonadal axis is assessed with FSH, luteinizing hormone (LH), estrogen, and antimullerian hormone (AMH) [48]. Biochemical elevation of FSH (>25 IU/I) with low estrogen is diagnostic of POI [50]. Elevated LH and low AMH are also typically seen [49]. AMH is a marker of ovarian follicular reserve but not of diagnostic value for POI [50]. FSH and estrogen levels fluctuate and if inconclusive, serum testing should be repeated in 4 to 6 weeks [50]. In the United States, many clinicians require 2 elevated FSH values before making a diagnosis of POI [14].

Management

Treatment objectives are to reduce sequelae, offer HRT for symptomatic relief, and counsel on contraception and fertility (Table 3) [54]. Early detection, diagnosis, and intervention are crucial as ovarian reserve loss is irreversible and adolescents have a critical window for bone accrual [53]. Estrogen replacement

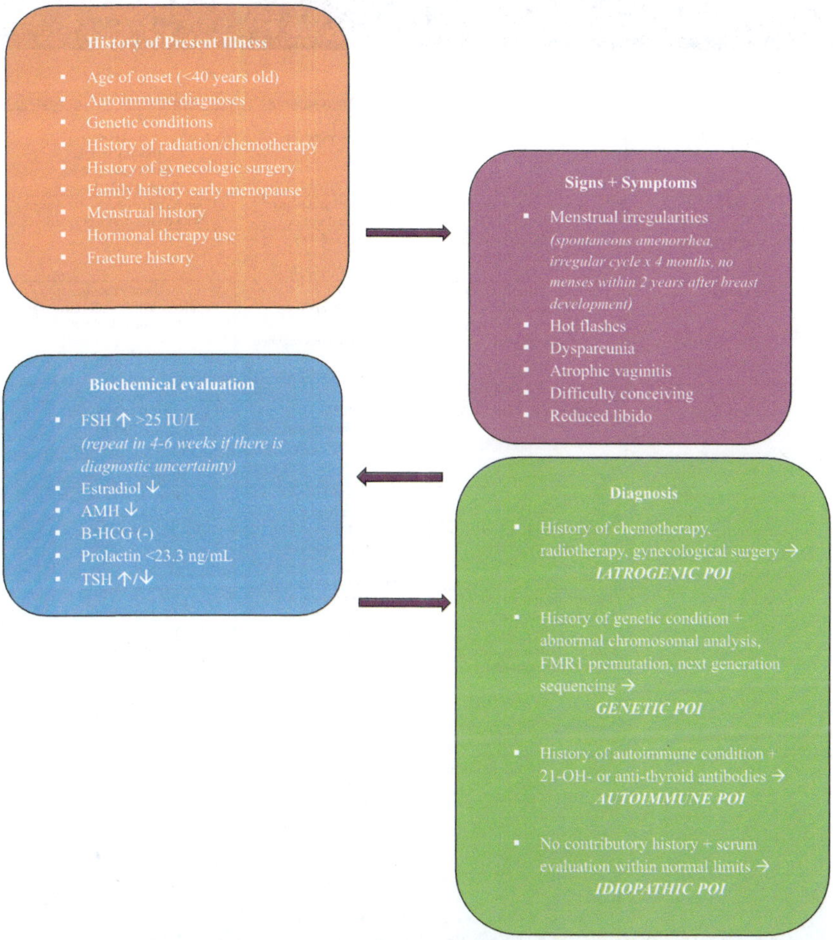

Fig. 2. Diagnosis of POI β-HCG, beta-human chorionic gonadotropin; FMR1, fragile X messenger ribonucleoprotein 1; hx, history; TSH, thyroid stimulating hormone; 21-OH-Abs, 21-hydroxylase autoantibodies. (*Data from* American Society for Reproductive Medicine, 2025 Mayo Foundation for Medical Education and Research, 2025.)

aids with pubertal progression, breast development, and uterine growth [14]. Pubertal induction and completion; menstruation induction and reinstitution, as well as vasomotor symptoms, are addressed with estrogen use [49]. Further, estrogen therapy for pubertal delay supports height potential, feminization, and bone mass accrual, with any delay in initiation of replacement treatment compromising final stature [46]. Cardiometabolic disease, osteoporosis, and neurologic dysfunction are prevented with HRT [46,50]. Transdermal formulations mimic physiologic release, avoiding the hepatic first-pass effect and are preferred. The recommended regimen includes:

Table 3
Sequelae of premature ovarian insufficiency and management

Sequalae		Rationale	Medical management	Non-medical management
Life expectancy Morbidity/mortality	↓	CV complications	HRT – *until menopause*	Healthy nutrition Exercise Healthy weight Smoking cessation Reduce ETOH intake
Fertility	↓	Low ovarian reserve	Preservation options Oocyte donation	Contraceptive options for patients who do not desire pregnancy
Obstetric complications	↑	Oocyte donation pregnancy Uterine radiation	High risk OB Specialty Cardiology	
Bone health	↓	Abnormal bone architecture Reduced BMD Increased risk of fractures and osteoporosis	HRT – *until menopause* COC – continuous regimen DXA – baseline	Dietary calcium Supplementation with calcium and cholecalciferol
Muscle mass	↓	Risk of sarcopenia		Resistance exercises
Cardiovascular	↑	Risk of CVD, HF, CVA	HRT – *until menopause*	Healthy nutrition Exercise Maintain healthy weight Smoking cessation Reduce ETOH intake
Psychological well-being + QOL	↓	Stressor of POI + impact on fertility	SSRI – if indicated	Psychosocial support Counselling
Sexual function	↓	Reduced libido due to hypo-estrogenic state	HRT – *until menopause* Transdermal testosterone	Counselling
Genitourinary	↑	Vaginal discomfort secondary to hypo-estrogenic state	Transvaginal estradiol Lubricants	
Cognition	↓	Risk of impairment, dementia, parkinsonism	HRT – *until menopause*	Healthy nutrition Exercise Maintain healthy weight Smoking cessation Reduce ETOH intake
Vasomotor	↑	Blood vessel constriction/dilation due to ↓ estrogen – hot flashes, night sweats	HRT – *until menopause* SSRI/anti-convulsant	Healthy nutrition Exercise Maintain healthy weight

Principles of HRT

- Options for therapy include 2 mg oral estradiol *or* up to 100 µg transdermal estradiol (as total adult dose).
- Pubertal induction should begin at 11 years with low dose estradiol and gradual dose increase over 2-3 years.
- Transdermal estrogen mimics physiologic release of estradiol and is the preferred option for therapy.
- Combined oral contraceptive pills are not appropriate for pubertal induction.
- Cyclical progesterone after 2 years of estrogen therapy or when breakthrough bleeding occurs, must be added to the regimen to reduce the risk of endometrial hyperplasia.

Abbreviations: COC, combined oral contraceptives; CV, cardiovascular; CVA, cerebrovascular accident; CVD, cardiovascular disease; DXA, dual-energy X-ray absorptiometry; ETOH, alcohol; HF, heart failure; HRT, hormone replacement therapy; OB, obstetric; QOL, quality of life.

Data from Yatsenko, et al, 2024 [14].

1. *Pubertal induction:* Low dose of 3 to 7 mcg/day—cut matrix patches (0.014–0.025 mg/24h) into quarters or eights [14].
2. Increase dose every 6 months until adult dose of 75-100 mg is reached over 2 to 3 years [14].
3. Add oral micronized progestin 100 to 200 mg daily for 12 days per month after 18 to 24 months, or if breakthrough bleeding occurs. Evaluate the endometrial stripe via sonography first, to assess its thickness [46].
4. *Pubertal arrest:* Higher doses of estrogen are indicated due to prior exposure at clinician discretion [46].

Adding progestin prevents endometrial hypoplasia, a significant risk of prolonged unopposed estrogen therapy, and minimizes thrombotic events when used with transdermal estrogen [49]. HRT does not provide contraceptive coverage so counseling is warranted [49]. Higher estrogen doses are avoided during growth to prevent premature epiphyseal closure and poor breast development [14]. Oral contraceptive pills with high estrogen doses are only appropriate after pubertal completion [14].

The risk of iatrogenic POI risk requires extensive discussion with patients before HSCT [54]. A multidisciplinary specialist team with pediatrics, reproductive endocrinology, oncology, surgery, and reproductive medicine represented can offer counsel to patients, help stratify risk and provide annual ovarian health monitoring [54,55]. Fertility preservation options need to be offered and assisted reproductive techniques completed before treatment, to support quality of life [47,48]. Ovarian tissue cryopreservation (OTC) is available for prepubertal females and oocyte retrieval for postpubertal females [47–49]. The American Society for Reproductive Medicine endorses OTC as a *medical procedure* that is no longer deemed experimental [49]. Recovery of AMH is possible one year after competition of use of any gonadotoxic therapies [56]. Comorbid mood disorders, anxiety, and poor self-esteem require psychosocial support and cognitive behavioral therapy. Patients should be counseled on adequate dietary calcium and vitamin D intake, with weight-bearing exercise to optimize bone health [14].

DISCUSSION

Medical advances have broadened the spectrum of HSCT use. Adolescents with malignancies, hemoglobinopathies, primary immunodeficiencies, and inborn errors of metabolism undergo this curative treatment. Transplant volume is rising, along with survivorship rates following transplant. The pre-transplant and post-transplant period requires use of agents including gonadotoxic conditioning regimens, immunosuppressants to promote graft acceptance, and supraphysiologic glucocorticoids to suppress inflammation. Secondary to use of these necessitated therapies, adolescents are at risk for endocrine sequelae. Treatment-related morbidity merits consideration as adolescents are transitioning through puberty and in a critical period for bone mineral acquisition. They are at high risk for iatrogenic AI secondary to glucocorticoid use; altered bone turnover, and consequently reduced BMD secondary to glucocorticoid use, immobility, compromised nutritional status, and primary chronic disease; hyperglycemia secondary to use of multiple diabetogenic medications and POI secondary to gonadal damage from reproductive toxicants. With raised awareness, early evaluation and immediate treatment initiation, health outcomes are preserved, and long-term sequelae are minimized.

SUMMARY

Adolescents following HSCT are at risk for endocrinopathies including iatrogenic AI, reduced BMD, medication-induced hyperglycemia, and POI. This is secondary to the use of essential therapies as part of the treatment process, which include gonadotoxic conditioning regimens, immunosuppressants, and supraphysiologic glucocorticoids. With broadened spectrum of use for HSCT and increasing transplant volume, early identification of endocrinopathies is crucial, to ensure prompt treatment and to minimize long-term sequelae.

CLINICS CARE POINTS

- Hematopoietic stem cell transplant (HSCT) has a broadened spectrum of use for malignant and nonmalignant conditions.
- Essential treatments include pre-transplant conditioning regimens, immunosuppressants, and glucocorticoids.
- These therapies cause endocrinopathies of iatrogenic adrenal insufficiency, reduced bone mineral density, medication-induced hyperglycemia, and premature ovarian insufficiency.
- Clinicians should evaluate endocrinopathies post-transplant and promptly start treatment if indicated.
- This minimizes long-term sequelae and preserves health for adolescents, who are in a critical period for growth and bone mass acquisition.

Disclosure

This work was supported by the Intramural Research Program of the National Institutes of Health, United States (NIH). The contributions of the NIH authors are considered Works of the United States Government. The findings and conclusions presented in this paper are those of the authors and do not necessarily reflect the views of the NIH or the U.S. Department of Health and Human Services.

References

[1] Organization WH. World Health Organization adolescent health. Available at: https://www.who.int/health-topics/adolescent-health#tab=tab_1.
[2] Explorer NCCR. Statistics in NCCR explorer. Available at: https://nccrexplorer.ccdi.cancer.gov/.
[3] Society LaL. Childhood and adolescent blood cancer facts and statistics. Available at: https://bloodcancerunited.org/childhood-and-adolescent-blood-cancer-facts-and-statistics.
[4] Board PPTE. Pediatric hematopoietic stem cell transplant and cellular therapy for cancer (PDQ®): health professional version. In: PDQ Cancer Information Summaries [Internet]. Bethesda (MD): National Cancer Institute (US); 2002.
[5] Olson TL, Pollack MM, Davila Saldana BJ, et al. Hospital survival following pediatric HSCT: changes in complications, ICU therapies and outcomes over 10 years. Front Pediatr 2023;11:1247792; https://doi.org/10.3389/fped.2023.1247792.
[6] Bense JE, Haverman L, von Asmuth EG, et al. Late effects in pediatric allogeneic hematopoietic stem cell transplantation for nonmalignant diseases: proxy-and patient-reported outcomes. Transplantation and Cellular Therapy 2023;29(3):186.e1-e10.
[7] Chevalley T, Rizzoli R. Acquisition of peak bone mass. Best Pract Res Clin Endocrinol Metabol 2022;36(2):101616.

[8] Phelan R, Chen M, Bupp C, et al. Updated trends in hematopoietic cell transplantation in the United States with an additional focus on adolescent and young adult transplantation activity and outcomes. Transplantation and cellular therapy 2022;28(7):409.e1-e10.
[9] Breehl L, Caban O. Physiology, puberty. In: StatPearls [Internet]. Treasure Island (FL): StatPearls Publishing; 2024. p. 202.
[10] Rattanaseksan K, Anurathapan U, Tanpowpong P. Features of gastrointestinal acute graft-versus-host disease in children undergoing hematopoietic stem cell transplantation. J Pediatr Gastroenterol Nutr 2025;80(2):271–81.
[11] Smallbone P, Mehta RS, Alousi A. Steroid refractory acute GVHD: the hope for a better tomorrow. Am J Hematol 2025;100:14–29.
[12] Bouliari A, Bullard F, Lin-Su K, et al. Current advances in the management of congenital adrenal hyperplasia. Adv Pediatr 2024;71(1):135–49.
13 Zemel BS, Winer KK, Kelly A, et al. Race-neutral pediatric reference ranges for bone mineral density predict prospective fractures in childhood. J Clin Endocrinol Metab 2025;110(11): 3034–48.
[14] Yatsenko SA, Witchel SF, Gordon CM. Primary amenorrhea and premature ovarian insufficiency. Endocrinol Metab Clin N Am 2024;53(2):293.
[15] Rosenfield RL. Normal and premature adrenarche. Endocr Rev 2021;42(6):783–814.
[16] Mouri M, Badireddy M. Hyperglycemia. In: StatPearls [Internet]. Treasure Island (FL): StatPearls Publishing; 2023.
[17] Lee SL-K, Nguyen Q-N, Ho C, et al. The late effects of hematopoietic stem cell transplants in pediatric patients: a 25-year review. The Journal of Clinical Endocrinology & Metabolism 2025;110(2):e347–62.
[18] Lewis A, Thant AA, Aslam A, et al. Diagnosis and management of adrenal insufficiency. Clin Med 2023;23(2):115–8.
[19] Martin-Grace J, Tomkins M, O'Reilly MW, et al. Iatrogenic adrenal insufficiency in adults. Nat Rev Endocrinol 2024;20(4):209–27.
[20] Khare S, Anjum F. Adrenocorticotropic hormone (cosyntropin) stimulation test. In: StatPearls [Internet]. StatPearls Publishing; 2023.
[21] Rushworth RL, Torpy DJ. The changing epidemiology of adrenal insufficiency: iatrogenic factors predominate. Journal of the Endocrine Society 2023;7(3):bvad017.
[22] Elshimy G, Chippa V, Kaur J, et al. Adrenal crisis. In: StatPearls [Internet]. StatPearls Publishing; 2025.
[23] Vance SJ, Horsley JT, Welch MP, et al. Educational case: adrenocortical insufficiency—Causes and pathogenesis. Academic Pathology 2022;9(1):100019.
[24] Pazderska A, Malchoff CD, Valassi E. Adrenal insufficiency: diagnostic approaches, treatments, and outcomes, volume II. Frontiers Media SA; 2025:1629881.
25 Development NIoCHaH. Stress Dose and Weaning Glucocorticoid Guidelines. Bethesda (MD): National Institutes of Health Clinical Center; 2025.
[26] Li T, Huang G, Hou D, et al. A comprehensive analysis of bone mineral density changes across the lifespan: insights from national surveys. Nutrients 2024;16(16):2804.
[27] Liang B, Burley G, Lin S, et al. Osteoporosis pathogenesis and treatment: existing and emerging avenues. Cellular & molecular biology letters 2022;27(1):72.
[28] Cipolla C, Sodero G, Cammisa I, et al. The impact of glucocorticoids on bone health and growth: endocrine and non-endocrine effects in children and young patients. Minerva Pediatrics 2022;75(6):896–904.
[29] Ward LM, Bakhamis SA, Koujok K. Approach to the pediatric patient with glucocorticoid-induced osteoporosis. Journal of Clinical Endocrinology & Metabolism 2025;110(2): 572–91.
[30] Guss CE, McAllister A, Gordon CM. DXA in children and adolescents. Journal of Clinical Densitometry 2021;24(1):28–35.
[31] Hong J, Sung H, Choi JO, et al. A prediction model of pediatric bone density from plain spine radiographs using deep learning. Sci Rep 2025;15(1):13039.

[32] Krugh M, Langaker MD. Dual energy x-ray absorptiometry. 2018.
[33] Philadelphia CsHo. Pediatric Z-Score calculator. Available at: https://zscore.research.chop.edu/calcpedbonedens.php.
[34] Health NIo. Calcium. Available at: https://ods.od.nih.gov/factsheets/Calcium-HealthProfessional/.
[35] Minkowitz B, Ristic J, Nadel L, et al. Bone health in pediatric fracture patients: a DEXA study. Open J Orthoped 2022;12(2):57–65.
[36] Akshaya N, Ravi K, Venkateswaramurthy N. Steroids induced hyperglycemia: its effects and management. J Drug Deliv Therapeut 2023;13(6).
[37] Cho J-H, Suh S. Glucocorticoid-induced hyperglycemia: a neglected problem. Endocrinology and Metabolism 2024;39(2):222–38.
[38] Liszka K, Marschollek P, Przystupski D, et al. Efficacy and safety assessment of antifungal prophylaxis with posaconazole using therapeutic drug monitoring in pediatric patients with oncohematological disorders—A single-centre study. J Fungi 2025;11(1):38.
[39] Shah P, Kalra S, Yadav Y, et al. Management of glucocorticoid-induced hyperglycemia. Diabetes, Metab Syndrome Obes Targets Ther 2022;1577–88.
[40] Li J-X, Cummins CL. Fresh insights into glucocorticoid-induced diabetes mellitus and new therapeutic directions. Nat Rev Endocrinol 2022;18(9):540–57.
[41] Barker HL, Morrison D, Llano A, et al. Practical guide to glucocorticoid induced hyperglycaemia and diabetes. Diabetes Therapy 2023;14(5):937–45.
[42] Jain AB, Lai V. Medication-induced hyperglycemia and diabetes mellitus: a review of current literature and practical management strategies. Diabetes Therapy 2024;15(9):2001–25.
[43] Fève B, Scheen AJ. When therapeutic drugs lead to diabetes. Diabetologia 2022;65(5):751–62.
[44] Struja T, Nitritz N, Alexander I, et al. Treatment of glucocorticoid-induced hyperglycemia in hospitalized patients-a systematic review and meta-analysis. Clinical Diabetes and Endocrinology 2024;10(1):8.
[45] Agbaje AO, Zachariah JP, Barker AR, et al. Persistent hyperglycemia and insulin resistance with the risk of worsening cardiac damage in adolescents: a 7-year longitudinal study of the ALSPAC birth cohort. Diabetes Care 2025;48(6):896–904.
[46] Cattoni A, Parissone F, Porcari I, et al. Hormonal replacement therapy in adolescents and young women with chemo-or radio-induced premature ovarian insufficiency: practical recommendations. Blood Rev 2021;45:100730.
[47] Chabut M, Schneider P, Courbiere B, et al. Ovarian function and spontaneous pregnancy after hematopoietic stem cell transplantation for leukemia before puberty: an LEA cohort study. Transplantation and Cellular Therapy 2023;29(6):378.e1-e9.
[48] Bender JD, Oquendo-del Toro H, Benoit J, et al. Reduced-intensity conditioning mitigates risk for primary ovarian insufficiency but does not decrease risk for infertility in pediatric and young adult survivors of hematopoietic stem cell transplantation. Transplantation and Cellular Therapy 2023;29(2):130.e1-e8.
[49] Foster KL, Lee DJ, Witchel SF, et al. Ovarian insufficiency and fertility preservation during and after childhood cancer treatment. J Adolesc Young Adult Oncol 2024;13(3):377–88.
[50] Panay N, Anderson RA, Bennie A, et al. Evidence-based guideline: premature ovarian insufficiency. Human reproduction open 2024;2024(4):hoae065.
[51] Koo J, Grom-Mansencal I, Howell JC, et al. Gonadal function in pediatric Fanconi anemia patients treated with hematopoietic stem cell transplant. Haematologica 2023;108(9):2358.
[52] Hou Y, Li Z, Bai L, et al. Fertility assessment in long-term young female survivors with hematological disease after allogeneic hematopoietic cell transplantation: a single-center real-life cross-sectional study. Ann Hematol 2025;104(3):1897–905.
53 Guo T, Liu H, Xu B, et al. Epidemiology, genetic etiology, and intervention of premature ovarian insufficiency. Endocr Rev 2025;46(5):621–51.

[54] Kim HK, Kim TJ. Current status and future prospects of stem cell therapy for infertile patients with premature ovarian insufficiency. Biomolecules 2024;14(2):242.
[55] Wikander I, Lundberg FE, Nilsson H, et al. A prospective study on fertility preservation in prepubertal and adolescent girls undergoing hematological stem cell transplantation. Front Oncol 2021;11:692834.
[56] Su H, Yang J, Pei L, et al. Gonadal function in pediatric female post-Allo-HSCT: a real-life prospective study from China. Gynecol Endocrinol 2025;41(1):2523420.

ELSEVIER

Advances in Pediatrics 73 (2026) 213–224

ADVANCES IN PEDIATRICS

Parathyroid Disorders in Children

Physiology, Pharmacology, and Practical Management Considerations

Ramin Jamshidi, MD[a,b,c,d,*]

[a]Department of Pediatric Surgery, Phoenix Children's, Phoenix, AZ, USA; [b]Department of Surgery & Child Health, Creighton University School of Medicine, Phoenix, AZ, USA; [c]Department of Surgery, University of Arizona School of Medicine, Phoenix, AZ, USA; [d]Department of Surgery, Mayo Clinic, Phoenix, AZ, USA

Keywords

• Parathyroid • Hyperparathyroidism • Hypoparathyroidism • Hypercalcemia • Hypocalcemia • PTH

Key points

- Parathyroid disorders are relatively uncommon in children but can have grave clinical consequences. Understanding underlying physiology and biochemistry is the foundation of disease management.
- In both hyperparathyroid and hypoparathyroid disorders, the pathology typically manifests as abnormal serum calcium. The priority of clinical management is the establishment of eucalcemia.
- Technological advances in parathyroid imaging/localization and intraoperative identification are evolving. The future may bring broader pharmacologic options and knowledge of relevant genetics.
- Pediatric-focused multidisciplinary endocrine care is optimal. In hyperparathyroidism, it is beneficial to consult early with an endocrine surgeon with higher operative volume.

PARATHYROID GLANDS

Parathyroids are endocrine glands which regulate calcium and phosphate homeostasis through production of parathyroid hormone. There are normally

*Department of Surgery, Mayo Clinic, Phoenix, AZ. *E-mail address:* rjamshidi@phoenixchildrens.com

https://doi.org/10.1016/j.yapd.2026.03.001

Abbreviations

4D	time-resolved
CT	computed tomography
HHM	humoral hypercalcemia of malignancy
PTHrp	PTH-related peptide

4 parathyroid glands, all located in the neck in close approximation to the thyroid. These are small glands, typically measuring 2 to 5 mm in each dimension, similar to a small pea. As they are so small, the glands were not discovered until 1850, when anatomist Sir Richard Owen noted them in an Indian rhinoceros [1,2]. Their exact location (relative anatomy) can be somewhat variable, particularly for the lower parathyroids. Variant anatomy is not so rare, with supernumerary glands in as many as one-sixth of patients and ectopic glands in as many as one-fourth of patients; common variant locations are within the thyroid, thymus, and mediastinum [3].

This article begins with an overview of parathyroid function and summary of relevant laboratory analyses, imaging and pharmacology. Parathyroid disorders are then grouped into hyperparathyroidism and hypoparathyroidism.

PARATHYROID PHYSIOLOGY

The glands are comprised of 2 cell types: chief cells and oxyphil cells. The former synthesize and secrete parathyroid hormone. The latter have no recognized endocrine function. Parathyroid hormone synthesis and secretion (and thus serum concentration) are regulated through inhibition by serum calcium and vitamin D concentrations. This negative feedback loop drives an inverse relationship between serum calcium and parathyroid hormone concentration [4,5]. Magnesium has a more subtle and often overlooked impact on parathyroid function. Low levels of magnesium promote parathyroid hormone secretion, but very low levels paradoxically inhibit parathyroid hormone (PTH) secretion and can exacerbate hypocalcemia [6,7].

There are 3 realms where end-organ effects of parathyroid hormone are observed: skeletal, renal, and intestinal [4].

- Bones: Inhibition of osteoblast activity and stimulation of osteoclast activity release calcium from bone into the bloodstream and limit formation of new bone. Vitamin D has similar effects.
- Kidneys: Calcium resorption is increased by upregulation of a calcium transporter. PTH also blocks phosphate reabsorption. This decreases urinary calcium excretion and increases phosphate excretion. At the proximal tubule, PTH upregulates translation of alpha-1-hydroxylase, which generates the biologically active form of vitamin D, the 1,-25-dihydroxy form. This is also known as calcitriol. In the kidney, vitamin D increases both calcium and vitamin D resorption.
- Intestines: PTH does not have direct effects on the intestine, but vitamin D increases calcium and phosphate absorption from the intestines. This is mediated by paracellular and transcellular mechanisms.

PARATHYROID-RELATED LABORATORY ASSAYS

A variety of biochemical assays are relevant to discussion of parathyroid function and there are subtleties which inform analysis of those results [8].

- Serum calcium is the sum of ionized calcium and calcium bound to bicarbonate, citrate, and protein. For every 1 g/dL decrease in serum albumin, total serum calcium is decreased by 0.8 mg/dL (ie, the total calcium level should be *corrected* by this amount for comparison with the lab's normal range). This does not affect the fraction of ionized calcium.
- Ionized calcium is the fraction which is unbound in the serum. This is the component that impacts nerve conduction, muscle contractility, myocyte stability, and hypocalcemic symptoms. Assays are not affected by hypoproteinemia but are more costly and require an anaerobic collection, transport on ice, and prompt processing.

At low pH, binding affinity of albumin to calcium is diminished and ionized calcium levels are increased. The converse explains the paresthesias that result from hyperventilatory acute respiratory alkalosis during a burst of physical activity (acute temporary decrease in ionized calcium).

- Parathyroid hormone has a half-life of less than 5 minutes. This makes it impractical to use as a long-term marker of parathyroid function. Meanwhile, the rapid metabolism makes it tremendously useful as a marker of nearly real-time parathyroid function. It is commonly used intraoperatively to aid parathyroidectomy by guiding extent of operation [9].
- PTH-related peptide (PTHrp) is really a group or class of endogenous proteins of multiple isoforms which bind to the PTH receptor and largely induce the same responses. PTHrp is produced by a wide variety of tissues in the body at a low, steady rate and half-life is similar to PTH. It becomes relevant when elevated levels are present in association with various malignancies, manifesting as hypercalcemia [10].
- Vitamin D assays typically evaluate the major storage form, 25-OH vitamin D, which is biologically inactive. The biologically active dihydroxy (1,25-OH) form has a half-life of just 4 to 6 hours [11,12].

PARATHYROID IMAGING

There are just a few imaging modalities relevant to evaluation of parathyroid disease. The goals of imaging are to identify the presence of abnormally enlarged or hyperfunctioning glands, determine the number of abnormal glands, and/or to facilitate surgery by anatomic localization (particularly detection of an ectopic gland) [13].

- Ultrasound is the primary modality for imaging of parathyroid glands. Normal parathyroid glands are commonly not visualized, but it is the first imaging modality used to look for enlarged parathyroids when evaluating hyperparathyroidism.
- Sestamibi is a nuclear medicine study which uses intravenous Technetium (Tc) 99m to identify parathyroid glands, imaging them based on differential Tc elimination compared to the adjacent thyroid. Intensity of signal can differentiate glandular hypertrophy or hyperplasia, which is useful in directing operative approaches, particularly selective versus complete (4-gland) exploration.

- Time-Resolved (4D) computed tomography (CT) (4D-CT) protocols have been increasingly used to aid in localization of enlarged parathyroid glands and plan operations in adult patients. Those caring for pediatric patients have generally avoided this because of the considerable radiation dose delivered directly over the thyroid gland (one of the most radiation-sensitive tissues in the body).
- MRI allows cross-sectional imaging without radiation but doesn't generally distinguish well between parathyroid glands and lymph nodes or thyroid. The author and colleagues have developed a 4D-MRI protocol for pediatric parathyroid localization. In initial evaluations, this has proven useful for localization of parathyroid glands and differentiation between adenomatous disease and hyperplasia (Fig. 1A–C) [14].
- PET with 18F-labeled fluorocholine is an evolving nuclear medicine modality which has undergone evaluation in last several years. Sensitivity of approximately 95% has been reported for detection of small or ectopic parathyroid adenomas. However, it is not universally available and can be confounded by false positives, particularly in the setting of thyroid nodules [15,16]. Optimal performance of this modality involves combination with CT, again raising consideration of ionizing radiation exposure in a pediatric patient, albeit much lower thyroid exposure than with 4D-CT.

PARATHYROID-RELATED PHARMACOLOGY

A relatively short list of medications and supplements are relevant to management of parathyroid disorders. There are subtleties about some of these which are worth summarizing before discussion of disorders of parathyroid function.

- Calcium supplements are central to management of parathyroid disease. Carbonate and citrate complexes are oral forms, while gluconate and chloride formulations are for intravenous administration. Carbonate complexes provide 40% by mass elemental calcium, while citrate complexes provide about 20% by mass elemental calcium. While more concentrated, carbonate complexes require normal gastric acid for proper absorption, is more associated with constipation, and can cause mild gastric irritation in those with digestive disorders like inflammatory bowel disease.

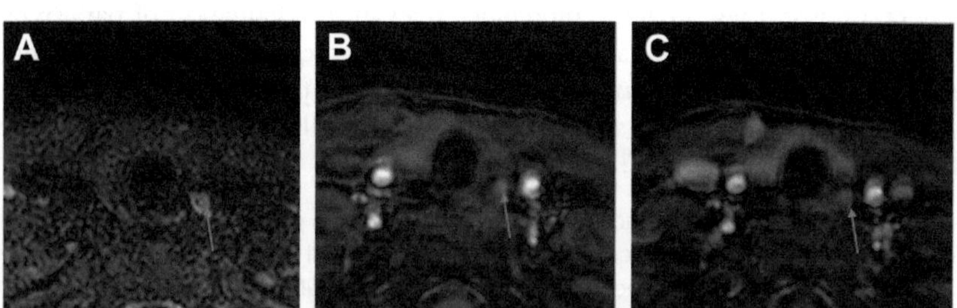

Fig. 1. 4-dimensional MRI for parathyroid localization. *Orange arrows* indicate location of parathyroid glands. (*A*) Parathyroid gland hyperintensity on T2 sequence. (*B*) Early arterial enhancement and (*C*) venous "washout" on 4D-DCE MR TRAK series.

- Cholecalciferol is the other name for the mono-hydroxy form of vitamin D (25-OH D3). This is the standard formulation used for dietary supplementation and repletion of deficiency.
- Calcitriol is the other name for the shorter-lasting but biologically active dihidroxy form of vitamin D (1,25-OH D3).
- Calcitonin is a natural product which lowers serum calcium by osteoclast inhibition and increasing renal calcium excretion. Endogenously made by the thyroid's chief cells, it can be administered by subcutaneous or intramuscular injection or nasal spray. Metabolized by renal and serum pathways, it has a duration of action of 6 to 8 hours. This makes it very useful for acute and subacute management of hypercalcemia.
- Cinacalcet is a calcimimetic which is used to lower PTH in hyperparathyroidism. It acts on the calcium-sensing receptors of the parathyroid's chief cells to lower PTH and calcium levels [17]. They are effective in secondary hyperparathyroidism, but not primary hyperparathyroidism (see below) [18].
- Bisphosphonates such as alendronate induce apoptosis of osteoclasts, reducing serum calcium as they reduce bone turnover and facilitate increases in bone density. Calcium lowering is seen within 48 hours, peaks at 5 to 7 days, and lasts for months to years [19].
- Synthetic parathyroid hormone is a long-term option for treatment of hypoparathyroidism, though no pediqtric-approved options exist to date. Teriparatide is a recombinant PTH approved in 2002 for treatment of postmenopausal osteoporosis and effects of long-term glucocorticoid therapy. Another recombinant PTH (Natpara , Takeda Pharmaceutical Company) was approved by the Federal Drug Administration for treatment of hypocalcemic hypoparathyroidism in 2015, but manufacturing issues resulted in recalls in 2019, and global manufacturing ceased in 2024. That same year, a synthetic PTH analogue palopegteriparatide (Yorvipath , Ascendis Pharma) was approved for treatment of chronic hypoparathyroidism. Neither of these medications have been evaluated for safety in pediatric patients; the presence of open epiphyses raises concerns about increased osteosarcoma risk [20]. It remains to be seen whether a parathyroid analogue is developed which can benefit pediatric patients with permanent hypoparathyroidism.

HYPERPARATHYROIDISM

The most common derangement of parathyroid function is excessive function (hyperparathyroidism), which causes hypercalcemia. A variety of symptoms result, including nephrolithiasis, constipation, and depressed mood; with greater severity and/or chronicity, bone mineral density diminishes (Fig. 2). Incidence of pediatric primary hyperparathyroidism is estimated at 2 to 5 per 100,000 population, while the incidence in adults is 100 times greater [21].

Acute hypercalcemia should be corrected to ease symptoms and prevent dysrhythmia. Loop diuretics such as furosemide augment calcium excretion, but their use must be preceded by hydration to maintain euvolemia. Bisphosphonates may be used for longer-lasting limitation of severe hypocalcemia, particularly if the calcium is above 12 and/or the patient has significant symptoms. Their effect can last for some time, which must be taken into

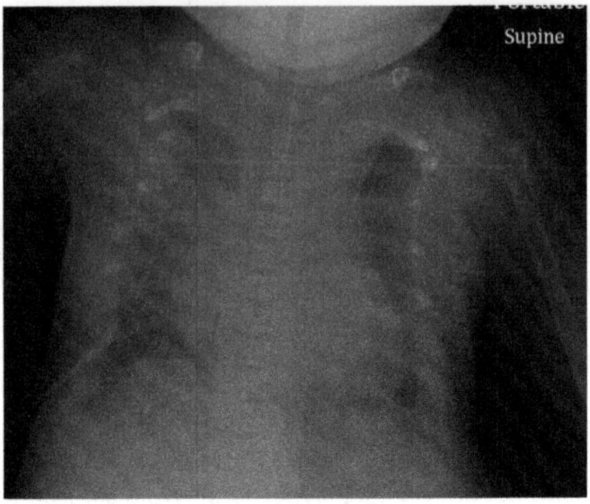

Fig. 2. Chest radiograph in an infant with severe primary hyperparathyroidism. Ribs demonstrate marked osteopenia and heterogeneous appearance.

consideration. The underlying cause can then be identified and addressed. It should be emphasized that in the case of severe hypercalcemia, corrective operation is not the critical or urgent issue. More important is the control of hypercalcemia and evaluation of underlying cause to properly plan longer-term and definitive treatment. Such treatment depends on the etiology, which is divided into the groups below, and can generally be delineated by medical history and laboratory analysis (Table 1).

Table 1
Laboratory assay values in differential diagnosis of hyperparathyroidism and hypercalcemia

	Hyperparathyroidism			Humoral hypercalcemia of malignancy	Familial hypocalciuric hypocalcemia
	Primary	Secondary	Tertiary		
Calcium	Elevated	Decreased	Elevated	Elevated	Elevated
PTH	Elevated/ normal	Elevated	Elevated	Decreased	Slightly elevated/ normal
Phosphate	Decreased	Elevated	Elevated	Decreased	Slightly decreased/ normal
Vitamin D		Decreased/ normal	Decreased	Decreased	
Other				Elevated PTHrp	Decreased urinary calcium & $U_{Ca/Cr}$

Abbreviations: PTH, parathyroid related hormone; PTHrp, PTH related peptide; $U_{Ca/Cr}$, urinary calcium-creatinine ratio.

Primary hyperparathyroidism reflects inherent hyperfunction of parathyroids, no longer responsive to inhibition by elevated serum calcium. This can be caused by adenoma, hyperplasia, or carcinoma. Parathyroid carcinoma is rare, and particularly rare in pediatric patients. It presents similarly to a single-gland adenoma, though typically causing more dramatic hypercalcemia. Whatever the histologic etiology, primary hyperparathyroidism results in elevated serum calcium, elevated or normal PTH, and reduced phosphate. Treatment requires resection of the pathologic glands, even when there are multiple adenomas. The remaining glands are typically suppressed and require several weeks to resume normal function and restore euthyroidism.

When generalized hyperplasia is present, subtotal parathyroidectomy is performed, preserving just one gland (or a portion of it) to avoid absolute hypoparathyroidism with severe permanent hypocalcemia. The preserved gland is either preserved in the original location or transplanted elsewhere in the neck or forearm. Whether partially preserved in situ or autotransplanted, the preserved parathyroid will invariably be stunned and may require weeks to months to produce PTH.

Genetic evaluation of primary hyperparathyroidism is an important consideration. Careful family history can elicit suggestion of entities arising from either somatic or germline mutations. Principal considerations are multiple endocrine neoplasia, familial isolated hyperparathyroidism, and hyperparathyroidism–jaw tumor syndrome [22]. Spontaneous mutations can also occur. These are important considerations which influence decision to proceed with minimally invasive parathyroidectomy versus 4-gland exploration and subtotal parathyroidectomy. There is no uniform approach or generalized guideline to genetic testing for pediatric primary hyperparathyroidism and genetic testing is not routinely performed in adults. This element of evaluation needs to be individualized.

Secondary hyperparathyroidism is a physiologic response to chronic hypocalcemia, as can result from chronic kidney disease or vitamin D deficiency. Vitamin D deficiency limits calcium absorption and calcium release from bone as summarized above, leading to chronic hypocalcemia. In chronic kidney disease, the failing kidneys are unable to produce 1-alpha-hydoxylase to convert vitamin D to its active form, resulting in the same end problem. These lower vitamin D levels result in hypocalcemia which stimulates PTH production. In chronic kidney disease, the failing kidneys are also unable to adequately excrete phosphate, and the elevated serum phosphate is itself a stimulus for PTH release. The end effect is elevated PTH, elevated phosphate, low calcium, and variable 25-OH vitamin D depending on the etiology.

Treatment of secondary hyperparathyroidism is aimed at correcting the underlying cause. For vitamin D deficiency, high-dose weekly supplements are prescribed, and hypomagnesemia should be addressed as well [23–25]. The effects of chronic kidney disease are curtailed by use of phosphate binders, calcitriol, and cinacalcet. The goal is to maintain normal electrolyte balance and prevent progression to tertiary hyperparathyroidism (see below). Operation (subtotal parathyroidectomy) is a very uncommon intervention, typically for severe hypercalcemia with calciphylaxis or extraskeletal calcification, advanced bone disease, or PTH elevation greater than 800 pg/mL for more than 6 months. Renal transplant can cure secondary hyperparathyroidism in 95% of patients, but the resolution occurs gradually [26,27].

Tertiary hyperparathyroidism results from chronic secondary hyperparathyroidism. The processes outlined above continue unabated and cause development of diffuse parathyroid hyperplasia. In this state, the parathyroid glands develop pathologic autonomous function, continuing to drive extremely high parathyroid hormone levels despite achieving elevated calcium. Phosphate levels remain high due to underlying kidney dysfunction.

Treatment of tertiary hyperparathyroidism fundamentally requires renal transplantation to abort the pathogenic signals and processes. However, renal transplant doesn't resolve all tertiary hyperparathyroidism, and parathyroidectomy is sometimes still needed. Some pediatric patients have such severe disease that it precludes candidacy for transplantation, and parathyroidectomy is required before transplantation [28]. Rates of PTH normalization following transplantation (without differentiating between secondary and tertiary) are approximately 30% at 1 year and 60% at 2 years following successful transplantation [29]. Data suggest similarity in these response rates between children and adults [26,27].

As most hyperparathyroidism is discovered in the evaluation of hypercalcemia, there are 2 other important elements of the differential diagnosis worthy of mention. Hypercalcemia of malignancy, specifically humoral hypercalcemia of malignancy (HHM) shares underlying physiology and initial stabilizing treatments with primary hyperparathyroidism [30]. HHM is typically caused by excessive secretion of PTHrp from tumor cells. While classically manifested by squamous cell lung carcinoma, it can occur in a wide variety of malignancies. This paraneoplastic phenomenon is more common in adult cancers, but has been observed in pediatric patients as well [31]. Elevated PTHrp levels cause increased calcium and suppressed PTH, vitamin D, and phosphate. Initial treatment is aimed at hydration and normalization of calcium, then definitive treatment is aimed at cure of malignancy.

Familial hypocalciuric hypercalcemia is a genetic condition in which decreased sensitivity of calcium receptors results in chronically elevated serum calcium. The degree of hypercalcemia is typically mild to moderate, and patients are typically asymptomatic. Because of the adjusted sensitivity to calcium, PTH is usually normal or just slightly elevated. Accordingly, phosphorus is either normal or slightly decreased. Distinction from primary hyperparathyroidism is achieved by urinary calcium excretion: low 24-hour urine calcium and calcium/creatinine clearance ratio. This is a benign hypercalcemia which usually does not require treatment. In rare cases, cinacalcet can be used to modulate the degree of hypercalcemia, but parathyroidectomy is not advised [32].

HYPOPARATHYROIDISM

Insufficient parathyroid function leads to reduced serum PTH and calcium levels and elevated phosphorus levels. This can present with muscle cramping and paresthesias (perioral and digital, in particular). When more severe, it can result in tetany and cardiac dysrhythmia. By far the most common cause of hypoparathyroidism is iatrogenic related to operations on or around the parathyroid glands and their vasculature. A commonly overlooked cause is hypomagnesemia. DiGeorge syndrome (22q11.2 deletion syndrome) is associated with inadequate function or absent parathyroid glands. With an incidence of 1 in 2000 to 4000 births, it is the most common human microdeletion syndrome. More rare genetic syndromes, PTH calcium receptor mutations, and hemochromatosis are also associated with hypoparathyroidism [33–35].

Hypoparathyroidism following neck surgery (particularly thyroidectomy and parathyroidectomy) is a well-recognized phenomenon. This can be related to inadvertent parathyroidectomy, parathyroid devascularization, or simply parathyroid *stun.* Most cases are temporary, but permanent hypoparathyroidism is possible. Pediatric patients are far more susceptible to these problems, with a notably higher incidence of postoperative parathyroid stun.

The greatest impact on postoperative hypoparathyroidism comes from a combination of experienced surgeons and preoperative metabolic optimization. Identification of vitamin D deficiency, hypocalcemia, and generalized nutritional deficiency (which impacts albumin, calcium, and magnesium) allows for preoperative correction. Studies have demonstrated that empiric preoperative vitamin D and calcium supplementation can also be beneficial. Postoperative support is centered on prescription of calcium supplements and calcitriol to maintain eucalcemia [36]. Most transient postoperative hypoparathyroidism resolves in 2 to 4 weeks.

Identification of parathyroid glands is essential to their preservation and protection to minimize postoperative hypoparathyroidism. Intraoperative management of threatened or injured parathyroid glands involves considerable subtlety. Historically, surgeon experience was the singular influential factor. In recent years, a variety of imaging technologies have been developed for intraoperative identification [4]. Some are based on perfusion and differential *wash-out* of an optical tracer like indocyanine green, and some are based on inherent autofluorescence of the tissue. The utility and impact of these devices is an active area of investigation. In the adult realm, some demonstrations of beneficial impact have been published, but there is paltry data in the pediatric realm. In the author's institution, we are actively conducting an evaluation of autofluorescence technology's impact on intraoperative parathyroid identification and postthyroidectomy parathyroid function.

Surgeon experience plays an important role in outcomes of thyroidectomy and minimization of complications. Increased annual surgeon volume has been demonstrated to decrease incidence of complications. This was studied in adult patients and assumed to translate to the pediatric realm [37]. The importance of the volume-outcome relationship is particularly relevant in the pediatric realm, where there is far less volume of thyroid and parathyroid disease requiring operation. Many adult surgeons are not familiar with pediatric management and have limited experience operating on pediatric anatomy. Meanwhile, many pediatric surgeons have lower volumes of thyroid and parathyroid operations which threaten maintenance of skills. Regionalization of care and cross-specialty collaboration helps address these challenges. Pediatric-focused multidisciplinary endocrine surgery programs use these approaches to offer the most robust care.

SUMMARY

Pediatric parathyroid disease is uncommon, but can have severe physiologic consequences. Medical history and laboratory evaluation differentiate into hyperparathyroidism and hypoparathyroidism. Imaging is not always indicated to inform a treatment plan. As uncommon as these disorders are in the pediatric population, physicians or centers with limited experience may benefit from consultation and collaboration with pediatric centers where multidisciplinary approaches are undertaken and greater experience can be shared.

CLINICS CARE POINTS

- Serum calcium, parathyroid hormone, and vitamin D levels can quickly determine the parathyroid pathology relevant to abnormal calcium.
- Immediate management of hypercalcemia should focus on hydration followed by calciuresis with a loop diuretic.
- When imaging is indicated, ultrasound is the initial and primary modality. Computed tomography should not routinely be obtained.
- Postoperative hypoparathyroidism is minimized by preoperative preparation with vitamin D and calcium and involvement of a surgeon who maintains consistent volume of thyroid and parathyroid surgery.

Disclosure

The author has no financial conflict of interest to disclose.

References

[1] Organ C. The history of parathyroid surgery, 1850-1996: the excelsior surgical society 1998 edward D churchill lecture. J Am Coll Surg 2000;191:284.
[2] Dorairajan N, Pradeep P. Vignette hyperparathyroidism: glimpse into its history. Int Surg 2014;99:528.
[3] Reitz R, Dreimiller A, Khil A, et al. Ectopic and supernumerary parathyroid glands in patients with refractory renal hyperparathyroidism. Surgery 2021;169:513.
[4] Jamshidi R, Egan J. Pediatric parathyroid disease. Semin Pediatr Surg 2020;29:150923.
[5] Lofrese J, Basit H, Lappin S. Physiology, parathyroid. In: StatPearls. Treasure Island (FL): StatPearls Publishing; 2025. Available at: https://www.ncbi.nlm.nih.gov/books/NBK482510/.

[6] Vetter R, Lohse M. Magnesium and the parathyroid. Curr Opin Nephrol Hypertens 2002;11:403.
[7] Rodriguez-Ortiz M, Canalejo A, Herencia C, et al. Magnesium modulates parathyroid hormone secretion and upregulates parathyroid receptor expression at moderately low calcium concentration. Nephrol Dial Transplant 2013;29:282.
[8] Candy T, Grey A, Reid I. Calcium, phosphate, and magnesium. In: Marshall W, Lapsley M, editors. Clinical Biochemistry: Metabolic and Clinical Aspects. Philadelphia (PA): Churchill-Livingstone; 2014. p. 93–123.
[9] Medas F, Cappellacci F, Canu G, et al. The role of rapid intraoperative parathyroid hormone (ioPTH) assay in determining outcome of parathyroidectomy in primary hyperparathyroidism: a systematic review and meta-analysis. Int J Surg 2021;92:106042.
[10] Brescia V, Fontana A, Lovero R, et al. Parathyroid hormone-related peptide (PTHrP): evaluation of pediatric, covariate-stratified reference intervals. Children 2022;9:896.
[11] Christakos S, Ajibade D, Dhawan P, et al. Vitamin D: metabolism. Endocrinol Metab Clin North Am 2010;39:243.
[12] Holick M. Vitamin D deficiency. New Engl J Med 2007;357:266.
[13] Morris M, Saboury B, Ahlman M, et al. Parathyroid imaging: past, present, and future. Front Endocrinol 2022;12:760419.
[14] Jamshidi R, Vaughn J. (2025, September 12) 4-dimensional MRI for radiation-reduced parathyroid localization in pediatric patients (Conference presentation). American Thyroid Association Annual Meeting, Scottsdale, AZ, USA.
[15] Cudeman A, Senica K, Rep S, et al. ^{18}F-Fluorocholine PET/CT in primary hyperparathyroidism: superior diagnostic performance to conventional scintigraphic imaging for localization of hyperfunctioning parathyroid glands. J Nuc Med 2020;61:577.
[16] Scerrino G, Paladino N, Graceffa G, et al. Primary hyperparathyroidism: 18F-fluorocholine PET/CT vs. 4D-CT for parathyroid identification: toward a comprehensive diagnostic Framework-An updated review and recommendations. J Clin Med 2025;14:5468.
[17] Junaid S, Patel P, Patel J. Cinacalcet. In: StatPearls. Treasure Island (FL): StatPearls Publishing; 2025. Available at: https://www.ncbi.nlm.nih.gov/sites/books/NBK557658/.
[18] Makras P, Anastasilakis A. Bone disease in primary hyperparathyroidism. Metabolism 2018;80:57.
[19] Ye Z, Silverberg S, Sreekanta A, et al. The efficacy and safety of medical and surgical therapy in patients with primary hyperparathyroidism: a systematic review and meta-analysis of randomized controlled trials. J Bone Miner Res 2022;37:2351.
[20] Khan S, Khan A. Hypoparathyroidism: diagnosis, management, and emerging therapies. Nat Rev Endocrinol 2025;21:360.
[21] Burke J, Chen H, Gosain A. Parathyroid surgery in children. Semin Pediatr Surg 2014;23:66.
[22] Marini F, Giusti Fbrandi M, Brandi ML. Molecular genetics of parathyroid tumors. Curr Opin Endocr Metab Res 2024;34:100510.
[23] Fischer P, Johnson C, Leopold K, et al. Treatment of vitamin D deficiency in children. Expert Rev Endocrinol Metab 2023;18:489.
[24] Holick M. The vitamin D deficiency pandemic: approaches for diagnosis, treatment, and prevention. Rev Endocr Metab Disord 2017;18:153.
[25] Corsello A, Spolidoro G, Milani G, et al. Vitamin D in pediatric age: current evidence, recommendations, and misunderstandings. Front Med 2023;10:1107855.
[26] Rene O, Andres L, Hernan L. Surgical management of renal hyperparathyroidism with total parathyroidectomy, autotransplantation, and cryopreservation with deferred autotransplantation: a 13-year experience. J Ped Surg 2026;61:162589.
[27] Kievit A, Tinnemans J, Groothoff J, et al. Outcome of total parathyroidectomy and autotransplantation as treatment of secondary and tertiary hyperparathyroidism in children and adults. Wrold J Surg 2010;34:993.

[28] Crepeau P, Chen X, Udyavar R, et al. Hyperparathyroidism at 1 year after kidney transplantation is associated with graft loss. Parathyroid 2023;173:138.
[29] Lou I, Foley D, Odorico SK, et al. How well does renal transplantation cure hyperparathyroidism? Ann Sug 2015;262:653.
[30] Guise T, Wysolmerski J. Cancer-associated hypercalcemia. N Engl J Med 2022;386:1443.
[31] Hirschfeld R, Welch J, Harrison D, et al. Two cases of humoral hypercalcemia of malignancy comlicating infantile fibrosarcoma. Pediatr Blood Cancer 2017;64.
[32] Lee J, Shoback D. Familial hypocalciuric hypercalcemia and related disorders. Best Pract Res Clin Endocrinol Metab 2018;32:609.
[33] Kim J, Shin Y, Yang S, et al. Diverse genetic aetiologies and clinical outcomes of paediatric hypoparathyroidism. Clin Endocrin 2015;83:790.
[34] Mantovani G, Elli F, Corbetta S. Hypothyroidism associated with parathyroid disorders. Best Pract Res Clin Endocrinol Metab 2017;31:161.
[35] Pasieka J, Wentworth K, Yeo C, et al. Etiology and pathophysiology of hypoparathyroidism: a narrative review. J Bone Miner Res 2022;37:2586.
[36] Gonsalves R, Jamshidi R, Newbern D, et al. A quality improvement project for managing hypocalcemia after pediatric total thyroidectomy. J Pediatr Endocrinol Metab 2020;33:1443.
[37] Adam M, Thomas S, Youngwirth L, et al. Is there a minimum numer of thyroidectomies a surgeon should perform to optimize patient outcomes? Ann Surg 2017;265:402.

Advances in Pediatrics 73 (2026) 225–237

ADVANCES IN PEDIATRICS

Fetal Surgery Today

Indications, Outcomes, and Future Innovations

Andrew P. Bain, MD[a,*], Mary T. Austin, MD, MPH[b]

[a]Department of Surgery, University of Texas Southwestern Medical Center, Dallas, TX, USA; [b]Division of Pediatric General Surgery, Department of Surgery, University of Washington Medicine, Seattle, WA, USA

Keywords

• Fetal surgery • Fetoscopy • Prenatal intervention • Congenital anomalies

Key points

- Fetal intervention can alter the natural history of select congenital anomalies, improving survival and long-term functional outcomes when applied to carefully selected candidates.
- Indications and contraindications vary significantly by anomaly, requiring multidisciplinary evaluation to balance fetal benefit with maternal risk.
- Maternal risks remain substantial, particularly with open hysterotomy, underscoring the importance of counseling, center expertise, and long-term obstetric considerations.
- Emerging therapies—including stem cell transplantation, gene therapy, and tissue engineering—represent the next frontier, offering the potential for regenerative or molecular correction of disease in utero.

INTRODUCTION

Maternal-fetal surgery is a therapeutic intervention for prenatally diagnosed conditions, with the underlying rationale that correction of anatomic abnormalities can lead to normalization of postnatal physiology. In 1981, the first open fetal surgical procedure was performed by Dr. Michael Harrison, who placed a fetal vesicoamniotic shunt for obstructive uropathy [1]. Modern fetal surgery

*Corresponding author. Department of Surgery, UT Southwestern Medical Center, 5323 Harry Hines Boulevard, Dallas, TX 75390-9159. *E-mail address:* Andrew.bain@utsouthwestern.edu

https://doi.org/10.1016/j.yapd.2025.12.010
0065-3101/26/

Abbreviations

BPS	bronchopulmonary sequestrations
CCAM	congenital cystic adenoid malformations
CDH	congenital diaphragmatic hernia
CPAM	congenital pulmonary airway malformations
CVR	CCAM volume ratio
EXIT	ex utero intrapartum treatment
FETO	fetoscopic endoluminal tracheal occlusion
LHR	lung-to-head ratio
MMC	myelomeningocele
MSCs	mesenchymal stem cells
o/e	observed to expected
TTTS	twin-twin transfusion syndrome

now includes open, fetoscopic, and image-guided interventions that can alter the natural history of multiple congenital diseases while continuing the pregnancy. The field's foundation rests on multidisciplinary collaboration among maternal-fetal medicine specialists, pediatric surgeons, anesthesiologists, neonatologists, and other medical and surgical subspecialists, all working together to push the boundaries of the field. Their work has led to maternal-fetal surgery becoming the standard of care for treating anomalies like myelomeningocele (MMC) and twin-twin transfusion syndrome (TTTS) [2].

Maternal-fetal surgery, by definition, involves 2 patients simultaneously undergoing an operation. Initially, indications for fetal intervention were limited to uniformly lethal conditions as they were deemed a justifiable risk to the pregnant woman. As surgical techniques and fetal access have improved, indications have broadened. Despite these advances, significant risks for the fetus and mother remain, and these risks must be weighed against potential fetal benefits [3].

The following review examines the current state of maternal-fetal intervention organized by anomaly, emphasizing the clinical indications, maternal considerations, and innovations shaping the field's future.

FETAL CONDITIONS AMENABLE TO SURGICAL INTERVENTION

Myelomeningocele

MMC remains one of the most common severe congenital anomalies, affecting roughly 1 in 3000 live births in the United States [4]. In MMC, incomplete closure of the neural results in exposed spinal cord tissue and cerebrospinal fluid leakage, resulting in progressive neurologic damage and hindbrain herniation. These patients develop a range of lifelong clinical consequences, including paralysis, bowel and bladder incontinence, and musculoskeletal deformities [5]. These patients also develop cerebral anomalies like Chiari II malformations, hydrocephalus, hypoplastic pons, and abnormal corpus callosum, which may lead to cognitive dysfunction [6].

The *two-hit hypothesis* posits that initial neural tube malformation is compounded by ongoing injury from amniotic fluid toxicity and mechanical trauma

[7]. Ideally, the first hit would be prevented. While folic acid supplementation has reduced the incidence of MMC, it has not eliminated the condition. In-utero closure of the defect aims to halt secondary damage. The landmark randomized trial, Management of Myelomeningocele (MOMS), compared open fetal repair of MMC or repair after delivery [8]. The investigators found that prenatal repair significantly reduced the need for cerebrospinal shunting (40% vs 82%) and improved motor outcomes at 30 months of age compared with postnatal repair. Secondary analysis of the study population has shown that these benefits persist into school age [9].

Candidates for fetal intervention include singleton pregnancies with isolated MMC between T1 and S1, evidence of hindbrain herniation, and no other major fetal abnormalities [10]. Typical gestational age at time of surgery is between 24 and 26 weeks. Contraindications relate primarily to maternal factors, including comorbidities, body mass index (BMI) ≥ 35, short cervix or previous preterm birth, placental abruption, or multifetal gestation [10].

The MOMS trial had no maternal deaths but found significant maternal morbidity in the prenatal intervention group, including oligohydramnios, chorioamniotic separation, placental abruption, and spontaneous rupture of membranes [8]. Open hysterotomy increased the risk of uterine rupture ($\approx$10% in subsequent pregnancies), and thus, cesarean delivery was mandated for the current and all future pregnancies [11,12]. Minimally invasive fetoscopic MMC repairs have been developed to mitigate these risks and allow for potential vaginal delivery. Uterine access techniques include total percutaneous access and laparotomy-assisted access [13]. While fetoscopic MMC repair is not associated with uterine rupture, it is associated with a higher rate of premature rupture of membranes than the open approach [13].

Prenatal repair of MMC has served as a key success in demonstrating the efficacy of maternal-fetal surgery for a nonlethal condition.

Sacrococcygeal teratoma

Sacrococcygeal teratoma (SCT) is one of the most common congenital tumors, and long-term outcomes for infants are typically excellent. However, SCTs can grow to extreme sizes in relation to the fetus, potentially leading to high-output cardiac failure and nonimmune hydrops via massive arteriovenous shunting. If fetal hydrops develops, mortality approaches 50% [14]. Additional complications of large SCT include internal or external hemorrhage, preterm labor, dystocia, or traumatic delivery, which could result in tumor rupture, neonatal hemorrhage, and/or neonatal demise.

Interventions for giant SCTs include open fetal resection, radiofrequency ablation, and ex utero intrapartum treatment (EXIT)-to-resection [15]. The EXIT approach allows for resection while maintaining uteroplacental circulation. The most common approach for fetal resection is via maternal laparotomy and hysterotomy with tumor resection or debulking. In managing solid tumors, open surgical intervention may be superior in terms of the number of interventions, lower failure rates, and survival to discharge compared with percutaneous interventions [16]. However, the reported literature is limited and heterogeneous. In cystic SCT, cyst decompression before delivery may decrease complications during delivery [16]. While outcomes vary by tumor type and the presence of absence of hydrops, intervention can salvage selected fetuses with an otherwise lethal physiology.

Indications for referral to a fetal surgery center include rapid tumor growth, large size, and early signs of hydrops. Tumor volume to fetal weight ratio greater than 0.12 before 24 weeks of gestation has been suggested as a cutoff for poor prognosis [14]. Hemorrhage remains a significant concern, and open surgical intervention carries the same obstetric risks, including preterm labor and future uterine rupture, as other hysterotomy procedures.

Fetal cervical masses

Fetal cervical masses can compress or obstruct the trachea and esophagus, leading to polyhydramnios, craniofacial abnormalities, preterm labor, and potential for high-output heart failure [17]. These masses include cervical teratomas, vascular malformations, and, more rarely, thymic cysts, or congenital neuroblastoma [18]. Diagnosis is typically made on prenatal ultrasound, with fetal MRI often used to characterize the mass and predict risk of a complicated airway [19,20].

In the EXIT-to-airway procedure, uteroplacental circulation is maintained during a partial delivery, facilitating direct laryngoscopy for endotracheal intubation [21]. Escalation to bronchoscopy or tracheostomy may be necessary. Resection of the mass on uteroplacental support can be performed if the airway cannot be secured.

Prenatal imaging can guide referral indications to fetal surgery centers. In addition to concerning findings like polyhydramnios, in-utero neck extension, and micrognathia, MRI can estimate fetal lung volumes and measure the degree of tracheoesophageal displacement, which helps predict the need for an EXIT procedure [19]. Unlike a cesarean section, the EXIT procedure requires deep anesthesia with complete relaxation of the uterine muscle. Postpartum hemorrhage is a risk and occurs in approximately 5% of cases based on a recent meta-analysis [21].

Congenital diaphragmatic hernia

Congenital diaphragmatic hernia (CDH) is often diagnosed prenatally by the hallmark diaphragmatic defect and associated herniation of abdominal viscera into the thorax [22]. This defect leads to pulmonary hypoplasia and persistent pulmonary hypertension. Prenatal diagnosis is associated with decreased survival, with larger defects more readily apparent on prenatal imaging [23]. In isolated cases, severity can be assessed in utero by measuring the lung-to-head ratio (LHR) and associated factors like intrathoracic herniation of the liver [23]. Using healthy fetal measurements from the same gestational age, the observed to expected LHR can be calculated (o/e LHR) [24]. These measurements allow for stratification into mild, moderate, or severe disease [25]. Mild severity refers to o/e LHR greater than 35% without liver herniation or

45% with liver herniation and carries an approximate postnatal survival of 85%. Moderate severity refers to o/e LHR of 25% to 34.9% regardless of liver position or 35% to 44.9% with liver herniation, with an approximate postnatal survival of 55%. Severe disease refers to an o/e LHR less than 25%, with less than 25% expected postnatal survival [26]. The observed to expected LHRs provide insight into early neonatal complications including length of stay in the intensive care unit, use of assisted ventilation, and need for supplemental oxygen [27].

Early trials in fetal repair of CDH did not improve survival or need for extracorporeal membranous oxygenation (ECMO) when compared to postnatal repair [28]. However, occlusion of the fetal trachea, which led to accumulating lung parenchymal fluid in the fetus was associated with lung growth [29].

Attempts at tracheal occlusion with a metallic clip increased risk of preterm labor along with tracheal stenosis and compromised airway at delivery [30]. Advances in fetoscopy enabled the placement of a balloon in the trachea, a procedure termed fetoscopic endoluminal tracheal occlusion (FETO) [31]. No survival benefit was incurred in early trials but the Tracheal Occlusion to Accelerate Lung Growth (TOTAL) trials reexamined this question [25,26]. While benefit was not seen in patients with moderate disease, in patients with severe CDH, the trial was stopped early with 40% of patients in the FETO groups surviving to discharge compared to 15% in the expectant care group [26]. Limitations of these 2 trials include their European setting and variability in CDH volume at the participating fetal centers. Compared to high volume North American centers, these trials had significantly lower use of ECMO and lower overall survival in both treatment and control arms [32].

FETO is offered at several fetal centers between 27 and 29 weeks for isolated severe CDH (o/e LHR $< 25\%$) and contraindicated in associated anomalies or chromosomal abnormalities. The balloon is retrieved fetoscopically or punctured at 34 weeks but can require retrieval via an EXIT procedure to secure a definitive airway at birth. FETO also carries an increased risk of preterm labor, rupture of membranes, and preterm birth, which compromises survival as gestational age at delivery is significant predictor of survival [27].

Congenital lung lesions

Congenital pulmonary airway malformations (CPAM) include bronchopulmonary sequestrations (BPS) and congenital cystic adenoid malformations (CCAM). Severity can range from asymptomatic with normal development to life-threatening hydrops [33]. CCAM can be either macro or microcystic. Microcystic CCAM growth typically plateaus at 28 weeks of gestation, while macrocystic CCAMs can enlarge abruptly and should be followed closely throughout pregnancy [34]. The risk of hydrops can be predicted by the CCAM volume ratio (CVR), which is calculated as the CCAM volume divided by the head circumference. CVR less than 1.6 has a less than 3% chance of developing hydrops [35].

In the setting of hydrops, large macrocystic lesions can be treated with minimally invasive drainage by either US-guided cyst aspiration or thoracoamniotic shunt placement, with the potential to reverse hydrops [36,37]. In predominantly microcystic lesions, maternal administration of steroids can be an effective treatment in the setting of hydrops and is commonly administered to any fetus with a CVR greater than 1.6 [38]. Open fetal resection is an option, but it is rarely indicated [38]. After 30 weeks of gestation, EXIT or EXIT-to-resection can be considered. Percutaneous sclerotherapy in CCAM or fetal laser ablation of the feeding artery in BPS has also been described as a potential therapy in select cases [39,40].

Lower urinary tract obstruction

Lower urinary tract obstruction is most commonly due to posterior urethral valves, and the rationale for fetal intervention is that obstruction can lead to both renal dysplasia and pulmonary hypoplasia from oligohydramnios [41]. Serial amnioinfusion can increase amniotic fluid levels, but repeated interventions carry risk and can be challenging to sustain [42]. A multicenter trial evaluating the efficacy of serial amnioinfusions is ongoing [43]. Bladder decompression can be performed via cystoscopy or percutaneous vesicoamniotic shunt placement [44]. Shunts are not fixed to the abdominal wall, so migration may occur after shunt placement. On systematic review and metanalysis of primarily observational data, pooled 2-year survival is similar in patients undergoing shunt placement and those undergoing conservative management, at approximately 40% [45]. However, the populations studied are heterogenous with inconsistent selection criteria for intervention. Fetal cystoscopy can also be performed through the abdominal wall and posterior urethral valves can be treated with laser fulguration, restoring urethral patency [46]. Criteria for candidacy for fetal intervention established via international Delphi consensus include absence of life-limiting structural or genetic anomalies, gestational age greater than or equal to 16 weeks, and oligohydramnios [47].

Twin-twin transfusion syndrome

In monochorionic twin pregnancies, twins share blood flow across arteriovenous connections, typically in a balanced fashion. In TTTS, this distribution is unbalanced. This can lead to oligohydramnios in the *donor* twin and polyhydramnios in the *recipient*, as well as growth restriction, cardiac failure, hydrops, and even death. 10% of monochorionic diamniotic twins, approximately 1 in 50 twin pregnancies, are affected [48]. Stages of TTTS are presented in Table 1.

The cornerstone of therapy is fetoscopic laser ablation of the intertwin placental vascular connections, typically performed between 16 and 26 weeks of gestation. This restores independent placental circulation. Randomized controlled trials have demonstrated clear superiority of laser ablation over serial amnioreduction, increasing survival of at least one twin from ~50% to 70% to 75% and decreased neurologic complications [49]. The procedure, however, carries risks of premature rupture of membranes and preterm delivery. Intervention does not appear to have a clear benefit in Stage I TTTS. However, patients can progress rapidly to more advanced stages and require urgent

Table 1
Quintero staging of twin-twin transfusion syndrome

Stage	Ultrasound assessment	Description
I	Amniotic fluid discordance	Maximal vertical pocket <2 cm in donor sac and >8 cm in recipient sac
II	Fetal bladder	Nonvisualization of donor fetal bladder over 60 min of observation
III	Doppler studies	Absent or reversed umbilical artery end-diastolic velocity, reversed ductus venous a-wave flow, or pulsatile umbilical vein flow
IV	Fetal ascites or hydrops	Presence of ascites or hydrops in one or both twins
V	Fetal cardiac activity	Fetal demise in one or both twins

From Quintero RA, Morales WJ, Allen MH, et al. Staging of twin-twin transfusion syndrome. J Perinatol. 1999;19(8 Pt 1):550–5. https://doi.org/10.1038/sj.jp.7200292.

intervention. Thus, patients should be monitored closely and have access to a fetal center experienced in performing these procedures [50].

Emerging and experimental therapies

The future of maternal-fetal surgery is bright, with many exciting developments on the horizon. In gastroschisis, exposure of amniotic fluid to the small intestine and other involved viscera is hypothesized to contribute to postnatal intestinal dysfunction [51]. Early animal studies show that in utero intervention is safe in fetal sheep models [52]. An ongoing Phase 1 feasibility study is evaluating fetoscopic in utero repair in the setting of complex gastroschisis [53].

The fetus exists in an inherent regenerative milieu, and the fetal immune system's tolerance provides a window for durable stem cell engraftment. Experimental in utero transplantation of hematopoietic stem cells for hemoglobinopathies (sickle cell disease and thalassemia) establishes chimerism without conditioning, allowing later *booster* transplants [54,55]. Mesenchymal stem cells (MSCs) from the placenta or amniotic fluid show promise for osteogenesis imperfecta and neural protection in MMC models [56,57]. In gastroschisis models, intraamniotic MSC delivery reduced bowel injury, leveraging the regenerative milieu of amniotic fluid [51]. Scaffold-based delivery of placental MSCs has restored ambulation in ovine MMC models [56,58], now advancing to early clinical trials (NCT04652908). Similarly, MSC-seeded diaphragmatic patches may improve outcomes in CDH [59].

Gene therapy aims to achieve durable correction of monogenic disease through viral vector delivery. In nonhuman primate models of hemophilia B, adeno-associated vector transfer achieved long-term factor IX expression [60]. CRISPR-Cas9–based intraamniotic delivery in mice has corrected pulmonary gene defects, representing a paradigm shift toward preventive genomic medicine [61]. Targeted delivery, maternal exposure avoidance, and ethical governance remain significant barriers to translating these advancing therapies into human use.

Table: Summary of major fetal anomalies amenable to fetal intervention

Anomaly	Fetal intervention(s)	Indications for referral/candidate selection	Contraindications	Maternal risks/considerations
MMC	Open fetal repair via hysterotomy; Fetoscopic (laparotomy-assisted or percutaneous) repair	Singleton pregnancy; Lesion between T1–S1 with hindbrain herniation; Gestational age (GA) 19–26 wk; Normal karyotype, absence of severe anomalies	Maternal comorbidities (hypertension and diabetes); BMI $\geq$35; Short cervix or prior preterm birth; Uterine anomaly or multiple gestation	Uterine rupture/dehiscence in future pregnancies ($\approx$10%); Preterm delivery ($\sim$34 wk); Mandatory cesarean for all future deliveries
SCT	Open fetal resection; RFA or laser coagulation; EXIT-to-resection at delivery	Rapid tumor growth; High tumor volume-to-fetal weight ratio; Early signs of hydrops or high-output cardiac failure	Extensive extrapelvic invasion or maternal mirror syndrome	Polyhydramnios, mirror syndrome; Maternal hemorrhage; Preterm labor, infection
Fetal cervical masses	EXIT-to-airway (intubation, bronchoscopy, tracheostomy); EXIT-to-resection for obstructing lesions	Large teratoma or lymphatic malformation with airway compression on imaging; Polyhydramnios, neck hyperextension, or hydrops	Severe maternal comorbidities; Late gestation with nonviable airway plan	Deep anesthesia with uterine relaxation; Postpartum hemorrhage ($\approx$7%); Prolonged operative time and anesthetic exposure
CDH	FETO with balloon placement/retrieval	Severe isolated left-sided CDH (o/e LHR <25%, liver up); GA 27–29 wk	Moderate or mild CDH (o/e LHR >35%); Major cardiac/chromosomal anomalies	PPROM (30%–40%); Preterm birth; Possible need for EXIT for balloon removal
TTTS	Fetoscopic laser ablation of placental anastomoses; Serial amnioreduction (historical)	Monochorionic diamniotic twins with Stage II–V TTTS; Rapidly progressive stage I disease; GA 16–26 wk	Discordant anomalies incompatible with survival; Anterior placenta limiting visualization; Maternal contraindications to anesthesia	Preterm rupture of membranes (25%–30%); Preterm delivery; Rare bleeding or infection; Tocolytic side effects

CPAM/ BPS	Thoracoamniotic shunt; Maternal corticosteroids (for microcystic CPAM); Laser ablation of feeding artery (for BPS)	CVR >1.6 or hydrops; Evidence of mediastinal shift or cardiac compression	Stable or regressing lesions; Advanced GA near term	Shunt dislodgement or blockage (up to 20%); Preterm labor; Infection risk
LUTO	Vesicoamniotic shunt placement; Fetal cystoscopy with laser ablation of posterior urethral valves	Isolated obstruction with preserved renal function markers; Absence of lethal anomalies	Renal dysplasia or anhydramnios before 16 wk; Aneuploidy or multisystem anomalies	Shunt migration/dislodgement; Infection, preterm labor; Procedural bleeding or amniotic fluid leak

Abbreviations: LUTO, Lower Urinary Tract Obstruction; RFA, radio frequency ablation.

Ethical considerations in maternal-fetal surgery

A unique hallmark of maternal-fetal surgery is that potential benefit accrues to the fetus, while maternal risk is substantial and without direct medical gain. The ethical framework thus balances beneficence for the fetus with autonomy and nonmaleficence toward the mother. In 1982, Harrison and colleagues established an early ethical framework that continues to guide practice: proceed only when fetal disease is severe, intervention has scientific justification, and maternal risk is acceptable [58]. The American College of Obstetricians and Gynecologists recommends multidisciplinary oversight with the inclusion of ethicists and psychologists alongside materal-fetal medicine (MFM) specialists, pediatric surgery, anesthesia, and neonatology [62].

Clinicians must weigh fetal benefit against maternal risk without coercion, and thorough informed consent involves a complete discussion of uncertain benefits, the need for cesarean delivery, and implications for future pregnancies [63].

SUMMARY

Fetal intervention and surgery now stand at the intersection of innovation, ethics, and compassion. From open repair of myelomeningocele to fetoscopic tracheal occlusion and emerging molecular therapies, the field continues to evolve toward safer, more precise, and ethically grounded care. Ongoing multidisciplinary collaboration and rigorous clinical trials remain the cornerstone of progress. The promise of the next decade is not only to treat the fetus but to redefine the boundaries of perinatal medicine itself.

CLINICS CARE POINTS

- Early referral to a high-volume fetal therapy center is critical once disease severity thresholds are met, as outcomes for conditions such as myelomeningocele, severe congenital diaphragmatic hernia, and twin–twin transfusion syndrome are strongly influenced by gestational age at intervention and institutional experience.
- Maternal risks often extend beyond the index pregnancy and must be explicitly addressed during counseling, particularly the lifelong implications of open hysterotomy, including mandatory cesarean delivery and increased risk of uterine rupture in subsequent pregnancies.
- Not all prenatally diagnosed anomalies benefit from intervention, and disease progression can be heterogeneous, highlighting the importance of standardized severity metrics (eg, o/e lung-to-head ratio, CCAM volume ratio, Quintero staging) to avoid unnecessary maternal risk in conditions likely to remain stable with expectant management.

Disclosure

The authors have nothing to disclose.

References

[1] Golbus MS, Harrison MR, Filly RA, et al. In utero treatment of urinary tract obstruction. Am J Obstet Gynecol 1982;142(4):383–8.
[2] Society for Maternal-Fetal M, Simpson LL. Twin-twin transfusion syndrome. Am J Obstet Gynecol 2013;208(1):3–18.
[3] Yamashiro KJ, Galganski LA, Hirose S. What you need to know about maternal-fetal medicine. Semin Pediatr Surg 2019;28(4):150822; https://doi.org/10.1053/j.sempedsurg.2019.07.005.
[4] Best BJ, Cabacungan ET, Cohen SS, et al. Trends in the early care of infants with myelomeningocele in the United States 2012-2018. Childs Nerv Syst 2023;39(9):2413–21.
[5] Adzick NS. Fetal myelomeningocele: natural history, pathophysiology, and in-utero intervention. Semin Fetal Neonatal Med 2010;15(1):9–14.
[6] Pollenus J, Lagae L, Aertsen M, et al. The impact of cerebral anomalies on cognitive outcome in patients with spina bifida: a systematic review. Eur J Paediatr Neurol 2020;28:16–28.
[7] Meuli MM-SC, Hutchins GM, Hutchins GM, et al. In utero surgery rescues neurological function at birth in sheep with spina bifida. Nat Med 1995;(1):342–7.
[8] Adzick NS, Thom EA, Spong CY, et al. A randomized trial of prenatal versus postnatal repair of myelomeningocele. N Engl J Med 2011;364(11):993–1004.
[9] Houtrow AJ, MacPherson C, Jackson-Coty J, et al. Prenatal repair and physical functioning among children with myelomeningocele: a secondary analysis of a randomized clinical trial. JAMA Pediatr 2021;175(4):e205674; https://doi.org/10.1001/jamapediatrics.2020.5674.
[10] Committee opinion no. 720: maternal–fetal surgery for myelomeningocele. Obstet Gynecol 2017;130(3).
[11] Goodnight WH, Bahtiyar O, Bennett KA, et al. Subsequent pregnancy outcomes after open maternal-fetal surgery for myelomeningocele. Am J Obstet Gynecol 2019;220(5):494.e1–7.
[12] Chmait RH, Kontopoulos EV, Quintero RA. Uterine legacy of open maternal-fetal surgery: preterm uterine rupture. Am J Obstet Gynecol 2019;221(5):535.
[13] Sanz Cortes M, Chmait RH, Lapa DA, et al. Experience of 300 cases of prenatal fetoscopic open spina bifida repair: report of the international fetoscopic neural tube defect repair consortium. Am J Obstet Gynecol 2021;225(6):678.e1–11.
[14] Akinkuotu AC, Coleman A, Shue E, et al. Predictors of poor prognosis in prenatally diagnosed sacrococcygeal teratoma: a multiinstitutional review. J Pediatr Surg 2015;50(5):771–4.
[15] Adzick NS. Open fetal surgery for life-threatening fetal anomalies. Semin Fetal Neonatal Med 2010;15(1):1–8.
[16] Menchaca AD, Olutoye OO, Cass DL, et al. Percutaneous versus open fetal surgical intervention for sacrococcygeal teratomas: is less really more? Fetal Diagn Ther 2023;50(5):313–31.
[17] Berge SJ, von Lindern JJ, Appel T, et al. Diagnosis and management of cervical teratomas. Br J Oral Maxillofac Surg 2004;42(1):41–5.
[18] Hirose S, Sydorak RM, Tsao K, et al. Spectrum of intrapartum management strategies for giant fetal cervical teratoma. J Pediatr Surg 2003;38(3):446–50 [discussion: 446–50].
[19] Cash H, Bly R, Masco V, et al. Prenatal imaging findings predict obstructive fetal airways requiring EXIT. Laryngoscope 2021;131(4):E1357–62.
[20] Paula Pinho Matos A, Teixeira Castro P, de Barros Duarte L, et al. Prenatal diagnosis of cervical masses by magnetic resonance imaging and 3D virtual models: perinatal and long-term follow-up outcomes. J Matern Fetal Neonatal Med 2020;33(13):2181–9.
[21] Novoa RH, Quintana W, Castillo-Urquiaga W, et al. EXIT (ex utero intrapartum treatment) surgery for the management of fetal airway obstruction: a systematic review of the literature. J Pediatr Surg 2020;55(7):1188–95.
[22] Wynn J, Krishnan U, Aspelund G, et al. Outcomes of congenital diaphragmatic hernia in the modern era of management. J Pediatr 2013;163(1):114–9.e1.

[23] Jancelewicz T, Brindle ME. Prediction tools in congenital diaphragmatic hernia. Semin Perinatol 2020;44(1):151165; https://doi.org/10.1053/j.semperi.2019.07.004.
[24] Peralta CF, Cavoretto P, Csapo B, et al. Assessment of lung area in normal fetuses at 12-32 weeks. Ultrasound Obstet Gynecol 2005;26(7):718–24.
[25] Deprest JA, Benachi A, Gratacos E, et al. Randomized trial of fetal surgery for moderate left diaphragmatic hernia. N Engl J Med 2021;385(2):119–29.
[26] Deprest JA, Nicolaides KH, Benachi A, et al. Randomized trial of fetal surgery for severe left diaphragmatic hernia. N Engl J Med 2021;385(2):107–18.
[27] Jani JC, Benachi A, Nicolaides KH, et al. Prenatal prediction of neonatal morbidity in survivors with congenital diaphragmatic hernia: a multicenter study. Ultrasound Obstet Gynecol 2009;33(1):64–9.
[28] Harrison MR, Adzick NS, Bullard KM, et al. Correction of congenital diaphragmatic hernia in utero VII: a prospective trial. J Pediatr Surg 1997;32(11):1637–42.
[29] Khan PA, Cloutier M, Piedboeuf B. Tracheal occlusion: a review of obstructing fetal lungs to make them grow and mature. Am J Med Genet C Semin Med Genet 2007;145c(2):125–38.
[30] Harrison MR, Adzick NS, Flake AW, et al. Correction of congenital diaphragmatic hernia in utero VIII: response of the hypoplastic lung to tracheal occlusion. J Pediatr Surg 1996;31(10):1339–48.
[31] Sydorak RM, Harrison MR. Congenital diaphragmatic hernia: advances in prenatal therapy. World J Surg 2003;27(1):68–76.
[32] Deprest J, Flake A. How should fetal surgery for congenital diaphragmatic hernia be implemented in the post-TOTAL trial era: a discussion. Prenat Diagn 2022;42(3):301–9.
[33] Downard CD, Calkins CM, Williams RF, et al. Treatment of congenital pulmonary airway malformations: a systematic review from the APSA outcomes and evidence based practice committee. Pediatr Surg Int 2017;33(9):939–53.
[34] Kunisaki SM, Barnewolt CE, Estroff JA, et al. Large fetal congenital cystic adenomatoid malformations: growth trends and patient survival. J Pediatr Surg 2007;42(2):404–10.
[35] Crombleholme TM, Coleman B, Hedrick H, et al. Cystic adenomatoid malformation volume ratio predicts outcome in prenatally diagnosed cystic adenomatoid malformation of the lung. J Pediatr Surg 2002;37(3):331–8.
[36] Cass DL, Olutoye OO, Ayres NA, et al. Defining hydrops and indications for open fetal surgery for fetuses with lung masses and vascular tumors. J Pediatr Surg 2012;47(1):40–5.
[37] Peranteau WH, Adzick NS, Boelig MM, et al. Thoracoamniotic shunts for the management of fetal lung lesions and pleural effusions: a single-institution review and predictors of survival in 75 cases. J Pediatr Surg 2015;50(2):301–5.
[38] Loh KC, Jelin E, Hirose S, et al. Microcystic congenital pulmonary airway malformation with hydrops fetalis: steroids vs open fetal resection. J Pediatr Surg 2012;47(1):36–9.
[39] Cruz-Martinez R, Martinez-Rodriguez M, Bermudez-Rojas M, et al. Fetal laser ablation of feeding artery of cystic lung lesions with systemic arterial blood supply. Ultrasound Obstet Gynecol 2017;49(6):744–50.
[40] Chon AH, Korst LM, Abdel-Sattar M, et al. Types II and III congenital pulmonary airway malformation with hydrops treated in utero with percutaneous sclerotherapy. Prenat Diagn 2018;38(7):493–8.
[41] Saccone G, D'Alessandro P, Escolino M, et al. Antenatal intervention for congenital fetal lower urinary tract obstruction (LUTO): a systematic review and meta-analysis. J Matern Fetal Neonatal Med 2020;33(15):2664–70.
[42] Warring SK, Novoa V, Shazly S, et al. Serial amnioinfusion as regenerative therapy for pulmonary hypoplasia in fetuses with intrauterine renal failure or severe renal anomalies: systematic review and future perspectives. Mayo Clin Proc Innov Qual Outcomes 2020;4(4):391–409.
[43] O'Hare EM, Jelin AC, Miller JL, et al. Amnioinfusions to treat early onset anhydramnios caused by renal anomalies: background and rationale for the renal anhydramnios fetal therapy trial. Fetal Diagn Ther 2019;45(6):365–72.

[44] Miller JL, Baschat AA, Atkinson MA. Fetal therapy for renal anhydramnios. Clin Perinatol 2022;49(4):849–62.
[45] Nassr AA, Shazly SAM, Abdelmagied AM, et al. Effectiveness of vesicoamniotic shunt in fetuses with congenital lower urinary tract obstruction: an updated systematic review and meta-analysis. Ultrasound Obstet Gynecol 2017;49(6):696–703.
[46] Farrugia MK, Braun MC, Peters CA, et al. Report on the society for fetal urology panel discussion on the selection criteria and intervention for fetal bladder outlet obstruction. J Pediatr Urol 2017;13(4):345–51.
[47] Mustafa HJ, Khalil A, Johnson S, et al. Fetal lower urinary tract obstruction: international Delphi consensus on management and core outcome set. Ultrasound Obstet Gynecol 2024;64 (5):635–50.
[48] Lewi LJJ, Boes AS, Boes AS, et al. OC112: the natural history of monochorionic twins and the role of prenatal ultrasound scan. Ultrasound Obstet Gynecol 2007;(30):401–2.
[49] Senat MV, Deprest J, Boulvain M, et al. Endoscopic laser surgery versus serial amnioreduction for severe twin-to-twin transfusion syndrome. N Engl J Med 2004;351(2):136–44.
[50] Stirnemann J, Slaghekke F, Khalek N, et al. Intrauterine fetoscopic laser surgery versus expectant management in stage 1 twin-to-twin transfusion syndrome: an international randomized trial. Am J Obstet Gynecol 2021;224(5):528.e1–12.
[51] Feng C, Graham CD, Connors JP, et al. Transamniotic stem cell therapy (TRASCET) mitigates bowel damage in a model of gastroschisis. J Pediatr Surg 2016;51(1):56–61.
[52] Stephenson JT, Pichakron KO, Vu L, et al. In utero repair of gastroschisis in the sheep (ovis aries) model. J Pediatr Surg 2010;45(1):65–9.
[53] Belfort M. Gastroschisis: prenatal repair – phase 1 study. presented at: 20th World Congress in Fetal Medicine; June 25, 2023 2023; Valencia, Spain. Session Oral Presentation.
[54] Peranteau WH, Hayashi S, Abdulmalik O, et al. Correction of murine hemoglobinopathies by prenatal tolerance induction and postnatal nonmyeloablative allogeneic BM transplants. Blood 2015;126(10):1245–54.
[55] Kreger EM, Singer ST, Witt RG, et al. Favorable outcomes after in utero transfusion in fetuses with alpha thalassemia major: a case series and review of the literature. Prenat Diagn 2016;36(13):1242–9.
[56] Watanabe M, Li H, Kim AG, et al. Complete tissue coverage achieved by scaffold-based tissue engineering in the fetal sheep model of myelomeningocele. Biomaterials 2016;76: 133–43.
[57] Gotherstrom C, Westgren M, Shaw SW, et al. Pre- and postnatal transplantation of fetal mesenchymal stem cells in osteogenesis imperfecta: a two-center experience. Stem Cells Transl Med 2014;3(2):255–64.
[58] Vanover M, Pivetti C, Lankford L, et al. High density placental mesenchymal stromal cells provide neuronal preservation and improve motor function following in utero treatment of ovine myelomeningocele. J Pediatr Surg 2019;54(1):75–9.
[59] Fauza DO. Tissue engineering in congenital diaphragmatic hernia. Semin Pediatr Surg 2014;23(3):135–40.
[60] Mattar CNZ, Gil-Farina I, Rosales C, et al. In utero transfer of adeno-associated viral vectors produces long-term factor IX levels in a cynomolgus macaque model. Mol Ther 2017;25(8): 1843–53.
[61] Alapati D, Zacharias WJ, Hartman HA, et al. In utero gene editing for monogenic lung disease. Sci Transl Med 2019;11(488); https://doi.org/10.1126/scitranslmed.aav8375.
[62] Committee opinion no. 501: maternal-Fetal intervention and fetal care centers. Obstet Gynecol 2011;118(2 Pt 1):405–10; https://doi.org/10.1097/AOG.0b013e31822c99af.
[63] Austin MT, Cole TR, McCullough LB, et al. Ethical challenges in invasive maternal-fetal intervention. Semin Pediatr Surg 2019;28(4):150819; https://doi.org/10.1053/j.sempedsurg.2019.07.002.

Advances in Pediatrics 73 (2026) 239–251

ADVANCES IN PEDIATRICS

Infant Jaundice

Updates in Biliary Atresia

Alyssa Stetson, MD, MPH, MMSc[a,b], Marissa Ray, MD, MS[b,c,*], Michael Rogers, DO, MPH[d], Gregory M. Tiao, MD[b,e]

[a]Department of Surgery, Brigham and Women's Hospital, 75 Francis Street, Boston, MA 02115, USA; [b]Division of Pediatric General and Thoracic Surgery, Cincinnati Children's Hospital Medical Center, Cincinnati, OH, USA; [c]Department of Surgery, University of Cincinnati College of Medicine, 231 Albert Sabin Way, ML 0558, Cincinnati, OH 45267-0558, USA; [d]Division of Gastroenterology, Hepatology, and Nutrition, UC Department of Pediatrics, 420 Albert Sabin Way, ML 2010, Cincinnati, OH 45229, USA; [e]Department of Surgery, Division of Gastroenterology, Hepatology, and Nutrition, Pediatric General and Thoracic Surgery, Liver Transplant Program, Cincinnati Children's Hospital Medical Center, Cincinnati, OH, USA

Keywords

• Biliary atresia • Jaundice • Direct hyperbilirubinemia • Diagnostic work-up • Kasai portoenterostomy • Liver transplantation

Key points

- Direct hyperbilirubinemia (>1.0 mg/dL) in a neonate should raise concern for a cholestatic pathology.
- No universal screening for biliary atresia exists in the United States, though some regions use bilirubin testing at birth or stool color cards.
- Novel diagnostic strategies include serum testing for matrix metalloproteinase-7 and genetic testing using jaundice chip microarrays.
- Kasai portoenterostomy (KPE) is the current standard of care to restore bile flow and delay need for transplantation, ideally performed before 45 days of life.
- Around half of patients who undergo KPE require liver transplantation within 5 years, and transplant remains the only definitive treatment of those who fail KPE.

*Corresponding author. 231 Albert Sabin Way, ML 0558, Cincinnati, OH 45267-0558. *E-mail address:* Marissa.ray@cchmc.org

https://doi.org/10.1016/j.yapd.2025.12.009
0065-3101/26/

Abbreviations

AUC	area under the curve
BA	biliary atresia
CMV	cytomegalovirus
ERCP	endoscopic retrograde cholangiopancreatography
HIDA	hepatobiliary iminodiacetic acid
ICG	indocyanine green
IOC	intraoperative cholangiogram
KPE	Kasai portoenterostomy
MMP-7	matrix metalloproteinase-7
MRCP	magnetic resonance cholangiopancreatography
NPV	negative predictive value
OLT	orthotopic liver transplant
PPV	positive predictive value
PTC	percutaneous transhepatic cholangiography

INTRODUCTION

Biliary atresia (BA) is a progressive, obstructive cholangiopathy characterized by fibrosis of the intrahepatic and extrahepatic biliary system leading to obstruction of bile flow. This leads to jaundice and direct hyperbilirubinemia in the early neonatal period. If untreated, it will eventually lead to cirrhosis, liver failure, and death by age 2 to 3 years old [1]. The incidence of BA varies across the world, with reported rates of around 1 in 5000 in Taiwan, 1 in 15,000 in United States, and around 1 in 20,000 in Europe and Canada [2,3]. Although rare, BA is the most common indication for pediatric liver transplantation [4]. There are at least 4 recognized phenotypes of BA: isolated, syndromic (most commonly BA splenic malformation syndrome), cystic variant with a co-occurring bile duct cyst at the porta hepatis, and cytomegalovirus (CMV)-associated [5,6]. By far the most common is the isolated form, occurring in 70% to 80% of cases [6]. Early identification, workup, and treatment are crucial for patients with BA.

JAUNDICE IN AN INFANT: WHEN TO WORRY

Jaundice is a nonspecific, common finding among newborns and can be due to a wide range of causes from self-limited physiologic conditions to pathologic conditions requiring intervention. Jaundice is caused by hyperbilirubinemia and typically becomes evident at total bilirubin levels of 2.5 to 3.0 mg/dL or greater [7]. Hyperbilirubinemia is classified as indirect or direct; common etiologies for each type can be found in Table 1.

In general, indirect hyperbilirubinemia results from increased indirect bilirubin production from red blood cells (eg, hemolysis), impaired uptake by the liver, or impaired conjugation in the liver. Direct hyperbilirubinemia typically results from obstruction of the hepatic bile ducts leading to a buildup of bilirubin that has been conjugated by the liver. Direct hyperbilirubinemia is defined as a direct bilirubin concentration higher than 1.0 mg/dL [7]. Jaundice poses a challenge to primary care providers who see infants in the newborn

Table 1
Most common causes of direct and indirect hyperbilirubinemia

Causes of indirect hyperbilirubinemia	Causes of direct hyperbilirubinemia
Physiologic	Structural
• Breastmilk jaundice	• Extrahepatic biliary atresia
• Breastfeeding jaundice	• Choledochal cyst/Caroli's disease
Hemolytic diseases	• Alagille's syndrome
• G-6-PD deficiency	• Biliary hypoplasia
• Sickle cell anemia	Infectious
• Thalassemia	• Viral: CMV, Herpesvirus, adenovirus, parvovirus B19, hepatitis B
• Hereditary spherocytosis	• Toxoplasmosis
Increased enterohepatic circulation	Metabolic
• Bowel obstruction	• Alpha-1 antitrypsin deficiency
○ Duodenal/ileal atresia	• Progressive familial intrahepatic cholestasis syndromes
○ Hirschsprung's disease	• Glactosemia
• Ileus	• Tyrosinemia
• Pyloric stenosis	• Glycogen storage diseases
Hereditary	Toxic
• Gilbert syndrome	• Drug induced
• Crigler-Najjar syndrome	• Total parenteral nutrition-associated cholestasis
Metabolic	Hereditary
• Hypothyroidism	• Dubin Johnson syndrome
• -Hypopituitarism	• Rotor's syndrome

period because while jaundice is most often physiologic and self-limited, around 1 in 2500 infants will have an underlying cholestatic liver disease, [8] which requires further evaluation and management.

Further workup for jaundice in an otherwise healthy infant should begin if it persists beyond 2 weeks [8–10]. Of note, persistent jaundice does not automatically indicate a pathologic process, as an estimated 15% of neonates will exhibit physiologic jaundice beyond the first month of life [10]. Initial workup should begin with a fractionated bilirubin test. If labs are consistent with direct hyperbilirubinemia (>1 mg/dL), then additional workup to rule out other causes of jaundice is required. Additional bloodwork should include a complete blood count, coagulation studies, serologies for TORCH infections (toxoplasmosis, rubella, cytomegalovirus, herpes simplex virus), thyroxine and thyroid-stimulating hormone levels, and iron studies [8].

SCREENING AND INITIATION OF EARLY WORKUP

Currently there is no widely adopted newborn screening approach to BA in the United States [11,12]. A few screening approaches currently in use are highlighted in Table 2. Novel screening approaches currently in development are discussed later in this article.

Table 2
Screening approaches

Screening method	Timing	Benefits	Barriers/limitations
Fractionated bilirubin levels	At birth or around 2–4 weeks old	Highly sensitive and specific Early detection	No universal direct bilirubin assay so each hospital has to establish their own reference levels Cost-benefit analysis not yet determined
Bile acid blood test [13]	At birth	Easy to implement if able to conduct with already established screenings for inborn errors of metabolism	Tests have not yet demonstrated better sensitivity or specificity compared to other detection methods
Physical examination- jaundice evaluation	2–4 weeks old	Already performed by pediatricians	Nonspecific and may not be present early Less-empiric than a laboratory test and subject to bias
Stool color card	2–4 weeks old	Simple, easy to implement Low cost	Acholic stools may be a late finding Need system in place for caregivers concerned for positive finding
Mobile phone application detecting acholic stools [14,15]	2–4 weeks old	Highly sensitive and specific	Difficult to widely implement Similar to stool color card, need a system in place for positive screening

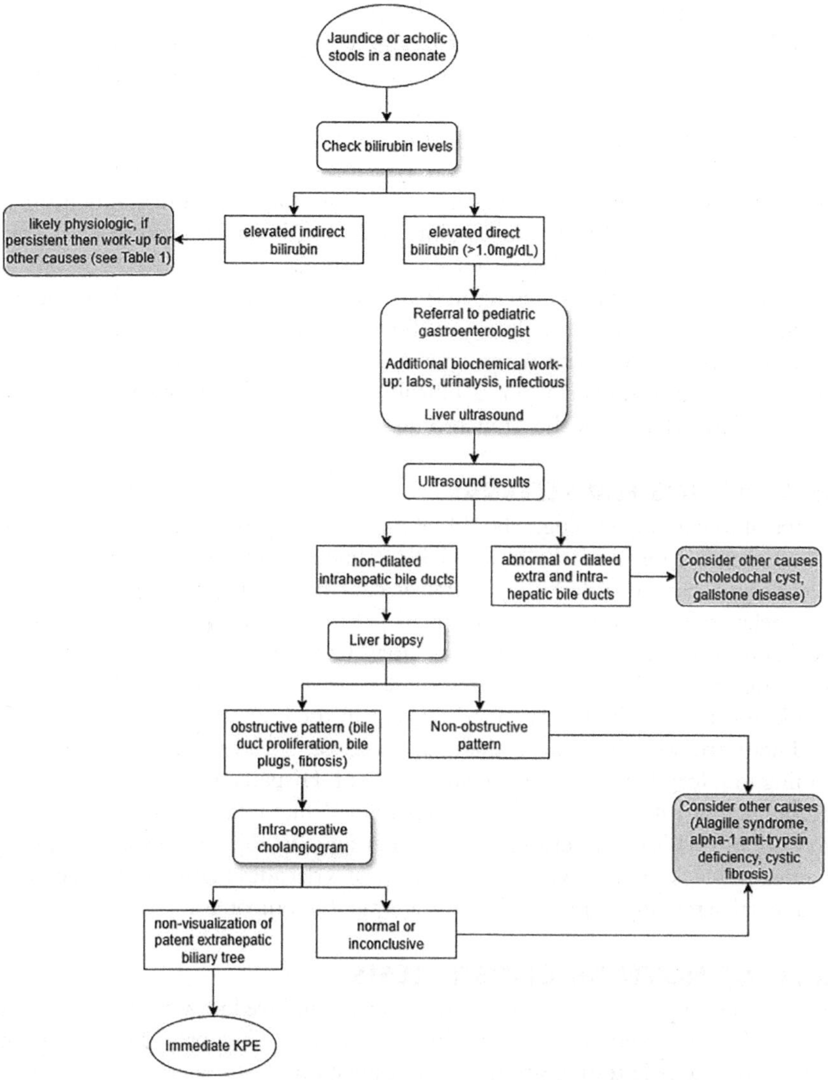

Fig. 1. Comprehensive diagram of the diagnostic workup for suspected BA.

Given the lack of universal newborn screening for BA and progressive nature of the condition, workup most commonly occurs in the outpatient setting. Thorough physical examination and timely laboratory evaluation are crucial for early detection and initiating appropriate workup.

The American Academy of Pediatrics recently published a guidance document for primary care providers to assist with early identification of patients with BA [9]. The 3-step strategy involves (1) assessing for jaundice through skin color and eye color, (2) screening for acholic stools by direct observation or caregiver report, and (3) obtaining hospital records to determine if an initial bilirubin was obtained and elevated (Fig. 1). Direct bilirubin levels may be elevated at birth in BA; however, many hospitals only check total bilirubin, and not all BA patients will have elevated levels at birth [16]. Absence of any one of these elements should not necessarily rule out BA.

Stool color evaluation has been a target for screening as caregivers may be able to alert providers of changes in stool before their scheduled appointment. Universal screening using stool color cards has been implemented in some countries with success [17–20]. For example, the stool color card program implemented as universal screening in Taiwan has led to more Kasai portoenterostomies (KPEs) performed before 60 days of life and improved 3-year jaundice-free survival with native liver [21,22]. This is also a cost-effective option compared to universal direct bilirubin screening [23]; however, it has not been widely adopted in the United States [12].

INDICATIONS FOR REFERRAL

Referral to gastroenterology should be made if direct bilirubin remains greater than1 mg/dL after 2 weeks of life [7,9]. While imaging such as an abdominal ultrasound can be ordered by primary care providers, these studies should not delay referral and may be obtained before or after referral occurs [9,24]. Referral to the emergency department may be warranted to expedite workup, particularly in patients who are already delayed in diagnosis. Ideally, however, workup can occur in an expedited fashion in the outpatient setting.

There are some notable disparities based on sociodemographic factors in timing to referral and subsequent surgery. Non-Hispanic Black infants and Hispanic infants with BA are referred later than White infants [25] and less likely to undergo KPE or undergo KPE at a later age [25,26]. The disparities in outcomes and lack of improvement over the past 3 decades highlight the need for a universal screening approach for more equitable outcomes.

ROLE OF NOVEL DIAGNOSTIC TESTS

Because no universal screening approach exists and we know the importance of early diagnosis and intervention in BA, various diagnostic tests including serum and genetic testing are under investigation.

Matrix metalloproteinase-7

Matrix metalloproteinase-7 (MMP-7) plays a role in the remodeling of the extracellular matrix, a phenomenon that occurs secondary to the liver damage and fibrosis caused by biliary atresia [27,28]. Over the last decade, multiple studies have demonstrated an association between elevated serum levels of MMP-7 and biliary atresia, allowing for diagnosis of BA among infants with cholestasis. In an observational study from China, using data from 3 tertiary pediatric centers, high serum concentrations of MMP-7 identified all but one patient with BA, with MMP-7 levels in BA patients increased on anaverage 10-fold more than those non-BA patients. Another study found a diagnostic value of 10.37 gave a sensitivity, specificity, positive predictive value (PPV), and negative predictive value (NPV) of 95.19%, 93.07%, 97.27%, and 91.43% respectively [29]. In a study by Pandurangi and colleagues, using a cut-off of 52.8 ng/m, the area under the curve (AUC) was 0.90, with a sensitivity of 90.55% (CI: 0.85–0.94), specificity of 84.34% (CI: 0.78–0.89), PPV of 71.25% (CI: 0.65–0.77), and NPV of 95.42% [30].

While MMP-7 is promising in many regards as a laboratory marker of BA, there remain limitations that need to be addressed before it becomes more widely used for diagnosis. First, the optimal cutoff has yet to be identified [30,31]. Second, research has yet to demonstrate that MMP-7 leads to more rapid diagnosis. There are many possible reasons for this–lack of test availability, the fact that a significant portion of the delay occurs in the prehospital phase, and appropriate hesitation to perform a major operation on the basis of a novel test [32].

Genetic testing using jaundice chip microarrays

Research has also been directed toward identifying genomic signatures that are associated with diagnosis of BA using microarray technology, otherwise known as *jaundice chips* [33]. The goal of genetic sequencing is 2-fold–to increase diagnostic accuracy and develop targeted, nonsurgical therapeutics. To date, identified genes include RRAS, VEGFA, MIF, HMGB1, and MAN1A2, which play a role in differential lymphocyte function, suppression of immunoglobulin genes, inflammation response, and reconstruction of the extracellular matrix [33–35]. Two other genes used in combination to diagnose BA, SPP1 and ANKRD1, were found to achieve an AUC of 0.830 with a sensitivity of 71.81% and a specificity of 80.18% [27]. Given the time required to perform these assays, genetic testing is not currently used as the primary mechanism to diagnose BA, and as of yet there are no targeted nonsurgical medical therapies for the disease.

BRIEF ALGORITHM FOR WORKUP

Variability exists in the work-up for patients with suspected BA. While there are several key components to the workup described later and depicted in Fig. 1, ultimately the decision to proceed with KPE depends on the expertise of a multidisciplinary team of specialists [7].

Laboratory markers

Direct bilirubin is required to establish the diagnosis of cholestasis [36,37]. Other commonly obtained laboratory markers include alanine aminotransferase, aspartate aminotransferase, alkaline phosphatase, gamma glutamyl transpeptidase, prothrombin time with the international normalized ratio, glucose, and albumin. Based on infant presentation, an infectious disease workup is also warranted [7,38].

Imaging

A fasting abdominal ultrasound with Doppler should be performed in all infants with concern for BA. Sonographic features associated with BA include a small or absent gallbladder, triangle cord sign, absence of common bile duct, and enlarged hepatic vasculature. Ultrasound can also visualize anomalies and malformations that are associated with BA [7,38]. However, it is important to note that ultrasound does not establish or rule out a diagnosis of BA.

Other imaging techniques that are less commonly used include hepatobiliary iminodiacetic acid (HIDA) scan, endoscopic retrograde cholangiopancreatography (ERCP), magnetic resonance cholangiopancreatography (MRCP), and percutaneous transhepatic cholangiography (PTC). However, these tests are not routinely performed due to a combination of factors [38]. HIDA, MRCP, and PTC have low sensitivity, while ERCP is invasive; it requires advanced endoscopists, and specialized equipment [7]. Furthermore, additional testing is expensive and can delay KPE [32,39].

Histopathology and intraoperative cholangiogram

Intraoperative cholangiogram (IOC), in combination with histopathology, is considered the gold-standard for diagnosis of BA. Biopsy can be performed percutaneously or surgically. The correct diagnosis on histopathology identified in 90% to 95% of cases [7,40,41]. Diagnosis with IOC is made if there is failure to visualize a patent extrahepatic biliary tree, although this can also be seen with Alagille syndrome and cystic fibrosis so preoperative testing of these conditions can help decrease rates of false-positive results [7].

More recently, indocyanine green (ICG) has been used to assist in the diagnosis of BA. ICG, once injected intravenously, is taken up by hepatocytes and cleared into the biliary tree. Intraoperative infrared light can then be used to better delineate biliary anatomy, or in the case of BA confirm its absence [42]. This method does not require cannulation of the bile duct, which can be challenging in patients with atretic gallbladders [43,44].

SURGICAL OPTIONS FOR BILIARY ATRESIA: KASAI PORTOENTEROSTOMY VERSUS LIVER TRANSPLANTATION

The Kasai portoenterostomy was first described by Professor Morio Kasai in the 1950s. The purpose of the procedure is to restore bile flow to the intestine: this is accomplished by resecting fibrotic biliary remnants at the hepatic plate and bringing up a loop of proximal jejunum to create a Roux-en-Y anastomosis, allowing the liver to drain bile directly into the jejunum. The current paradigm is to offer KPE as the primary treatment to all patients with BA unless there is clear evidence of liver failure, which is generally associated with diagnosis after 100 days of age [45]. The reported range of successful KPE, defined as biliary clearance at 2 months, is 34% to 64% [46–50]. While younger age at time of KPE has been shown to be associated with improved clearance, the precise cut-off–and to what extent age plays a role–remains a subject of investigation [7,32,48,51–53].

When the KPE procedure was first developed, orthotopic liver transplant (OLT) had not yet been performed and even into the 1980s OLT was not widely available for children with BA [45]. However, as it becomes more commonly performed, the question arises as to whether it should be used as the first line surgery for patients with biliary atresia given the moderate success rates of KPE. There are several reasons why KPE remains the initial operation of choice. First, liver transplant is associated with a defined significant mortality: children undergoing OLT have a 20-year overall survival rate of 69% and graft survival of 53%, which does not account for waitlist-associated mortality [54,55]. Second, liver transplant requires a life of immunosuppressive medication, which is not without risk [45]. Third, it appears that OLT after KPE does not confer worse survival, and in fact perhaps is associated with improved outcomes as it gives children a chance to grow [56,57]. Lastly, organ availability is an issue, with more than 40% of children spending more than a year on the waitlist [55]. Given these reasons, KPE remains the primary surgery for most patients with BA [45].

LONG-TERM OUTCOMES

While KPE remains the best early option for treatment of BA, progressive fibrosis following KPE means that even those with initially successful KPE may require transplantation: approximately 50% to 60% of patients require OLT by 5 years, with this number rising to almost 70% to 75% by 20 years [46–48]. The overall survival rate of patients with BA ranges from 76% to 87% [58,59]. One significant risk following KPE is cholangitis, which occurs in 40% to 93% patients and likely contributes to failure of KPE [58,60,61]. Patients with biliary atresia are also at risk of other long-term complications related to sequelae of liver disease including portal hypertension, hypersplenism, varices, and impaired bone health [58,60,62].

Although significant progress has been made in the diagnosis and management of biliary atresia, this condition remains a challenging paradigm for pediatricians, pediatric gastroenterologists, and pediatric surgeons. While promising new screening tools or programs are under development, our current management relies on early identification through patient history and physical examination followed by laboratory testing and imaging to rule out other causes of jaundice or hyperbilirubinemia. KPE remains the mainstay of initial management with liver transplantation as the final definitive treatment.

CLINICS CARE POINTS

- Early recognition: direct hyperbilirubinemia (>1.0 mg/dL) in a neonate is pathologic and warrants evaluation for cholestasis. Symptoms such as acholic stools and jaundice may develop later and their absence does not rule out biliary atresia.
- Screening: Fractionated bilirubin is the first-line test; if direct bilirubin is elevated, proceed with expanded labs (CBC, coagulation, TORCH serologies, thyroid studies, iron studies).

- Referral: Refer to pediatric gastroenterology if direct bilirubin >1 mg/dL after 2 weeks of life. Expedite referral rather than waiting for imaging results, which may delay definitive management.
- Novel diagnostics: Serum MMP-7 shows high sensitivity and specificity for BA and genetic microarray "jaundice chips" are emerging tools, however cutoffs are not yet standardized and availability is still limited.
- Imaging and histopathology: Ultrasound can suggest BA (absent gallbladder, triangular cord sign) but cannot confirm diagnosis. IOC with histopathology remains the gold standard.
- Surgical management: Kasai portoenterostomy (KPE) is most effective if performed before 45–60 days of life. Early surgery improves native liver survival.

Disclosures

The authors have nothing to disclose.

References

[1] Bezerra JA, Wells RG, Mack CL, et al. Biliary atresia: clinical and research challenges for the twenty-first century. Hepatology 2018;68(3):1163–73.
[2] Schreiber RA, Harpavat S, Hulscher JBF, et al. Biliary atresia in 2021: epidemiology, screening and public policy. JCM 2022;11(4):999.
[3] Jimenez-Rivera C, Jolin-Dahel KS, Fortinsky KJ, et al. International incidence and outcomes of biliary atresia. J Pediatr Gastroenterol Nutr 2013;56(4):344–54.
[4] Spada M, Riva S, Maggiore G, et al. Pediatric liver transplantation. World J Gastroenterol 2009;15(6):648–74.
[5] Asai A, Miethke A, Bezerra JA. Pathogenesis of biliary atresia: defining biology to understand clinical phenotypes. Nat Rev Gastroenterol Hepatol 2015;12(6):342–52.
[6] Davenport M, Muntean A, Hadzic N. Biliary atresia: clinical phenotypes and aetiological heterogeneity. J Clin Med 2021;10(23):5675.
[7] Fawaz R, Baumann U, Ekong U, et al. Guideline for the evaluation of cholestatic jaundice in infants: joint recommendations of the north American Society for pediatric gastroenterology, hepatology, and nutrition and the European Society for pediatric gastroenterology, hepatology, and nutrition. J Pediatr Gastroenterol Nutr 2017;64(1):154–68.
[8] Gilmour SM. Prolonged neonatal jaundice: when to worry and what to do. Paediatr Child Health 2004;9(10):700–4.
[9] Harpavat S, Aucott SW, Karpen SJ, et al. Guidance for the primary care provider in identifying infants with biliary atresia by 2–4 weeks of life: clinical report. Pediatrics 2025;155 (3):e2024070077.
[10] Hussein M, Howard ER, Mieli-Vergani G, et al. Jaundice at 14 days of age: exclude biliary atresia. Arch Dis Child 1991;66(10):1177–9.
[11] Rabbani T, Guthery SL, Himes R, et al. Newborn screening for biliary atresia: a review of current methods. Curr Gastroenterol Rep 2021;23(12):28.
[12] Corrado MM, Mack CL. Diagnostic tools for early detection of biliary atresia: is a newborn screen attainable? Clin Liver Dis 2022;19(1):25–8.
[13] Zhou K, Lin N, Xiao Y, et al. Elevated bile acids in newborns with biliary atresia (BA). In: Rota R, editor. PLoS One 2012;7(11):e49270.
[14] Angelico R, Liccardo D, Paoletti M, et al. A novel mobile phone application for infant stool color recognition: an easy and effective tool to identify acholic stools in newborns. J Med Screen 2021;28(3):230–7.
[15] Hoshino E, Hayashi K, Suzuki M, et al. An iPhone application using a novel stool color detection algorithm for biliary atresia screening. Pediatr Surg Int 2017;33(10):1115–21.

[16] Harpavat S, Finegold MJ, Karpen SJ. Patients with biliary atresia have elevated direct/conjugated bilirubin levels shortly after birth. Pediatrics 2011;128(6):e1428–33.
[17] Gu YH, Yokoyama K, Mizuta K, et al. Stool color card screening for early detection of biliary atresia and long-term native liver survival: a 19-Year cohort study in Japan. J Pediatr 2015;166(4):897–902.e1.
[18] Hsiao C, Chang M, Chen H, et al. Universal screening for biliary atresia using an infant stool color card in Taiwan. Hepatology 2008;47(4):1233–40.
[19] Tseng JJ, Lai MS, Lin MC, et al. Stool color card screening for biliary atresia. Pediatrics 2011;128(5):e1209–15.
[20] Wildhaber BE. Screening for biliary atresia: swiss stool color card. Hepatology 2011;54 (1):368.
[21] Lee M, Chen SCC, Yang HY, et al. Infant stool color card screening helps reduce the hospitalization rate and mortality of biliary atresia: a 14-Year nationwide cohort study in Taiwan. Medicine 2016;95(12):e3166.
[22] Lien TH, Chang MH, Wu JF, et al. Effects of the infant stool color card screening program on 5-year outcome of biliary atresia in Taiwan. Hepatology 2011;53(1):202–8.
[23] Masucci L, Schreiber RA, Kaczorowski J, et al. Universal screening of newborns for biliary atresia: cost-Effectiveness of alternative strategies. J Med Screen 2019;26(3):113–9.
[24] Harpavat S, Lupo PJ, Liwanag L, et al. Factors influencing time-to-diagnosis of biliary atresia. J Pediatr Gastroenterol Nutr 2018;66(6):850–6.
[25] Bonn J, Gamm K, Ambrosino T, et al. Distinct effects of racial and socioeconomic disparities on biliary atresia diagnosis and outcome. J Pediatr Gastroenterol Nutr 2024;78(5): 1038–46.
[26] Lee H, Lewis J, Schoen BT, et al. Kasai portoenterostomy: differences related to race. J Pediatr Surg 2001;36(8):1196–8.
[27] Jiang J, Dong R, Du M, et al. Serum matrix metalloproteinase-7 for discriminating biliary atresia: a diagnostic accuracy and validation study. J Transl Med 2024;22(1):636.
[28] Rohani P, Mirrahimi SB, Bashirirad H, et al. Serum matrix metalloproteinase-7 levels in infants with cholestasis and biliary atresia. BMC Pediatr 2022;22(1):351.
[29] Jiang J, Wang J, Shen Z, et al. Serum MMP-7 in the diagnosis of biliary atresia. Pediatrics 2019;144(5):e20190902.
[30] Pandurangi S, Mourya R, Nalluri S, et al. Diagnostic accuracy of serum matrix metalloproteinase-7 as a biomarker of biliary atresia in a large North American cohort. Hepatology 2024;80(1):152–62.
[31] Yang L, Zhou Y, Xu P, et al. Diagnostic accuracy of serum matrix Metalloproteinase-7 for biliary atresia. Hepatology 2018;68(6):2069–77.
[32] Farooqui ZA, Hartman SJ, Stetson AE, et al. Real-world multi-institutional data from the midwest pediatric surgery consortium (MWPSC) to assess the effect of delayed Kasai procedure on biliary drainage in patients with biliary atresia. J Pediatr Surg 2025;60(5):162250.
[33] Bezerra JA, Tiao G, Ryckman FC, et al. Genetic induction of proinflammatory immunity in children with biliary atresia. Lancet 2002;360(9346):1653–9.
[34] Zhao R, Li H, Shen C, et al. RRAS: a key regulator and an important prognostic biomarker in biliary atresia. WJG 2011;17(6):796.
[35] Wu LN, Zhu ZJ, Sun LY. Genetic factors and their role in the pathogenesis of biliary atresia. Front Pediatr 2022;10:912154.
[36] Harpavat S, Ramraj R, Finegold MJ, et al. Newborn direct or conjugated bilirubin measurements as a potential screen for biliary atresia. J Pediatr Gastroenterol Nutr 2016;62(6): 799–803.
[37] Harpavat S, Garcia-Prats JA, Anaya C, et al. Diagnostic yield of newborn screening for biliary atresia using direct or conjugated bilirubin measurements. JAMA 2020;323(12): 1141.
[38] El-Guindi MAS, Sira MM, Sira AM, et al. Design and validation of a diagnostic score for biliary atresia. J Hepatol 2014;61(1):116–23.

[39] Lim YZ, Chaudhary U, Issioui Y, et al. Kasai portoenterostomy delays: is a HIDA scan worth the wait? J Pediatr Surg 2023;58(8):1476–82.
[40] Ali KM, Zalata KR, Barakat T, et al. Pathologic approach to neonatal cholestasis with a simple scoring system for biliary atresia. Virchows Arch 2024;484(1):93–102.
[41] Chen G, Xue P, Zheng S, et al. A pathological scoring system in the diagnosis and judgment of prognosis of biliary atresia. J Pediatr Surg 2015;50(12):2119–23.
[42] Hollington P, Mawdsley J, Lim W, et al. An 11-year experience of enterocutaneous fistula. Br J Surg 2004;91(12):1646–51.
[43] Shirota C, Hinoki A, Togawa T, et al. Intraoperative indocyanine green fluorescence cholangiography can rule out biliary atresia: a preliminary report. Front Pediatr 2022;10:1005879.
[44] Zhao J, Zhao Y, Zhang Y, et al. Preliminary exploration of the efficacy of laparoscopic fluorescence cholangiography (LFC) in the diagnosis of biliary atresia compared with intraoperative cholangiography (IOC). Photodiagnosis Photodyn Ther 2023;41:103241.
[45] Davenport M, Superina R. Primary liver transplant in biliary atresia: the case for and against. J Pediatr Surg 2024;59(8):1418–26.
[46] De Vries W, Homan–Van Der Veen J, Hulscher JBF, et al. Twenty-year transplant-free survival rate among patients with biliary atresia. Clin Gastroenterol Hepatol 2011;9(12): 1086–91.
[47] Pakarinen MP, Johansen LS, Svensson JF, et al. Outcomes of biliary atresia in the Nordic countries – a multicenter study of 158 patients during 2005–2016. J Pediatr Surg 2018;53(8):1509–15.
[48] Fanna M, Masson G, Capito C, et al. Management of biliary atresia in France 1986 to 2015: long-term results. J Pediatr Gastroenterol Nutr 2019;69(4):416–24.
[49] Wildhaber BE, Majno P, Mayr J, et al. Biliary atresia: Swiss National Study, 1994–2004. J Pediatr Gastroenterol Nutr 2008;46(3):299–307.
[50] Bezerra JA, Spino C, Magee JC, et al. Use of corticosteroids after hepatoportoenterostomy for bile drainage in infants with biliary atresia: the START randomized clinical trial. JAMA 2014;311(17):1750.
[51] Lemoine CP, Melin-Aldana H, Brandt KA, et al. Identification of early clinical and histological factors predictive of Kasai portoenterostomy failure. JCM 2022;11(21):6523.
[52] Uecker M, Kuebler JF, Schukfeh N, et al. Kasai procedure in patients older than 90 days: worth a cut. Eur J Pediatr Surg 2022;32(01):080–4.
[53] Serinet MO, Wildhaber BE, Broué P, et al. Impact of age at Kasai operation on its results in late childhood and adolescence: a rational basis for biliary atresia screening. Pediatrics 2009;123(5):1280–6.
[54] Venick RS, Farmer DG, Soto JR, et al. One thousand pediatric liver transplants during thirty years: lessons learned. J Am Coll Surg 2018;226(4):355–66.
[55] Perito ER, Roll G, Dodge JL, et al. Split liver transplantation and pediatric waitlist mortality in the United States: potential for improvement. Transplantation 2019;103(3):552–7.
[56] Stetson A, Bondoc A, Tiao G. Revision Kasai portoenterostomy: a review of indications and outcomes. Semin Pediatr Surg 2024;33(6):151476.
[57] Bondoc AJ, Taylor JA, Alonso MH, et al. The beneficial impact of revision of Kasai portoenterostomy for biliary atresia: an institutional study. Ann Surg 2012;255(3):570–6.
[58] Jung E, Park WH, Choi SO. Late complications and current status of long-term survivals over 10 years after Kasai portoenterostomy. J Korean Surg Soc 2011;81(4):271.
[59] Witt M, Van Wessel DBE, De Kleine RHJ, et al. Prognosis of biliary atresia after 2-year survival with native liver: a nationwide cohort analysis. J Pediatr Gastroenterol Nutr 2018;67 (6):689–94.
[60] Chung PHY, Chan EKW, Yeung F, et al. Life long follow up and management strategies of patients living with native livers after Kasai portoenterostomy. Sci Rep 2021;11 (1):11207.

[61] Calinescu AM, Madadi-Sanjani O, Mack C, et al. Cholangitis definition and treatment after Kasai hepatoportoenterostomy for biliary atresia: a Delphi process and international expert panel. JCM 2022;11(3):494.
[62] Hukkinen M, Ruuska S, Pihlajoki M, et al. Long-term outcomes of biliary atresia patients surviving with their native livers. Best Pract Res Clin Gastroenterol 2022;56-57: 101764.

Advances in Pediatrics 73 (2026) 253–267

ELSEVIER

ADVANCES IN PEDIATRICS

Updates on Lymphatic Malformations

Medical Therapies, Sclerotherapy, and Surgery

Michelle Hough, MD*, Dean Anselmo, MD

Division of Pediatric Surgery, Department of Surgery, Children's Hospital Los Angeles, Los Angeles, CA, USA

Keywords

• Lymphatic malformations • Vascular anomalies • Multi-disciplinary

Key points

- Lymphatic malformations (LMs) are rare, nonneoplastic, slow-flow vascular malformations with diverse clinical manifestations.
- Treatment focuses on restoring function, preserving anatomy, and improving symptoms.
- Management requires a multidisciplinary and multimodal approach dependent on cystic type and anatomic location.
- Therapies include pharmacologic agents, such as sirolimus and alpelisib, percutaneous procedures including sclerotherapy, and surgical intervention.

INTRODUCTION

Lymphatic malformations (LMs), previously termed "lymphangiomas" or "cystic hygromas," are a type of vascular malformation within the classification system of vascular anomalies. LMs, and vascular anomalies in general, often present a clinical challenge given their rarity, diverse presentations, and historically variable and confusing naming conventions [1,2].

The International Society for the Study of Vascular Anomalies (ISSVA) divides vascular malformations by flow: fast-flow, slow-flow, and developmental anomalies of named vessels. LMs are classified as slow-flow malformations, similar to capillary and venous malformations, and are distinct from

*Corresponding author. Division of Pediatric Surgery, Department of Surgery, Children's Hospital Los Angeles, 4650 Sunset Boulevard, MS #100, Los Angeles, CA 90027. *E-mail address:* michelleamiehough@gmail.com

https://doi.org/10.1016/j.yapd.2025.12.002

Abbreviations

APSA	American Pediatric Surgical Association
CFLM	cervicofacial lymphatic malformation
CT	computed tomography
ISSVA	International Society for the Study of Vascular Anomalies
LM	lymphatic malformation
mTOR	mammalian target of rapamycin
PROS	PIK3CA overgrowth syndrome
PI3K	phosphoinositide 3-kinase/protein kinase B
RFA	radiofrequency ablation
STS	sodium tetradecyl sulfate
US	ultrasound

arteriovenous malformations, which are fast-flow, as well as from combined vascular malformations. Despite advances in nomenclature, the spectrum of lymphatic disorders remains clinically complex owing to their heterogeneous presentation, unpredictable growth, and overlap with other vascular entities [3] (Fig. 1).

LMs can be categorized as isolated, complex, or lymphedematous forms. Isolated LMs are mass lesions further subdivided by cyst size (macro, micro, mixed). Complex lymphatic anomalies encompass a broader range of systemic disorders, including *generalized lymphatic anomaly*, *kaposiform lymphangiomatosis*, *Gorham-Stout disease*, *central conducting lymphatic anomaly*, and *generalized lymphatic dysplasia* [4]. Lymphedema, the most common lymphatic abnormality, may be primary (genetic, idiopathic, developmental, or congenital) or secondary

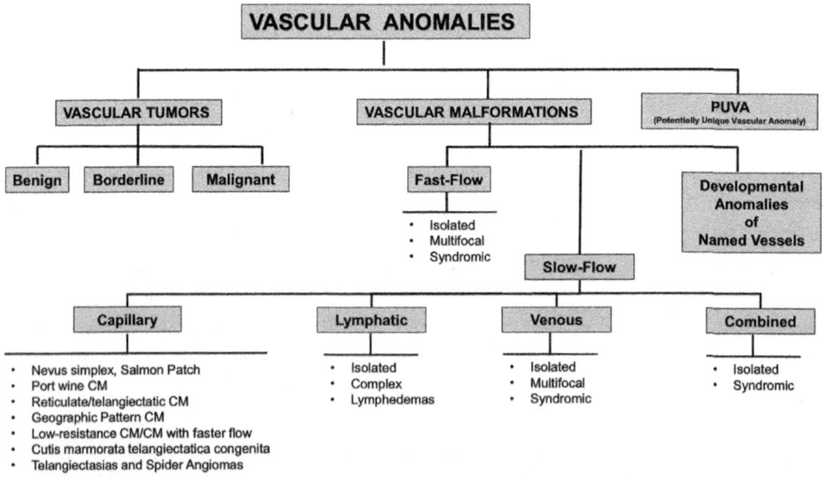

Fig. 1. ISSVA classification of vascular anomalies. CM, capillary malformation. (ISSVA Classification of Vascular Anomalies ©2025 International Society for the Study of Vascular Anomalies Available at "issva.org/classification" Accessed 27 Feb 2026.)

(acquired). Lymphedema occurs secondary to impaired lymphatic drainage and results in interstitial fluid accumulation leading to engorgement, and over time, fibrosis with persistent limb enlargement [1,2,4] (Fig. 2).

Most LMs fall within PIK3CA Overgrowth Syndrome (PROS), a group of somatic overgrowth disorders caused by activating mutations of the PIK3CA gene, although PROS vary greatly depending on the tissue type, associated vascular malformation (which does not have to be an LM), and their affected anatomy. PROS includes Klippel-Trenaunay syndrome, CLOVES (congenital lipomatous overgrowth, vascular malformations, epidermal nevi, and scoliosis/skeletal/spinal anomalies) syndrome, and macrocephaly-capillary malformation syndrome [5]. Recognition of these molecular underpinnings has not only clarified classification but also introduced targeted molecular therapies.

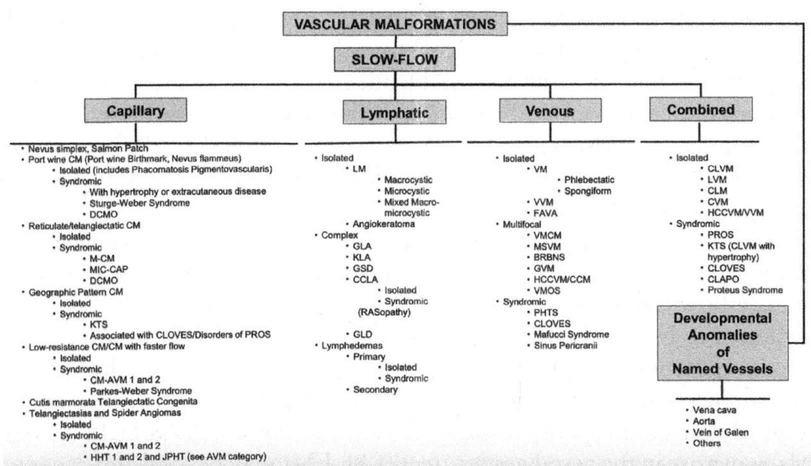

Fig. 2. ISSVA classification of vascular malformations. BRBNS, blue rubber bleb nevus syndrome; CCLA, central conducting lymphatic anomaly; CLAPO, capillary malformation of the lower lip, Lymphatic malformations of the head and neck, Asymmetry and Partial or generalized Overgrowth: Pathognomonic lower lip capillary malformation associated to intraoral and neck lymphatic and venous malformations; CLOVES, congenital lipomatous overgrowth, vascular malformations, epidermal nevi, and scoliosis/skeletal/spinal anomalies; CM-AVM, capillary malformation-arteriovenous malformation; CLM, capillary-lymphatic malformation; CLVM, capillary-lymphatic-venous malformation; FAVA, fibroadipose vascular anomaly; GLA, generalized lymphatic anomaly; GLD, generalized lymphatic dysplasia; GSD, Gorham-Stout disease; GVM, glomuvenous malformation; HHT, hereditary hemorrhagic telangectasia; HCCVM/CCM, hyperkeratotic cutaneous capillary-venous malformation/cerebral cavernous malformation; HCCVM/VVM, hyperkeratotic cutaneous capillary-venous-venous malformation/verrucous venous malformation; JPHT, juvenile polyposis hemorrhagic telangectasia; KLA, kaposiform lymphangiomatosis; LVM, lymphatic-venous-malformation; MSVM, multifocal sporadic venous malformation; PHTS, PTEN hamartoma tumor syndrome; VM, venous malformation; VMCM, venous malformation cutaneous-mucosal; VMOS, familial intraosseous vascular malformation. (ISSVA Classification of Vascular Anomalies ©2025 International Society for the Study of Vascular Anomalies Available at "issva.org/classification" Accessed 27 Feb 2026.)

This review summarizes the current understanding of LM subtypes, their pathophysiology, diagnostic evaluation, and multidisciplinary management, emphasizing recent advances in medical therapy, sclerotherapy, and surgery.

EPIDEMIOLOGY AND PATHOPHYSIOLOGY

LMs are nonneoplastic congenital malformations of the lymphatic system [1,2,5]. Although the embryology of the lymphatic system is incompletely defined, LMs have been theorized to arise from aberrant budding of the primordial lymph sac with failure to communicate with the venous plexus [2,6,7] and defective lymphatic endothelial cells [8]. Proposed mechanisms include mutations of the PIK3CA gene, which upregulate the phosphoinositide 3-kinase/protein kinase B/mammalian target of rapamycin (PI3K/mTOR) pathway leading to disordered lymphangiogenesis through upregulation of lymphatic endothelial cell proliferation [5,8,9]. Thus, these pathways have become targets in medical therapy. Most LMs occur secondary to somatic genetic mutations in growth factor signal transduction pathways, although germline gene variants have also been identified [5,9]. LMs are also found in syndromes, such as Turner, Proteus, and Milroy disease, which are associated with lymphangiogenesis secondary to gene activation in the PIK3K/protein kinase B (AKT)/mTOR pathway, and also linked to mutations in vascular endothelial growth factor C signaling [4,10].

Clinically, most LMs are recognized early in life, with approximately 60% present at birth and up to 90% diagnosed by 2 years of age [6], although they can be identified in older adolescents or even adults [2,5,8,10]. Incidence is reported to be 1 to 2000 to 16,000 births [6,8,11,12] with no clear gender or ethnic predilection [6,8,10]. Although they can occur anywhere in the body, the head and neck region is the most common site, followed by the axilla, mediastinum, abdomen/retroperitoneum, groin, and extremities [1,2,8,11,12]. Rarely, LMs may arise in the aerodigestive tract [1,8]. LMs may be focal and contained to one area or expand across anatomic regions, such as the neck, axilla, and chest wall [2].

LMs generally exhibit growth that is commensurate with growth of the child, although acute enlargement can occur in response to infection, trauma, or hormonal changes, such as puberty [13]. Histologically, LMs are thin-walled vascular spaces lined with endothelial cells and filled with protein-rich fluid and immune cells [4,7]. Pathologically, malformed lymphatic channels are prone to leakage, infection, hemorrhage, and inflammation, leading to tissue expansion and functional impairment [2,12].

CLINICAL PRESENTATION, WORKUP, AND DIAGNOSIS

The clinical spectrum of LMs varies widely depending on anatomic location, cyst type, and extent of disease. Isolated LMs are divided morphologically by cyst size: macrocystic, microcystic, or combined types. Macrocystic LMs contain cystic spaces greater than 1 to 2 cm filled with lymph and are typically located in the mediastinum, cervical, and axillary region. Comparatively, microcystic LMs consist of smaller, interwoven cysts embedded within connective tissue and tend to arise in the tongue, mouth, cheek, thorax, retroperitoneum, and extremities. Combined variants can arise in any location. There is no clearly defined cystic size criteria, although an important differentiation of macrocystic disease is if the size of the cyst allows needle decompression or injection to be performed [1,2,5,12].

LMs may be detected on prenatal imaging, such as ultrasound (US) or fetal MRI [4], on physical examination throughout childhood, and often after complications [2,11]. Deep-seated lesions can remain indolent until adolescence or adulthood [2]. Although LMs are highly variable in anatomy, they may be palpated as a swelling or mass lesion that is partially compressible or ballotable. They may have a blue, amber, or reddened hue and may have associated cutaneous vesicles or vascular stains [2,4,5,9]. Lesions may be spongy and fluctuant if macrocystic or firm if microcystic, with variable size [2,10]. Associated morbidities secondary to LMs include lymphatic leak, infections, bleeding, intralesional hemorrhage, coagulopathies, disfigurement, functional impairment, and compression [2,12]. Head and neck LMs can lead to airway compromise, and oral LMs may affect feeding. Mediastinal LMs can cause cardiopulmonary compromise, and abdominal LMs can cause constipation, intestinal obstruction, or genitourinary dysfunction [10]. Periorbital and orbital LMs pose a particular challenge given they are locally invasive and are difficult to resect [7,10]. Complex thoracic or abdominal LMs are further associated with chylothorax, chylopericardium, ascites, protein-losing enteropathy, or chylous reflux. The lymphatic vessels within LMs may leak, accumulate fluid, cause localized inflammation or infection, and during acute periods may enlarge given they are immune-reactive [2,7,9,10].

Cervicofacial LMs can be prenatally diagnosed as a collection of abnormal lymphatic fluid in the posterior cervical midline. The FASTER (First and Second Trimester Evaluation of Risk) Trial identified 134 cases out of 38,167 screened patients with "cystic hygromas" diagnosed at 10 to 14 weeks and noted associated chromosomal anomalies, including trisomy 21, Turner syndrome, and trisomy 18, along with major structural malformations. These posterior cervical LMs are distinct from more classically known LMs in the head and neck that are commonly detected postnatally and are not associated with chromosomal anomalies. Large cervicofacial malformations in utero risk airway obstruction after delivery and may require ex utero intrapartum treatment with partial delivery to ensure securing the airway [2,4,5,7,10].

Simple LMs may be differentiated on examination, although imaging modalities of choice include US and MRI. US is typically the initial study, given it is relatively accessible, is noninvasive, and does not require sedation or ionizing radiation. Duplex US can detect flow speed and differentiate LMs as slow-flow lesions compared with high-flow malformations, such as arteriovenous malformations. US describes macrocystic LMs as lobulated cystic lesions with thin septations and microcystic LMs as more solid with hypoechoic tiny microcysts or only tissue edema. MRI further characterizes LMs in anatomic detail and dimensions and is typically obtained to assist in procedural planning. Macrocystic lesions are multiseptated and hyperintense on T2 MRI scan, which importantly show the depth and invasion of malformations [5,9,12], whereas microcystic lesions are more solid and heterogenous on T1/T2-weighted signal [10]. Computed tomography (CT) scans are not recommended for diagnosis or surveillance of LMs; however, CT may be obtained during acute complications, such as infection or bleeding, and to identify bony involvement [5,10]. The differential for cystic lesions on imaging includes branchial cleft cysts and abscesses, as well as cystic malignancies and visceral cysts. Lymphatic scintigraphy has been used historically in the evaluation of lymphedema to localize sites of lymphatic obstruction, although it seldom yields findings that meaningfully guide therapy. Suspected complex lymphatic anomalies can be detected with whole-body MRI, as well as MR lymphangiography. MRI plays a role in fetal diagnosis and also posttreatment follow-up [5].

If the diagnosis of LM is not clear, fine-needle aspiration for cytology may be obtained to differentiate from brachial cleft cysts or visceral (biliary, pancreatic, urinary) cysts. Tissue biopsy combined with genetic testing can also delineate superficial LM [9].

Genetic testing

Most isolated LMs arise from somatic activating or gain-of-function mutations in PIK3CA [14], a gene encoding the catalytic subunit of lipid kinase PI3K-alpha, which drives various cellular processes and vascular development. Differing degrees of activation lead to changes in downstream signaling of serine-threonine protein kinase AKT and mTORC1 [8,14,15], which then affect disease conditions [12]. Somatic activating mutations in BRAF and KRAS have also been identified [16]. Tests must be sensitive enough to detect low-level somatic mosaicism given mutated cells within tissue may be low [12,14]. Next-generation sequencing and digital droplet polymerase chain reaction (ddPCR) have enabled detection of somatic mutations using amplified cell-free DNA from plasma and cyst fluid, assisting diagnostics to target medical therapies [12,17].

MANAGEMENT

A multidisciplinary approach to management of LMs is of paramount importance and is tailored to each patient according to clinical manifestation, size, anatomic location, cyst type, and severity of condition. Treatment focuses on reducing morbidity, improving function, and improving quality of life [4,9,11]. Aesthetics and reducing social stigma also play a role in multidisciplinary treatment. The vascular anomalies team may consist of diagnostic and interventional radiologists, surgeons (pediatric, otolaryngology, plastics, orthopedics), dermatologists, hematologist-oncologists, speech pathologists, and psychologists [4]. Traditionally, surgical resection has been the mainstay of therapy if technically feasible; however, other treatment options, such as medical management and percutaneous therapy, are used in conjunction with or in lieu of surgical management. As time progresses, these more minimally invasive options have become prevalent [2,4,9,11].

Watchful waiting and conservative management are considered for mild presentations and use modalities like compression garments [10] and antibiotics during periods of infection. Up to 45% of LMs have been reported to regress spontaneously under observation if mild in presentation [4]. Corticosteroids have been used in the past to reduce inflammation, particularly following infectious or inflammatory events [9].

Current medical management of LMs includes the mTOR inhibitor, sirolimus, or the direct PIK3CA inhibitor, alpelisib (Vijoice, Novartis Pharmaceuticals). In the past, oral phosphodiesterase inhibitors (sildenafil) were used to relax the smooth muscle with modest radiographic improvement and improvement of symptoms; however, some studies have shown no effects. Eppikajutsuto (TJ-28) is a Japanese Kampo herbal medication studied mostly for cervicofacial LMs, noting an 87% to 100% radiographic response. Propranolol, an oral beta-blocker, has also been studied to decrease vascular endothelial growth factor signaling with mild radiographic response, likely more effective with mixed vascular anomalies, as well as oral acetylsalicylic acid and cyclophosphamide in refractory cases. Medical therapies now focus on genetic targets in mTOR/PI3K inhibitors to decrease size of LMs and improve function, although no therapies are considered curative. Macrocystic lesions seem to respond better to medical therapy in comparison to microcystic and mixed lesions. Medical therapy for macrocystic lesions should be considered for macrocystic lesions that are complex and extensive, which may not be suitable for surgery or sclerotherapy [9,11].

Sirolimus

Sirolimus (rapamycin) binds to an intracellular protein called FKBP12 (FK506-binding protein). The sirolimus-FKBP12 complex inhibits mTOR, a kinase that plays a central role in cell growth, proliferation, and immune function, blocking a key downstream effector of PI3K/AKT signaling [4], which is often overactivated in LMs [5,18–21]. Sirolimus is the best-studied pharmacologic agent and is considered first-line medical therapy. A systematic review by the American Pediatric Surgical Association (APSA) found 80% to 97% of patients achieved partial radiographic or clinical response to sirolimus, particularly in head and neck lesions. Complete resolution is uncommon, but volume reduction and symptom improvement are typical [11].

Oral sirolimus treatment is often used in combination with sclerotherapy or surgery to improve outcomes. Studies suggest initial dosing target trough levels 5 to 15 ng/mL [9,21]. It is generally safe and well-tolerated, although it does have adverse events, including oral ulcers, hyperlipidemia, neutropenia, liver dysfunction, nausea, and diarrhea [9].

Alpelisib

Alpelisib (BLY719) is a selective PI3Kα inhibitor that directly counteracts PIK3CA gain-of-function mutations [14,17,22–26]. It was initially approved for adjuvant therapy use in breast cancer and subsequently received Food and Drug Administration approval in 2022 for PROS [12,27]. A prospective case series studied alpelisib in 3 children with gain-of-function mutations refractory to sirolimus who all had partial radiographic response without complications [11]. A prospective trial in 19 PROS patients who had refractory lesions also showed improvements [27]. Side effects have been described as mucositis, diarrhea, and hyperglycemia [9,27]. Ongoing phase II/III clinical trials will clarify optimal dosing and long-term safety [9].

Sclerotherapy

Percutaneous sclerotherapy is a cornerstone of LM management and often serves as primary monotherapy or as an adjunct to surgery or medical treatment. The technique involves aspiration of cyst contents followed by injection of a sclerosing agent to induce endothelial injury, fibrosis, and lesion collapse. Common agents include bleomycin, OK-432 (picibanil), doxycycline, sodium tetradecyl sulfate (STS), ethanol, pingyangmycin, polidocanol, acetic acid, and hypertonic saline. Each varies in potency, side-effect profile, and suitability for specific anatomic sites [4,9,11,13,28,29]. Fifty percent of patients studied in APSA's systematic review had complete response (>90% clinical or radiographic reduction), and 44.2% had partial response. Macrocystic lesions appear to respond better compared with mixed or microcystic lesions, although microcystic lesions may still respond partially. It is relatively well tolerated, although has variable effectiveness and often requires multiple treatment sessions [11]. Side-effect profiles between agents differ, but generally include periprocedural inflammatory response with tissue necrosis, fever, fatigue, erythema, infection, bleeding, skin pigmentation, and swelling, although cervicofacial LMs may have symptoms like dysphagia, obstruction, and speech issues [9,11]. Bleomycin has lower rates of postprocedural swelling so is preferred in head and neck cases with airway concerns [5].

Radiofrequency ablation (RFA), or coblation, has also been trialed for treatment of superficial, microcystic LMs of the mouth and aerodigestive tract, which are difficult to treat [10]. RFA destroys tissue by transmitting high-frequency energy to deep tissues and is thought to have less damage to adjacent structures. Carbon dioxide lasers, Nd:YAG lasers, fractionated erbium lasers, and pulsed dye lasers have also been trialed although are not widely used [4,9].

Surgical management

Surgical intervention remains an essential component of LM management, particularly for mass lesions that are localized, symptomatic, or obstructive, and for those that fail to respond to sclerotherapy or medical therapy. Complete resection is often not necessary given that LMs are benign, nonneoplastic, and nonproliferative lesions. The goal of surgery is debulking and functional restoration with improvement in quality of life. Surgical resections can be performed across various anatomic locations, although there is a lack of prospective, randomized data on surgery for specific subtype or anatomy [6,7,9,10]. More complex lesions may require a staged surgical approach and the use of closed suction drainage system postoperatively [4]. Studies on surgical management focus on resolution, residual disease, and recurrence rates. Sclerotherapy, which has emerged as first-line therapy for macrocystic disease, has resolution rates as high as 95%. Surgery, which has historically been preferred for microcystic disease, has reported resolution rates of 66% [30]. Some studies report success with US-guided liposuction for large microcystic extremity LMs and vascularized lymph node transfer for treating secondary lymphedema [4].

Published reports on postoperative complications have classically been small series focused on cervicofacial or intra-abdominal LMs, and most complications reported are acute postoperative fluid collections, nerve injury, and infection. A 20-year single-center review of short-term postoperative complications at a large quaternary referral center found that out of 109 surgical procedures across various anatomic locations (extremities, head/neck, trunk, thoracic, and abdominal), subtypes included 24% macrocystic, 28% microcystic, 36% mixed, and 11% unknown. Indications for surgery were debulking or planned complete resection. The most common complications were seroma (18%), infection (18%), and wound dehiscence (13%). Infrequent complications (5% or less) were nerve palsy, lymphedema, hematoma, and abscess. Seven percent of patients required an additional procedure, such as drainage/aspiration by interventional radiology, and 7% required return to the operating room. Of those with attempted complete resection, 32% recurred. However, subjective improvement in quality of life was 70% in the complete cohort. Fourteen percent of patients had preoperative sclerotherapy without a difference in complication profile. Ultimately, this study reflected that despite emerging first-line roles of pharmacotherapy and sclerotherapy, surgery remains important in treatment of all subtypes of LMs with a manageable side-effect profile and improved patient satisfaction [30]. Although only 3% of patients were on sirolimus therapy at the time of surgery, other studies have not found an increase in postoperative complications while on this immunosuppressive therapy [31].

Anatomic considerations

Cervicofacial lymphatic malformations (CFLMs) are the most common and best-studied anatomic LM subtype. Cyst type correlates with location–midline and oral cavity lesions tend to be microcystic, whereas parotid and submandibular lesions have also been described as macrocystic and mixed [6,7,32]. Some studies report more macrocystic lesions occur below the level of the mylohyoid compared with microcystic lesions, which occur above the mylohyoid [7]. Pretreatment imaging and clinicoradiologic staging include consideration of laterality and involvement of critical structures, which predicts operative risk and surgical outcome [33]. Endoscopy may be used to evaluate the airway along with US and MRI [34].

Traditional management has favored surgical resection with indications such as palpable mass, rapid growth, cosmesis, dysphagia, macroglossia, nerve palsy, dysphonia, malocclusion, bleeding, infection, and airway compromise [11,34].

However, sclerotherapy has emerged as an equally effective and less morbid alternative for management of CFLMs [35–38]. The 2021 systematic review and meta-analysis of Embrechts and colleagues [6] reviewed 1573 patients with CFLM and did not find differences in volume reduction between sclerotherapy and surgery; however, linear regression did show positive predictors for volume reduction with surgery and macrocystic lesions compared with sclerotherapy and microcystic lesions. This is likely because the feasibility of sclerotherapy depends on the size of cystic lesions–if the cyst is small and cannot be drained, then the sclerosant is diluted, and if injected into discontinuous cysts, the sclerosant may not propagate. Given this challenge, the Vascular Anomalies Center at Children's Hospital Los Angeles after institutional review describes a multidisciplinary treatment algorithm for treating CFLM (Fig. 3) [34].

This group recommends upfront sclerotherapy for most lesions and as first-line for macrocystic disease; however, upfront surgical debulking for neonates with massive CFLM should be considered to reduce disease burden [34]. If the anatomy of the CFLM involves the facial nerve, expert consensus opinion also recommends upfront surgical resection without preoperative sclerotherapy given increased risk of scarring, complicated dissection, and facial nerve palsy. Macrocystic lesions are preferentially treated with doxycycline, and microcystic lesions are preferentially treated with bleomycin. Larger and deep lesions may undergo drain placement for serial treatments. If lesions fail to improve, sirolimus therapy is considered, and then surgical resection can be performed if lesion burden is persistent [34].

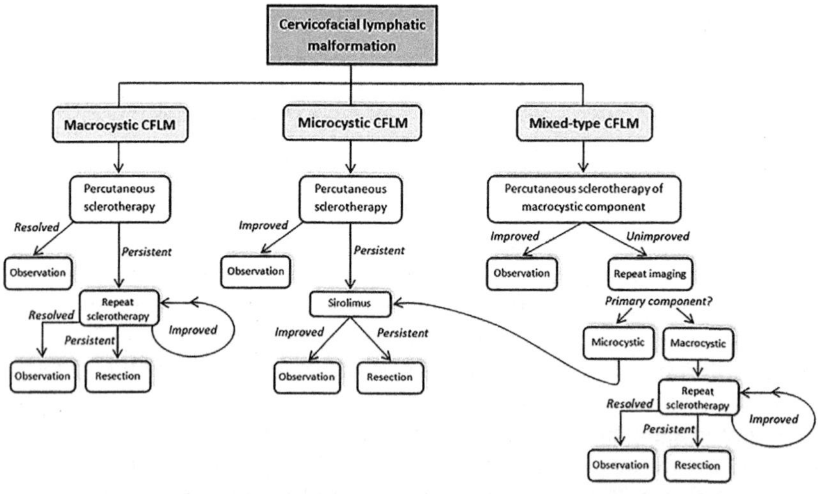

Fig. 3. Treatment algorithm: a multidisciplinary treatment algorithm based on the type of CFLM. (*From* Zobel MJ, Nowicki D, Gomez G, et al. Management of cervicofacial lymphatic malformations requires a multidisciplinary approach. J Pediatr Surg. 2021;56(5):1062–7. https://doi.org/10.1016/j.jpedsurg.2020.09.017.)

CFLM complications and mortality, noted to be 3.4% to 5.7%, increase with complex, extensive, multifocal disease, with microcystic and mixed lesions, and particularly with those that involve the airway. Permanent nerve injury has been reported along with long-term complications specific to the head and neck anatomy, such as malocclusion, dysphagia, and permanent tracheostomy [6,9,11]. Sirolimus has been shown to improve symptoms and volume reduction for large, complicated lesions [39].

Abdominal and retroperitoneal LMs have also been managed historically with surgical resection, although staging and completeness of resection vary. Symptoms can include abdominal pain, nausea/vomiting, palpable mass, obstruction, volvulus, and intralesional hemorrhage [40]. Complete resection may not be possible with extensive retroperitoneal involvement. Complications from resection include mortality, chylous ascites, obstruction, bleeding, and infection. A multidisciplinary approach and algorithm for abdominal LMs are summarized in Fig. 4. Macrocystic lesions are managed with sclerotherapy as a first-line treatment, with options to repeat sclerotherapy treatment if indicated or surgical resection if LM fails to improve and remains symptomatic. Symptomatic microcystic LMs are treated best with medical therapy (sirolimus or alpelisib); however, surgical resection may be needed if medical treatment is unsatisfactory. For mixed lesions, management depends on the dominant cystic type, with sclerotherapy recommended for the macrocystic component, and

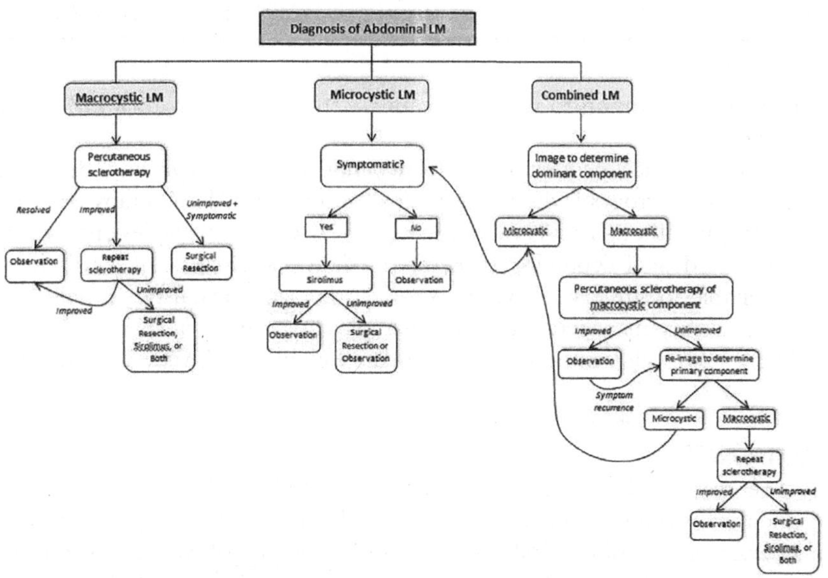

Fig. 4. Treatment algorithm: proposed abdominal LM treatment algorithm using a multidisciplinary approach. (*From* Zamora AK, Barry WE, Nowicki D, et al. A multidisciplinary approach to management of abdominal lymphatic malformations. J Pediatr Surg. 2021;56 (8):1425–9. https://doi.org/10.1016/j.jpedsurg.2020.10.007.)

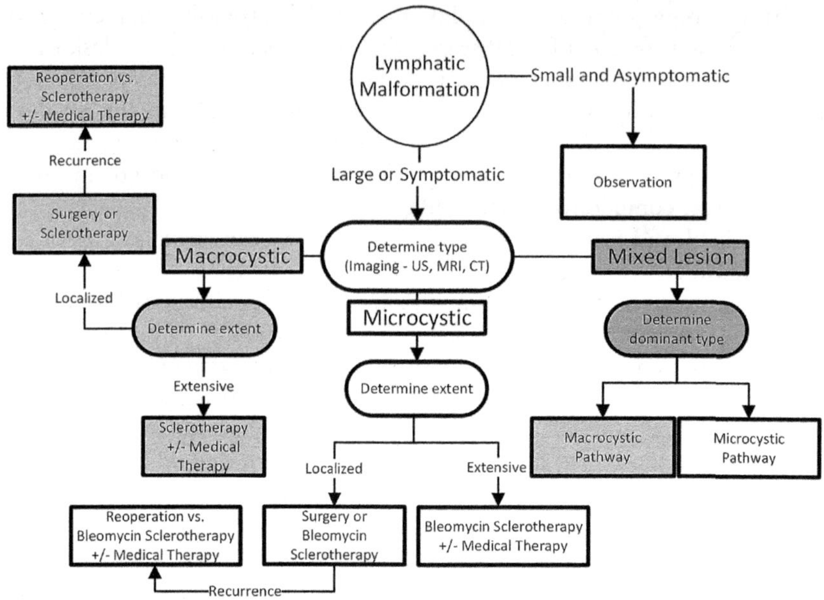

Fig. 5. Treatment algorithm: algorithm for management of LMs in children. (*From* Huerta CT, Beres AL, Englum BR, et al. Management and Outcomes of Pediatric Lymphatic Malformations: A Systematic Review From the APSA Outcomes and Evidence-Based Practice Committee. J Pediatr Surg. 2024;59(10):161589. https://doi.org/10.1016/j.jpedsurg.2024.05.019.)

ultimately, progression to medical treatment, resection, or both if LM fails to improve [41].

Ultimately, management of LMs depends on cyst type and degree of localization. Macrocystic disease responds favorably to sclerotherapy and medical therapy, although surgical resection can be beneficial for lesions that are well localized or if debulking is required. Microcystic disease if localized can be amenable to surgery; however, again, if disease is extensive, it will likely be concurrently managed with sclerotherapy and/or medical therapy.

APSA's 2024 algorithm for management of childhood LMs [11] is shown in Fig. 5.

SUMMARY

LMs represent a diverse group of congenital lymphatic disorders whose management has evolved dramatically with the advent of molecularly targeted therapies. Recognition of the PI3K/AKT/mTOR signaling pathway as a key driver of pathogenesis has transformed treatment, with sirolimus and alpelisib now complementing traditional procedural options.

Successful management demands multidisciplinary collaboration, integrating medical, interventional, and surgical involvement, and expertise. Treatment selection should consider lesion type, anatomic site, and symptom burden, with the goal of preserving function and quality of life rather than achieving radiographic cure. Continued research into genotype-driven therapy, biomarker development, and long-term outcomes will further refine care for this complex and heterogeneous disease.

CLINICS CARE POINTS

- Pearls: Presentations are variable: Lymphatic malformations (LMs) vary widely by location and cyst type and may present as soft, compressible masses, skin discoloration, oral lesions, or incidental radiographic findings making diagnosis challenging. A high index of suspicion is required, particularly for slowly enlarging or intermittently inflamed lesions.
- Early referral matters: Patients benefit from early referral to specialized vascular anomalies centers, where multidisciplinary teams can guide appropriate imaging, surveillance, and treatment planning. Early involvement may prevent complications such as airway compromise, functional impairment, or disfigurement.
- Use the right imaging: Ultrasound is an appropriate initial study while MRI is preferred for definitive diagnosis, subtype characterization and procedural planning. Routine CT should be avoided.
- Rapid growth is usually inflammatory: Acute enlargement is commonly triggered by infection, trauma, or hemorrhage rather than malignant transformation.
- Airway and feeding symptoms are urgent: Cervicofacial LMs associated with stridor, dysphagia, or feeding difficulty require prompt multidisciplinary evaluation.
- Treatment is not surgical by default: Surgery is no longer first-line therapy for many LMs. Medical therapy (eg, sirolimus, alpelisib) and sclerotherapy often offer effective, less invasive options, particularly for extensive or complex disease.
- Pitfalls: Misdiagnosis is common: LMs are frequently mistaken for infection, hematoma, or branchial cleft cyst. Recurrent swelling or poor response to antibiotics should prompt reconsideration of the diagnosis.
- Observation requires judgment: While some LMs remain stable, progressive symptoms, recurrent infection, or functional impairment warrant more urgent intervention.

Disclosure

The authors have no commercial or financial disclosures.

References

[1] Steiner JE, Drolet BA. Classification of vascular anomalies: an update. Semin Interv Radiol 2017;34(3):225–32.
[2] Fishman SJ, Young AE. Slow-flow vascular malformations. In: Mulliken JB, Burrows PE, Fishman SJ, editors. Mulliken and young's vascular anomalies. Oxford University Press; 2013. p. 562–94; https://doi.org/10.1093/med/9780195145052.003.0014.

[3] ISSVA Classification of Vascular Anomalies ©2025 International Society for the Study of Vascular Anomalies. Available at: "issva.org/classification". Accessed October 1 2025.
[4] Defnet AM, Bagrodia N, Hernandez SL, et al. Pediatric lymphatic malformations: evolving understanding and therapeutic options. Pediatr Surg Int 2016;32(5):425–33.
[5] Snyder EJ, Sarma A, Borst AJ, et al. Lymphatic anomalies in children: update on imaging diagnosis, genetics, and treatment. Am J Roentgenol 2022;218(6):1089–101.
[6] Embrechts JLA, Hiddinga S, Bot JC, et al. Surgery versus sclerotherapy versus combined therapy in head and neck lymphatic malformations in the pediatric population: systematic review and meta-analysis. Eur Arch Oto-Rhino-Laryngol Off J Eur Fed Oto-Rhino-Laryngol Soc EUFOS Affil Ger Soc Oto-Rhino-Laryngol - Head Neck Surg 2024;281(9):4529–39.
[7] Elluru RG, Balakrishnan K, Padua HM. Lymphatic malformations: diagnosis and management. Semin Pediatr Surg 2014;23(4):178–85.
[8] Zhang C, Liu J, Wang Y, et al. Lymphatic malformation: classification, pathogenesis, and therapeutic strategies. Ann Vasc Surg 2025;121:35–46.
[9] Fransén J, Frisk S, Ghaffarpour N. Lymphatic malformations revisited: genetics, clinics and future directions. Presse Med 2025;54(3):104293; https://doi.org/10.1016/j.lpm.2025.104293.
[10] Kulungowski AM, Patel M. Lymphatic malformations. Semin Pediatr Surg 2020;29(5):150971; https://doi.org/10.1016/j.sempedsurg.2020.150971.
[11] Huerta CT, Beres AL, Englum BR, et al. Management and outcomes of pediatric lymphatic malformations: a systematic review from the APSA outcomes and evidence-based practice committee. J Pediatr Surg 2024;59(10):161589; https://doi.org/10.1016/j.jpedsurg.2024.05.019.
[12] Petkova M, Ferby I, Mäkinen T. Lymphatic malformations: mechanistic insights and evolving therapeutic frontiers. J Clin Investig 2024;134(6):e172844; https://doi.org/10.1172/JCI172844.
[13] Burrows PE, Mason KP. Percutaneous treatment of low flow vascular malformations. J Vasc Interv Radiol JVIR 2004;15(5):431–45.
[14] Luks VL, Kamitaki N, Vivero MP, et al. Lymphatic and other vascular malformative/overgrowth disorders are caused by somatic mutations in PIK3CA. J Pediatr 2015;166(4):1048–54, e1-5.
[15] Zenner K, Cheng CV, Jensen DM, et al. Genotype correlates with clinical severity in PIK3CA-associated lymphatic malformations. JCI Insight 2019;4(21):129884; https://doi.org/10.1172/jci.insight.129884:e129884.
[16] Zenner K, Jensen DM, Dmyterko V, et al. Somatic activating BRAF variants cause isolated lymphatic malformations. HGG Adv 2022;3(2):100101; https://doi.org/10.1016/j.xhgg.2022.100101.
[17] Zenner K, Jensen DM, Cook TT, et al. Cell-free DNA as a diagnostic analyte for molecular diagnosis of vascular malformations. Genet Med Off J Am Coll Med Genet 2021;23(1):123–30.
[18] Maruani A, Tavernier E, Boccara O, et al. Sirolimus (Rapamycin) for slow-flow malformations in children: the observational-phase randomized clinical PERFORMUS trial. JAMA Dermatol 2021;157(11):1289–98.
[19] Ji Y, Chen S, Yang K, et al. A prospective multicenter study of sirolimus for complicated vascular anomalies. J Vasc Surg 2021;74(5):1673–81.e3.
[20] Hammill AM, Wentzel M, Gupta A, et al. Sirolimus for the treatment of complicated vascular anomalies in children. Pediatr Blood Cancer 2011;57(6):1018–24.
[21] Adams DM, Trenor CC, Hammill AM, et al. Efficacy and safety of sirolimus in the treatment of complicated vascular anomalies. Pediatrics 2016;137(2):e20153257; https://doi.org/10.1542/peds.2015-3257.
[22] Canaud G, Lopez Gutierrez JC, Irvine AD, et al. Alpelisib for treatment of patients with PIK3CA-related overgrowth spectrum (PROS). Genet Med Off J Am Coll Med Genet 2023;25(12):100969; https://doi.org/10.1016/j.gim.2023.100969.

[23] Wenger TL, Ganti S, Bull C, et al. Alpelisib for the treatment of PIK3CA-related head and neck lymphatic malformations and overgrowth. Genet Med Off J Am Coll Med Genet 2022;24(11):2318–28.
[24] Delestre F, Venot Q, Bayard C, et al. Alpelisib administration reduced lymphatic malformations in a mouse model and in patients. Sci Transl Med 2021;13(614):eabg0809; https://doi.org/10.1126/scitranslmed.abg0809.
[25] Venot Q, Blanc T, Rabia SH, et al. Targeted therapy in patients with PIK3CA-related overgrowth syndrome. Nature 2018;558(7711):540–6.
[26] Shaheen MF, Tse JY, Sokol ES, et al. Genomic landscape of lymphatic malformations: a case series and response to the PI3Kα inhibitor alpelisib in an N-of-1 clinical trial. eLife 2022;11: e74510; https://doi.org/10.7554/eLife.74510.
[27] Mäkinen T, Boon LM, Vikkula M, et al. Lymphatic malformations: Genetics, mechanisms and therapeutic strategies. Circ Res 2021;129(1):136–54.
[28] Motz KM, Nickley KB, Bedwell JR, et al. OK432 versus doxycycline for treatment of macrocystic lymphatic malformations. Ann Otol Rhinol Laryngol 2014;123(2):81–8.
[29] Smith MC, Zimmerman MB, Burke DK, et al. Efficacy and safety of OK-432 immunotherapy of lymphatic malformations. Laryngoscope 2009;119(1):107–15.
[30] Keane OA, O'Guinn ML, Adams S, et al. Short-term postoperative complications of lymphatic malformation surgical excision: a 20-Year institutional review. J Pediatr Surg 2025;60(3):162146; https://doi.org/10.1016/j.jpedsurg.2024.162146.
[31] Mehl SC, Whitlock RS, Ortega RM, et al. No association of sirolimus with wound complications in children with vascular anomalies. J Pediatr Surg 2023;58(8):1555–9.
[32] de Serres LM, Sie KC, Richardson MA. Lymphatic malformations of the head and neck. A proposal for staging. Arch Otolaryngol Head Neck Surg 1995;121(5):577–82.
[33] Perkins JA, Manning SC, Tempero RM, et al. Lymphatic malformations: review of current treatment. Otolaryngol–Head Neck Surg Off J Am Acad Otolaryngol-Head Neck Surg 2010;142(6):795–803, 803.e1.
[34] Zobel MJ, Nowicki D, Gomez G, et al. Management of cervicofacial lymphatic malformations requires a multidisciplinary approach. J Pediatr Surg 2021;56(5):1062–7.
[35] De Maria L, De Sanctis P, Balakrishnan K, et al. Sclerotherapy for lymphatic malformations of head and neck: systematic review and meta-analysis. J Vasc Surg Venous Lymphat Disord 2020;8(1):154–64.
[36] Cahill AM, Nijs E, Ballah D, et al. Percutaneous sclerotherapy in neonatal and infant head and neck lymphatic malformations: a single center experience. J Pediatr Surg 2011;46(11):2083–95.
[37] Cheng J. Doxycycline sclerotherapy in children with head and neck lymphatic malformations. J Pediatr Surg 2015;50(12):2143–6.
[38] Nehra D, Jacobson L, Barnes P, et al. Doxycycline sclerotherapy as primary treatment of head and neck lymphatic malformations in children. J Pediatr Surg 2008;43(3):451–60.
[39] Wiegand S, Dietz A, Wichmann G. Efficacy of sirolimus in children with lymphatic malformations of the head and neck. Eur Arch Oto-Rhino-Laryngol Off J Eur Fed Oto-Rhino-Laryngol Soc EUFOS Affil Ger Soc Oto-Rhino-Laryngol - Head Neck Surg 2022;279(8):3801–10.
[40] Lin JI, Fisher J, Caty MG. Newborn intraabdominal cystic lymphatic malformations. Semin Pediatr Surg 2000;9(3):141–5.
[41] Zamora AK, Barry WE, Nowicki D, et al. A multidisciplinary approach to management of abdominal lymphatic malformations. J Pediatr Surg 2021;56(8):1425–9.

ELSEVIER

Advances in Pediatrics 73 (2026) 269–282

ADVANCES IN PEDIATRICS

Pediatric Brain Tumors

Simone M. Chang, MBBS[a,*],
Michael Angelo C. Huang, MD[b], Mustafa Barbour, MD[c]

[a]Department of Pediatrics, Division of Pediatric Hematology–Oncology, University of South Florida Morsani School of Medicine, Tampa, FL, USA; [b]The Brain Tumor Center at Siteman Cancer Center, Washington University Medical Center, St. Louis, MO, USA; [c]Department of Pediatrics, Division of Pediatric Hematology–Oncology and Stem Cell Transplant, University of Louisville School of Medicine, Louisville, KY, USA

Keywords

• Brain tumors • Low-grade glioma • Medulloblastoma • Targeted therapy

Key points

- Brain tumors are the most common solid malignancy and the leading cause of cancer-related death in children.
- Clinical presentation varies by age and tumor location. Persistent headaches, vomiting, visual and neurologic deficits should heighten suspicion for consideration of a brain tumor.
- A team-based, multidisciplinary approach is ideal for diagnosis and management.
- Treatment and prognosis depend on tumor type, molecular features, and extent of resection.
- Long-term follow-up is critical to monitor for recurrence and late effects. Survivors require structured surveillance and multidisciplinary care.

INTRODUCTION

Pediatric brain tumors are the most common solid malignancy in children, with an incidence of 6.05 per 100,000 in the United States. There has been dramatic progress in the overall survival for children with cancer due to the decline in leukemia mortality over the last several decades. However, patients with primary central nervous system (CNS) tumors have only seen a modest improvement in survival. Not only have they emerged as the leading

*Corresponding author. Department of Pediatrics, Division of Pediatric Hematology-Oncology, University of South Florida Morsani College of Medicine, 13101 Bruce B. Downs Boulevard, Tampa, FL 33612. *E-mail address:* schang2@usf.edu

https://doi.org/10.1016/j.yapd.2025.11.002
0065-3101/25/

Abbreviations

CNS	central nervous system
CSF	cerebrospinal fluid
ICP	intracranial pressure
MTOR	mammalian target of rapamycin
PFS	progression-free survival
pLGG/GNTs	pediatric low-grade gliomas and glioneuronal tumors
RT	radiation therapy
SHH	Sonic Hedgehog
WHO	World Health Organization

cause of cancer-related mortality for children but also the treatment of these tumors results in significant morbidity with a decrease in the quality of life for both patients and their families [1].

Making the initial diagnosis of a brain tumor can be difficult, as signs and symptoms can be highly variable and mistaken for more commonly seen disorders. There are also cases where these lesions are effectively undetectable and may go unrecognized until a tumor is large or disseminated [2]. Our goal is for this review to be a practical overview of pediatric CNS tumors for pediatricians, and we hope to create a greater awareness of clinical manifestations and red flag symptoms that may allow for earlier referral and diagnosis. It will also provide updates regarding classification, targeted treatments, and early and late effects associated with management.

EPIDEMIOLOGY AND RISK FACTORS

In the United States, the incidence of childhood brain tumors varies with age, sex, race, and ethnicity. The highest incidence is in the adolescent population (7.26 per 100,000), which is closely followed by children aged less than 14 years (5.61 per 100,000). There is a slight male predominance, and the incidence is highest in the Caucasian population [1].

The etiology of most childhood brain tumors remains unknown; however, there are 2 established risk factors for the development of a CNS tumor in children:

1. Exposure to ionizing radiation [3].
2. Genetic predisposition syndromes [3,4] (Table 1).

CLINICAL PRESENTATION

The clinical manifestations of pediatric CNS tumors are often subtle, nonspecific, with no single clinical finding that is pathognomonic. Signs and symptoms can vary according to the child's age and location of the tumor, and it may be the direct result of tumor infiltration into an adjacent structure or as a result of impaired cerebrospinal fluid (CSF) flow leading to increased intracranial pressure (ICP) [5].

Table 1
Genetic predisposition syndromes and associated brain tumors

Genetic Syndromes	Associated Brain Tumors	Genes Involved
Neurofibromatosis type 1	Low-grade glioma including optic pathway gliomas	NF1
Neurofibromatosis type 2	Spinal ependymoma	NF2
Tuberous sclerosis	Subependymal giant cell astrocytoma	TSC1 and TSC2
Li Fraumeni	High grade glioma Sonic Hedgehog (SHH) medulloblastoma	TP53
Rhabdoid tumor predisposition syndrome 1/2	Atypical teratoid rhabdoid tumor and extracranial malignant rhabdoid tumor	SMARCB1 and SMARCA4
Retinoblastoma	Pineoblastoma	RB1
DICER-1 related tumor predisposition		DICER
Familial adenomatous polyposis	Medulloblastoma • Wingless medullo-blastoma (WNT-MB)	Adenomatous polyposis coli (APC)
Gorlin syndrome (nevoid basal cell carcinoma syndrome)	• SHH-Medulloblastoma	Patched 1 (PTCH1) and suppressor of fused homolog (SUFU)

Data from Hansford, J. R., et al. (2024). *Update on Cancer Predisposition Syndromes and Surveillance Guidelines for Childhood Brain Tumors. Clinical Cancer Research, 30*(11), 2342–350 [4].

Infants

Infants pose unique challenges for diagnosis. Unfused cranial sutures allow for the accommodation of rising ICP without acute changes in neurologic status; these patients frequently present with macrocephaly and a tense fontanelle. Infants and young children have difficulty expressing the source of their discomfort and are more likely to present with irritability. Other symptoms that may arise in infancy are failure to thrive, developmental delay or regression, and seizures [2,5].

Rare presentations in infancy include the *diencephalic syndrome*, which is characterized by profound failure to thrive despite normal or only slightly reduced caloric intake; this syndrome is typically accompanied by preserved or even accelerated linear growth, hyperactivity and euphoria. This is usually associated with hypothalamic tumors, and often they are low-grade gliomas [6–8]. *Parinaud syndrome* (another rare presentation) is a constellation of neuro-ocular findings that are associated with pineal or midbrain tumors, which include the setting-sun sign (seemingly forced downward deviation of the eyes), pupils that are middilated and poorly reactive to light, convergence or retraction nystagmus, and eyelid retraction [9].

Children

Headache is the most common manifestation of CNS tumors, occurring in approximately one-third of affected children. Headaches associated with CNS tumors generally are attributed to increased ICP. These headaches are typically described as an early morning headache that is relieved by vomiting. Depending on the location, the mass effect of the tumor may lead to impaired CSF drainage and increased ICP that is exacerbated while recumbent. This increase in ICP is responsible for the well-described diurnal variation in headache, which will usually improve throughout the day as the patient is upright [10].

Interestingly, many children do not present with these classic symptoms. Wilne and colleagues [2,5] showed that in children with brain tumors presenting with headaches, approximately 40% of headaches occurred during the daytime, early evening, or were continuous. Importantly, pediatricians should also remain mindful of headaches that remain persistent over time and increase in severity and frequency, as this is also a red flag symptom.

Other clinical manifestations include problems with balance, coordination and walking, abnormal eye movements with and without head tilt, visual disturbances, behavioral changes/educational difficulties, and seizures.

Teenagers

Because adolescents and young adults have less contact with their parents than younger children, early diagnosis can be problematic. Similar to children, they typically have persistent or recurrent headaches and vomiting, problems with balance, coordination and/or walking, abnormal eye movements and blurred/double vision, behavioral changes and seizures. Delayed or arrested puberty and slow growth are more specific to this age group [2,5].

Table 2 shows presentations based upon location.

DIAGNOSTIC APPROACH AND MOLECULAR PROFILING

For an unstable child who presents in the ER and for whom there is concern for a brain tumor, a computed tomographic scan is the most appropriate first choice to rule out emergencies such as acute hydrocephalus with impending herniation or hemorrhage. However, conventional MRI with and without contrast is the cornerstone for initial evaluation. MRI allows for a more accurate characterization of the tumor itself and the surrounding anatomy, and it does not expose children to ionizing radiation. In selected cases, spine imaging and lumbar puncture are performed to determine if metastatic disease is present.

Advanced MRI techniques can help to characterize pediatric brain tumors and can be useful for neurosurgical planning [11]; however, biopsy and tissue analysis are needed for establishing a diagnosis in most cases.

The use of next-generation sequencing and methylation profiling can now provide insight into the broad molecular heterogeneity of pediatric brain tumors, and it has become pivotal in identifying important genes and signaling pathways that drive tumor proliferation. This integration of novel molecular diagnostic tools has revolutionized the diagnosis of pediatric CNS tumors

Table 2
Clinical signs and symptoms of brain tumors in children based upon the location

Location	Constellation of Signs and Symptoms
Cerebral cortex	Seizures, headaches, focal signs of hemiparesis, hemisensory deficits, visual field disturbances, and language dysfunction
Midline (hypothalamus, pituitary, optic pathway, and pineal region)	Precocious puberty, short stature, diabetes insipidus, visual acuity abnormalities, and field defects Parinaud syndrome (impaired upward gaze, pupillary light-near dissociation, and convergence-retraction nystagmus) Diencephalic syndrome
Posterior fossa	Headache, nausea and vomiting, gait ataxia and coordination problems, papilledema. Dysarthria and nystagmus
Brainstem	Cranial nerve palsies, pyramidal signs, gait and coordination disturbances, nystagmus, focal motor weakness, headaches and papilledema
Spinal cord	Back pain, abnormal gait or coordination, spinal deformity, urinary or stool incontinence, and extremity weakness

Data from "The presenting features of brain tumors: a review of 200 cases," by S. H. Wilne, R. C. Ferris, A. Nathwani, et al, 2006, Archives of Disease in Childhood, 91(6), 502–06. https://doi.org/10.1136/adc.2005.090266 [2].

and is now critical for classification and for identifying potential targets for treatment. Due to these advancements in molecular analyses, pediatric tumors are now covered in separate sections of the fifth edition of the *WHO Classification of Tumors of the Central Nervous System* and in the inaugural World Health Organization (WHO) classification of Pediatric Tumors [12].

PRINCIPLES OF MANAGEMENT

Treatment involves a multidisciplinary team and includes pediatric neuro-oncology, neurosurgery, radiation oncology, pathology, neurology, endocrinology, ophthalmology, neuropsychology, genetic counseling, physical medicine and rehabilitation, palliative care, and social work.

Surgery

The goal of surgery usually involves maximal safe resection, as the degree of tumor resection correlates with improvement in outcomes, and surgery allows relief of hydrocephalus if present [13]. However, gross total resection is not always feasible if tumors are present in eloquent regions (primary motor and sensory cortices, cortical language areas [Broca's area and Wernicke's area]), visual cortex, internal capsule, basal ganglia and thalamus [14]) as resection may lead to significant morbidity and mortality. In these cases, biopsy is strongly recommended to verify histology and perform molecular testing. Fig. 1 displays the locations of common subtypes of pediatric tumors.

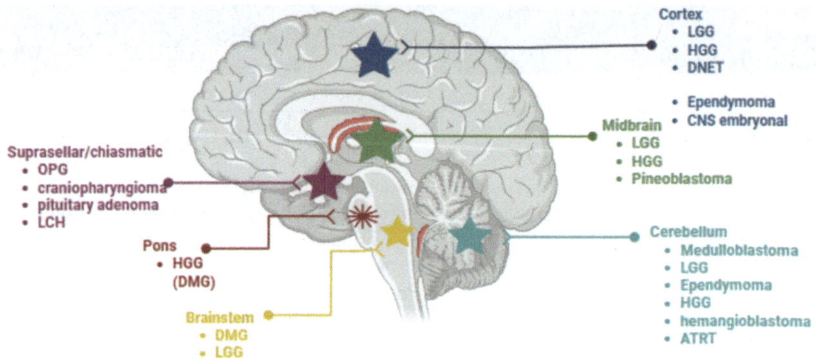

Fig. 1. Common pediatric brain tumor subtypes according to location. (Created in BioRender. Maharaj, S. (2026) https://BioRender.com/im211hl)

Surgical complications can include hemorrhage, infection, hydrocephalus, ischemic injury, and seizures. Neuroendocrine disorders and vision impairment may be seen after resection of supratentorial tumors, while cerebellar mutism can be seen in up to 25% of children after resection of midline posterior fossa tumors. Cerebellar mutism consists of absence of speech, emotional lability, hypotonia and ataxia, usually beginning 1 or 2 days after tumor resection. It can be partially or completely reversible over weeks to months [15].

Radiation therapy

Radiation therapy (RT) is a vital component of curative as well as palliative therapy. RT is typically avoided in children aged less than 3 years because of the risk of severe neurocognitive sequelae on the developing brain.

Efforts to mitigate the serious long-term side effects associated with RT have led to the development of novel agents, dosages, and delivery strategies. The 2 major forms of RT for pediatric brain tumors are high-energy photons and, more recently, protons.

Adverse effects are divided temporally as follows:

- Acute: occur during treatment and include headaches, nausea, and drowsiness.
- Subacute: occur a few weeks to 2 months after RT and include somnolence syndrome (extreme sleepiness, signs of increased ICP, headaches, nausea, vomiting and irritability [16], and focal neurologic defects).
- Late: occur several months to years after RT and are generally irreversible, and usually include diffuse white matter injury, vasculopathy and secondary malignancies, impaired neurocognitive function, and social and behavioral deficits.

Due to these adverse effects, the use of RT is cautiously considered in pediatric patients with CNS tumors. Proton therapy has emerged as a preferred RT modality for some pediatric CNS tumors. The delivery of proton therapy allows for lower doses/less scatter to surrounding normal tissues and has thus resulted in reductions in some of the acute and long-term effects:

- Reduction in acute effects by increased tolerance of concurrent and adjuvant chemotherapy (eg, decrease in hematologic and gastrointestinal toxicities) [17].
- Reduction in long-term effects by decreasing the risk of neurocognitive, endocrine, vascular, and developmental sequelae, as well as the risk of secondary malignancies due to RT [17,18].

Chemotherapy

Adjuvant chemotherapy also plays an important role in the management of childhood brain tumors and has become essential for improving the treatment of some tumors. Chemotherapeutic agents have been extensively evaluated, and enrollment in an open clinical trial is considered standard of care. Chemotherapeutic and novel targeted agents are constantly evolving with the changing landscape of our understanding of these tumors in recent years.

- Conventional chemotherapy: targets various phases of the cell cycle to interfere with DNA synthesis and mitosis.
- High-dose chemotherapy with stem cell rescue: uses myeloablative chemotherapy to achieve greater CNS penetration at the cost of irreversible bone marrow failure. Autologous stem cell support prevents lethal bone marrow toxicity. Used in children aged less than 3 years to forgo RT.
- Metronomic chemotherapy: the use of frequent, repetitive, low-dose, orally administered medications that target tumor angiogenesis.
- Targeted therapy: targets specific molecular alterations that drive the neoplastic process.

Current chemotherapy protocols focus on maximizing the therapeutic benefits while minimizing the toxicities associated with these medications. With growing knowledge of signaling pathways driving tumor proliferation, targeted therapies aimed at specific mutations may help replace some medications and decrease both acute and long-term adverse effects associated with chemotherapy [19].

Complications of chemotherapy regimens can include

- Myelosuppression: neutropenia, thrombocytopenia, anemia with need for transfusions, and increased risk for infection.
- Gastrointestinal toxicities: nausea, vomiting, and diarrhea.
- Ototoxicity: secondary to platinum-based chemotherapy.
- Nephrotoxicity: secondary to platinum-based chemotherapy. Appropriate hydration and avoidance of concurrent nephrotoxic agents must be provided.
- Neuropathy: vincristine-induced motor and sensory polyneuropathy.

PEDIATRIC LOW-GRADE GLIOMAS

Pediatric low-grade gliomas and glioneuronal tumors (pLGG/GNTs) account for about a third of pediatric CNS neoplasms, thus representing the largest subset of brain tumors in children [20]. pLGG can occur in any location in the brain and spinal cord but they are most commonly localized to the diencephalon (32%), cerebral hemispheres (27%), and cerebellum (26%) [1]. Over the past decades, the development of novel molecular techniques has led to revolutionary insights into the genetic drivers of these tumors, and it has improved our understanding of LGGs as a diverse group of tumors that still have significant morphologic overlap. In the 2021 WHO, the pLGG/GNTs group has been subclassified into 3 different families: pediatric-type diffuse low-grade gliomas, circumscribed astrocytic gliomas, and glioneuronal and neuronal tumors [21,22].

The mainstay of therapy for progressive or symptomatic pLGG is complete surgical resection whenever feasible. Many LGGs, however, are in areas where they cannot be safely resected without resulting in substantial morbidity. Tumors that progress after resection or residual tumors and that result in symptoms often require adjuvant therapy. While overall survival rates are excellent, progression-free survival (PFS) varies significantly depending on the extent of tumor resection. Ten-year PFS exceeds 85% in patients with tumors that have undergone gross total resection but drops to less than 50% in patients with residual disease.

Although RT is an effective treatment option for pLGG, it can lead to significant morbidities, including cognitive decline, endocrinopathies, growth retardation, vasculopathies, and secondary malignancy. This is especially true for patients with the NF1 gene in whom the risk of secondary malignancies and vasculopathy is higher [23]. Since the 1980s, chemotherapy has been used to avoid or delay the need for RT for these patients. However, RT should still be considered in patients with rapidly worsening clinical symptoms that may be difficult to control with other therapies [24]. RT can be used for recurrent or residual pLGG with improved PFS, but it comes at the cost of associated long-term toxicities [25–27]. Moreover, chemotherapy is currently used as upfront therapy for young children with pLGG that requires treatment in an effort to avoid or delay the use of RT.

Traditional chemotherapy regimens include either vincristine/carboplatin or a combination of thioguanine, procarbazine, lomustine, and vincristine as first-line therapy. Investigations of the molecular underpinnings of pLGG show that the majority is defined by alterations in the mitogen-activated protein kinase pathway through KIAA1549-BRAF fusions or through BRAFV600E point mutations. Additional pathways affected include the mammalian target of rapamycin (MTOR); pLGGs can also harbor fibroblast growth factor receptor alterations. This has led to the investigation of numerous novel treatment agents targeting these pathways in children with recurrent or newly diagnosed pLGGs.

Examples of targeted treatments include

- *MEK* inhibitors: for example, selumetinib and mirdametinib for the treatment of plexiform neurofibromas in NF1 [28,29] and trametinib monotherapy for recurrent and progressive pLGG [30,31].
- *BRAF* inhibitors: dabrafenib, vemurafenib, tovorafenib—approved for combination therapy with mitogen-activated protein kinase kinase (MEK) inhibitors in pLGG harboring BRAFV600E mutations [32].

- *MTOR* inhibitors: everolimus for the treatment of tuberous sclerosis complex associated-subependymal giant cell astrocytomas [33].

HIGH-GRADE GLIOMAS

Pediatric diffuse high-grade glioma represents approximately 9.5% of all primary malignant and nonmalignant brain and other CNS tumors diagnosed in children and adolescents aged 19 years or younger [1]. Pediatric-type diffuse high-grade gliomas are now broadly subdivided into 4 different entities:

- Diffuse midline glioma, H3 K27-altered
- Diffuse hemispheric glioma, H3 G34-mutant
- Diffuse pediatric-type high-grade glioma, H3-wildtype and IDH-wildtype
- Infant-type hemispheric glioma

All of these tumors represent novel entities, which were first included in the 2021 WHO classification of CNS tumors [22]. The prognosis for aggressive diffuse high-grade gliomas is dismal, despite the use of combined modality therapies of surgery, RT, and systemic therapy.

Management relies heavily on safe maximal resection, which would allow for tissue diagnosis, molecular profiling, and relief of any symptoms from mass effect. This is followed by adjuvant therapy adapted to age, location and molecular features, with enrollment in a clinical trial as the standard of care when possible. If safe maximal resection is not feasible due to the location of the tumor, biopsy is still warranted. Management is multimodal and consists of radiation with or without temozolomide followed by adjuvant chemotherapy or targeted treatment (dordaviprone or inhibitors of murine sarcoma viral oncogene homolog B [BRAF], neurotrophic tyrosine receptor kinase [NTRK], or anaplastic lymphoma kinase [ALK] fusions) or enrollment in a clinical trial [12].

EPENDYMOMAS

Ependymomas are the third most common brain tumors of childhood and account for 5% to 10% of CNS tumors in children. Approximately 90% are intracranial, with about two-thirds occurring in the posterior fossa; the remaining 10% are spinal. The classification is based on a combination of clinical, histologic, immunohistochemical, and molecular features and subdivides ependymal tumors into 3 main groups, according to their location:

- Supratentorial: zinc finger translocation associated 1 (ZFTA1) fusion, yes-associated protein 1 (YAP1) fusion or supratentorial ependymoma NEC.
- Infratentorial: posterior fossa A and posterior fossa B.
- Spinal: spinal ependymoma, myelocytomatosis viral related oncogene, neuroblastoma derived (MYCN) amplified, myxopapillary [22].

The majority of pediatric ependymomas falls into the category of PF-A, which is associated with the worst outcomes. Safe maximal resection is the cornerstone of treatment. Older children with grade 2 or 3 tumors receive adjuvant conformal focal RT, while chemotherapy is used to delay irradiation in infants (<12 months) [34,35]. A role for maintenance chemotherapy has not been established after RT, but clinical trials are underway. Despite multimodal treatment, prognosis remains guarded with 10 year overall survival rates of 50% to 75%.

CENTRAL NERVOUS SYSTEM EMBRYONAL TUMORS

Medulloblastomas

Medulloblastomas are the most common malignant brain tumor of childhood, with approximately 324 children diagnosed each year in the United States [1]. The median age of diagnosis is around 7 years with a slight male predominance [1]. Patients commonly present with signs and symptoms of increased ICP due to a mass arising in the cerebellum and compressing the fourth ventricle.

Risk of disease is based upon the extent of disease, volume of postoperative residual tumor and the age of the patient at diagnosis [36].

The 2021 CNS WHO now recognizes that molecularly defined medulloblastomas contain 4 subtypes (Table 3).

Management consists of gross total resection; however, safe maximal resection is best if gross total resection is not an option. Families are encouraged to enroll their children in a molecular classification-based clinical trial, if available. Treatment of all different risk categories of disease consists of chemoradiation followed by maintenance chemotherapy [12]. For children aged less than 4 years, management consists of multiagent chemotherapy paired with autologous stem cell rescue as part of a clinical trial protocol. This regimen aims to

Table 3
Subtypes of Medulloblastoma and their characteristics

Subtype	Incidence	Location	Prognosis	Treatment Caveats
Wingless/ integrated WNT	10%	Cerebellar midline Peduncles and brainstem	10 y event free survival (EFS) >95%	Clinical trials exploring reduced dose craniospinal irradiation (CSI)
Sonic hedgehog SHH	3%–6%	Cerebellar hemisphere	TP53 mutated portend a poor prognosis	Potential for smoothened inhibitors (vismodegib)
Sonic hedgehog SHH	24%–27%	Cerebellar hemisphere	TP53 wildtype	
Non-WNT, Non SHH Group 3/4	60%	Cerebellar midline	5 y overall survival (OS) 50% 5 y OS 70%	May be some benefit to concurrent carboplatin with chemoRT

Data adapted from "Molecular subgroups of medulloblastoma: The current consensus," by M. D. Taylor, C. F. Northcott, A. Rutka, and colleagues, *Acta Neuropathologica* 2012, 123(4), 465–72. https://doi.org/10.1007/s00401-011-0922-z

delay or obviate RT, allowing the nervous system to develop and improving overall survival.

LONG-TERM MANAGEMENT AND SURVIVORSHIP

With improvement in treatments and outcomes for patients with brain tumors, pediatricians now care for many pediatric brain tumor survivors. Improved survival is, however, associated with considerable morbidity in long-term outcomes (health, neurocognitive, psychosocial, and adaptive behavior), with late effects emerging over time [37]. These children are often followed by the pediatrician along with long-term follow-up by an oncologist. They work together with other specialties, not just for surveillance and periodic evaluations, but to focus on promoting wellness and positive health behaviors (exercise and avoidance of smoking), addressing modifiable health risk factors and addressing barriers to care while fostering resilience [37].

Neurocognitive defects are among the most common adverse effects and can range from mild to severe. Survivors often experience deficits in intelligence quotient, processing speed, working memory, and academic performance. This leads to difficulties with educational and occupational functioning along with impaired independence in adulthood. Survivors are also at an increased risk for long-term psychological morbidities including depression, anxiety, suicidal ideation, and behavioral problems [38].

Endocrinological dysfunction is also prevalent in survivors after receiving cranial/spinal irradiation. They are also frequent in patients who have suprasellar masses. Hypothalamic–pituitary dysfunction is seen in a range of brain tumors in childhood with almost half having at least 1 endocrinopathy; the most common are hypothyroidism, growth hormone deficiency, precocious puberty, gonadotrophin-releasing hormone deficiency, and central adrenal insufficiency [39].

Neurologic late effects can include cerebrovascular disorders, stroke, moyamoya disease, and vasculopathies, as well as late occurring seizures. Motor impairment as well as hearing loss and vision problems are also increased compared to the general population.

Secondary malignancies are also increased in survivors, especially in patients exposed to radiation and alkylating agents [37].

Survivors of pediatric brain tumors require multidisciplinary care with surveillance for neurocognitive, endocrine, neurologic, psychosocial, and secondary cancers. Childhood cancer guidelines focused on late effects help provide a framework for surveillance, but ongoing collaboration among cancer specialists and general pediatricians is critical. Optimal management must promote the development of competencies to manage complex health care needs as well as support transitioning to adulthood.

SUMMARY

Pediatric brain tumors are the most common solid malignancy in children and adolescents and the leading cause of cancer-related mortality in this population.

Children present with headaches in combination with neurologic deficits. Pediatricians should have a high index of suspicion in children who have persistent and/or worsening headaches over time. Management requires a multidisciplinary approach, with treatment and prognosis determined by tumor type, molecular features, and extent of resection. Ongoing multidisciplinary follow-up is essential to monitor for recurrence, late effects, optimize quality of life, and integrate advances in molecularly targeted agents as the field continues to evolve.

CLINICS CARE POINTS

- Maintain a high index of suspicion in children with persistent and/or progressive neurologic symptoms (headaches, nausea, vomiting, visual changes, seizures, ataxia, or personality changes) that are accompanied by developmental regression in infants.
- Prompt neuroimaging is essential for children with concerning symptoms. MRI with and without contrast is the preferred modality of imaging.
- A team-based, multidisciplinary approach is ideal for diagnosis and management. Treatment and prognosis will depend on tumor type, molecular features, and extent of resection.
- Long-term follow-up is critical to monitor for recurrence and late effects. Survivors require structured surveillance and multidisciplinary care.

DECLARATION OF ARTIFICIAL INTELLIGENCE AND ARTIFICIAL INTELLIGENCE-ASSISTED TECHNOLOGIES IN THE WRITING PROCESS

During the preparation of this article, the authors used Gen AI. After using this tool/service, the authors reviewed and edited the content as needed and take full responsibility for the content of the publication.

References

[1] Price M, Ballard CAP, Benedetti JR, et al. CBTRUS statistical report: pediatric brain tumor foundation childhood and adolescent primary brain and other central nervous system tumors diagnosed in the United States in 2017-2021. Neuro Oncol 2025;27 (Supplement_1):i1–42.

[2] Wilne SH, Ferris RC, Nathwani A, et al. The presenting features of brain tumours: a review of 200 cases. Arch Dis Child 2006;91(6):502–6.

[3] Ostrom QT, Adel Fahmideh M, Cote DJ, et al. Risk factors for childhood and adult primary brain tumors. Neuro Oncol 2019;21(11):1357–75.

[4] Hansford JR, Das A, McGee RB, et al. Update on cancer predisposition syndromes and surveillance guidelines for childhood brain tumors. Clin Cancer Res 2024;30(11):2342–50.

[5] Wilne SH, Dineen RA, Dommett RM, et al. Identifying brain tumours in children and young adults. Br Med J 2013;347:f5844.

[6] Poussaint TY, Barnes PD, Nichols K, et al. Diencephalic syndrome: clinical features and imaging findings. AJNR Am J Neuroradiol 1997;18(8):1499–505.

[7] Stival A, Lucchesi M, Farina S, et al. An infant with hyperalertness, hyperkinesis, and failure to thrive: a rare diencephalic syndrome due to hypothalamic anaplastic astrocytoma. BMC Cancer 2015;15:616.
[8] Fleischman A, Brue C, Poussaint TY, et al. Diencephalic syndrome: a cause of failure to thrive and a model of partial growth hormone resistance. Pediatrics 2005;115(6):e742–8.
[9] Ivakhnitskaia E, Bhagat D. Neuro-ophthalmic sequelae of pediatric brain tumors. Semin Pediatr Neurol 2025;53:101182.
[10] The epidemiology of headache among children with brain tumor. Headache in children with brain tumors. The childhood brain tumor consortium. J Neuro Oncol 1991;10(1):31–46.
[11] Nikam RM, Yue X, Kaur G, et al. Advanced neuroimaging approaches to pediatric brain tumors. Cancers (Basel) 2022;14(14).
[12] Gajjar A, Mahajan A, Bale T, et al. Pediatric central nervous system cancers, version 2.2025, NCCN Clinical Practice Guidelines in oncology. J Natl Compr Canc Netw 2025;23(3):113–30.
[13] Souweidane MM. The evolving role of surgery in the management of pediatric brain tumors. J Child Neurol 2009;24(11):1366–74.
[14] Rammeloo E, Schouten JW, Krikour K, et al. Preoperative assessment of eloquence in neurosurgery: a systematic review. J Neuro Oncol 2023;165(3):413–30.
[15] Tailor J, Jackson EM. Brain and spinal cord tumors in children. Pediatr Clin North Am 2021;68(4):811–24.
[16] Pascoe M, Byrne E, King A, et al. Sleep disorders associated with cranial radiation—A systematic review. Neuro Oncol 2024;27(1):63–76.
[17] McGovern SL, Okcu MF, Munsell MF, et al. Outcomes and acute toxicities of proton therapy for pediatric atypical teratoid/rhabdoid tumor of the central nervous system. Int J Radiat Oncol Biol Phys 2014;90(5):1143–52.
[18] Sienna J, Kahalley LS, Mabbott D, et al. Proton therapy mediates dose reductions to brain structures associated with cognition in children with medulloblastoma. Int J Radiat Oncol Biol Phys 2024;119(1):200–7.
[19] Kulubya ES, Kercher MJ, Phillips HW, et al. Advances in the treatment of pediatric brain tumors. Children 2023;10(1):62.
[20] Childhood Brain Tumor C. A study of childhood brain tumors based on surgical biopsies from ten North American institutions: sample description. J Neuro Oncol 1988;6(1):9–23.
[21] Bale TA, Rosenblum MK. The 2021 WHO classification of tumors of the central nervous system: an update on pediatric low-grade gliomas and glioneuronal tumors. Brain Pathol 2022;32(4):e13060.
[22] Louis DN, Perry A, Wesseling P, et al. The 2021 WHO classification of Tumors of the Central Nervous System: a summary. Neuro Oncol 2021;23(8):1231–51.
[23] Sharif S, Ferner R, Birch JM, et al. Second primary tumors in neurofibromatosis 1 patients treated for optic glioma: substantial risks after radiotherapy. J Clin Oncol 2006;24(16):2570–5.
[24] Merchant TE, Kun LE, Wu S, et al. Phase II trial of conformal radiation therapy for pediatric low-grade glioma. J Clin Oncol 2009;27(22):3598–604.
[25] Merchant TE, Conklin HM, Wu S, et al. Late effects of conformal radiation therapy for pediatric patients with low-grade glioma: prospective evaluation of cognitive, endocrine, and hearing deficits. J Clin Oncol 2009;27(22):3691–7.
[26] Garcia DM, Marks JE, Latifi HR, et al. Childhood cerebellar astrocytomas: is there a role for postoperative irradiation? Int J Radiat Oncol Biol Phys 1990;18(4):815–8.
[27] Pierce SM, Barnes PD, Loeffler JS, et al. Definitive radiation therapy in the management of symptomatic patients with optic glioma. Survival and long-term effects. Cancer 1990;65(1):45–52.
[28] Fangusaro J, Onar-Thomas A, Young Poussaint T, et al. Selumetinib in paediatric patients with BRAF-aberrant or neurofibromatosis type 1-associated recurrent, refractory, or progressive low-grade glioma: a multicentre, phase 2 trial. Lancet Oncol 2019;20(7):1011–22.

[29] Moertel CL, Hirbe AC, Shuhaiber HH, et al. ReNeu: a pivotal, phase IIb trial of mirdametinib in adults and children with symptomatic neurofibromatosis type 1-Associated plexiform neurofibroma. J Clin Oncol 2025;43(6):716–29.
[30] Manoharan N, Choi J, Chordas C, et al. Trametinib for the treatment of recurrent/progressive pediatric low-grade glioma. J Neuro Oncol 2020;149(2):253–62.
[31] Selt F, van Tilburg CM, Bison B, et al. Response to trametinib treatment in progressive pediatric low-grade glioma patients. J Neuro Oncol 2020;149(3):499–510.
[32] Bouffet E, Hansford JR, Garrè ML, et al. Dabrafenib plus trametinib in pediatric glioma with BRAF V600 mutations. N Engl J Med 2023;389(12):1108–20.
[33] Krueger DA, Care MM, Holland K, et al. Everolimus for subependymal giant-cell astrocytomas in tuberous sclerosis. N Engl J Med 2010;363(19):1801–11.
[34] Howe GN, Edmonston DY, Dirks GC, et al. Conformal radiation therapy for ependymoma at age ≤3 years: a 25-Year experience. Int J Radiat Oncol Biol Phys 2023;116(4):869–77.
[35] Boop SH, Shimony N, Boop FA. Review and update on pediatric ependymoma. Childs Nerv Syst 2023;39(10):2667–73.
[36] Packer RJ, Cogen P, Vezina G, et al. Medulloblastoma: clinical and biologic aspects. Neuro Oncol 1999;1(3):232–50.
[37] Rey-Casserly C, Diver T. Late effects of pediatric brain tumors. Curr Opin Pediatr 2019;31(6):789–96.
[38] Patel T, Johar P, Kanisetti V, et al. Long-term neurocognitive and behavioral outcomes in survivors of pediatric brain tumors: a systematic review. Front Neurosci 2025;19:1587059.
[39] Aktekin EH, Kütük MÖ, Sangün Ö, et al. Late effects of medulloblastoma treatment: multidisciplinary approach of survivors. Childs Nerv Syst 2024;40(2):417–25.

Advances in Pediatrics 73 (2026) 283–294

ADVANCES IN PEDIATRICS

Current Management of Food Allergies in Pediatric Patients

Alexandra Ha, DO[a,b], Ami Takei Yuen, MD[a,b], Charles Song, MD[a,b,*]

[a]Department of Pediatrics, Harbor-UCLA Medical Center, Torrance, CA, USA; [b]Department of Allergy and Immunology, David Geffen School of Medicine at UCLA, Los Angeles, CA, USA

Keywords

• Food allergy • Anaphylaxis • Epinephrine • Oral immunotherapy • Biologics • Component-resolved diagnostics • Alarmin

Key points

- The pathophysiology of food allergy is now understood to involve a complex interplay of genetic susceptibility, epithelial barrier dysfunction, the gut microbiome, and the release of "alarmins" (eg, TSLP, IL-33) as key upstream events that initiate the allergic cascade.
- Diagnosis relies on a convincing clinical history supported by sensitization testing (skin prick or specific IgE), but the oral food challenge remains the gold standard for a definitive diagnosis. Component-resolved and epitope-based diagnostics are improving risk stratification for select allergens.
- Management is shifting from a reactive model of avoidance and emergency epinephrine to proactive immunomodulatory therapies designed to induce desensitization and increase a patient's threshold of reactivity.
- A new era of Food and Drug Administration (FDA)-approved therapies has begun. The anti-IgE biologic omalizumab was approved in 2024 for reducing the risk of allergic reactions from accidental exposure to multiple foods, transforming the therapeutic landscape.
- The use of biologics as adjuncts to oral immunotherapy is a major advance for improving the safety and efficacy of desensitization, with agents targeting IL-4Rα (dupilumab) also showing significant promise.

*Corresponding author. 1000 W. Carson Street, Torrance, CA 90502. *E-mail address:* CSong3@dhs.lacounty.gov

https://doi.org/10.1016/j.yapd.2025.12.003

Abbreviations

AGS	alpha-gal syndrome
CRD	component resolved diagnostics
EGID	eosinophilic gastrointestinal disease
EoE	eosinophilic esophagitis
FPIES	food protein-induced enterocolitis syndrome
IM	intramuscular
OIT	oral immunotherapy
SIgE	serum-specific IgE
SPT	skin prick test
SU	sustained unresponsiveness

INTRODUCTION

Adverse reactions to foods encompass any undesirable clinical response following ingestion. This broad category is first divided into 2 distinct groups: reactions that are *nonimmune-mediated* (often called food intolerances) and those that are *immune-mediated.* Nonimmune reactions include metabolic issues like lactase deficiency, pharmacologic effects from substances like caffeine, and toxic reactions such as food poisoning.

This article focuses on the *immune-mediated reactions*, which are correctly termed *food allergies.* A food allergy is an objectively reproducible, adverse health effect arising from a specific immune response that occurs upon exposure to a given food [1]. The most common food allergies are driven by IgE antibodies, which involve a 2-step process: a *sensitization phase*, where allergen-specific IgE is produced and primes mast cells and basophils, and an *elicitation phase*, where re-exposure triggers these cells to release inflammatory mediators, causing rapid-onset symptoms.

A key concept related to the development of IgE-mediated food allergies is *atopy*, which refers to the genetic predisposition to develop IgE antibodies to common environmental allergens. However, it is important to note that not all food allergies are atopic, as non-IgE-mediated forms do not require this predisposition. The different immunologic mechanisms of food allergy are summarized in Table 1.

Table 1
Different immunologic mechanisms of food allergy

Mechanism	Key features	Examples
IgE-mediated	Rapid onset (minutes to 2 h) after allergen exposure	Anaphylaxis, pollen–food allergy syndrome, contact urticaria
Non–IgE-mediated	Delayed onset (hours to days); primarily gastrointestinal involvement	FPIES, food protein-induced proctocolitis, Heiner syndrome, Celiac disease (an autoimmune enteropathy triggered by gluten)
Mixed IgE and non–IgE	Combination of immediate and delayed features	Atopic dermatitis, eosinophilic esophagitis, some forms of cow's milk allergy

Food allergies have become a major public health concern, affecting approximately 7.6% of children and 10.8% of adults in the United States due to their increasing prevalence and the risk of life-threatening anaphylaxis [2]. While acknowledging the broad landscape of adverse food reactions, this article will provide an overview of the field with a primary focus on recent advances in the pathophysiology, diagnosis, and management of IgE-mediated food allergy.

EPIDEMIOLOGY AND RISK FACTORS

The prevalence of food allergies has risen significantly, now affecting up to 8% of children in developed countries. Over 90% of IgE-mediated reactions are caused by the "Top 9" allergens: milk, egg, peanut, tree nuts, soy, wheat, fish, crustacean shellfish, and sesame [3]. While allergies to milk, egg, soy, and wheat are often outgrown, those to peanut, tree nuts, and seafood are typically lifelong [4]. In the United States, a greater burden of food allergy is seen among non-Hispanic Black and other non-White subpopulations compared to those who identify as White [5].

Food allergy is a complex disease influenced by a critical interplay of genetic and environmental factors.

An emerging entity: alpha-gal syndrome

A notable emerging food allergy with a distinct epidemiology is alpha-gal syndrome (AGS). This unique, delayed IgE-mediated allergy is not to a protein but to the carbohydrate galactose-α-1,3-galactose (alpha-gal) found in mammalian meat [6]. The most significant recent advance concerning AGS is epidemiologic; the expanding habitat of its primary vector in the United States, the Lone Star tick (*Amblyomma americanum*), has led to a notable increase in cases beyond its traditional southern regions, making it a growing public health concern [3].

Key risk factors

- *Genetic Predisposition:* Food allergy is a polygenic disease with a strong hereditary component. Genome-wide association studies have identified risk loci in genes central to immune function, such as the human leukocyte antigen region, and those related to barrier integrity, like loss-of-function mutations in the filaggrin (*FLG*) gene, which impairs skin barrier function [7].
- *Atopic Dermatitis (Eczema):* An impaired skin barrier from early-life eczema is a major risk factor for developing food allergy. According to the "outside-in" hypothesis, sensitization can occur when food proteins are first encountered through inflamed skin (epicutaneous sensitization) rather than through the gut, leading to an allergic response.
- *Environmental and Dietary Factors:* The timing of allergen introduction is critical; landmark studies have shown that delayed introduction of allergenic foods increases risk, while early and regular oral exposure promotes tolerance [8]. Furthermore, factors like early-life antibiotic use have been linked to a higher food allergy risk, likely by disrupting the gut microbiome, which is essential for educating the immune system [9].

PATHOGENESIS

The development of food allergy is a multistep process involving the breakdown of oral tolerance. The underlying mechanisms can be broadly divided into IgE-mediated (Type 2) and non-IgE-mediated pathways.

IgE-mediated and type 2 inflammatory reactions

The classic food allergic reaction is a *Type I hypersensitivity response* that occurs in 2 distinct phases: sensitization and elicitation.

1. *The Sensitization Phase:* This is the initial, asymptomatic exposure to a food allergen. In a predisposed individual, this exposure leads to a Th2-polarized immune response, where T cells produce cytokines like IL-4 and IL-13 that instruct B cells to create allergen-specific IgE antibodies. This IgE then binds to high-affinity receptors (FcεRI) on the surface of mast cells and basophils, effectively "priming" them for future encounters.
2. *The Elicitation (Effector) Phase:* Upon re-exposure, the food allergen cross-links the specific IgE antibodies on the surface of the primed mast cells and basophils. This triggers rapid degranulation, releasing a flood of inflammatory mediators (like histamine and leukotrienes) that cause the immediate clinical symptoms of an allergic reaction .[10].

Recent advances have profoundly expanded this model to a broader understanding of Type 2 inflammation.

The paradigm has now shifted to begin at the *epithelial barrier* (skin or gut). Barrier disruption leads to the release of "alarmins" (eg, TSLP, IL-33), which activate innate lymphoid cells (ILC2s). These cells rapidly produce IL-4 and IL-13, creating a cytokine environment that powerfully drives naïve T-cells toward the Th2 phenotype. *The central role of this epithelial barrier dysfunction has led some immunologists to propose it as a distinct form of hypersensitivity, sometimes referred to as "Type V"* [11]. A key example of this is the "outside-in" hypothesis, where an impaired skin barrier from early-life atopic dermatitis is a major risk factor for epicutaneous sensitization to food allergens, leading to the development of a clinical food allergy.

In the subsequent adaptive response, T follicular helper cells are essential for generating the high-affinity, pathogenic IgE that drives severe reactions [12]. Groundbreaking work has also revealed that intestinal mast cells are the primary drivers of food-induced anaphylaxis, releasing leukotrienes as the critical mediators, rather than histamine [13], and the cast of effector cells has expanded to include neutrophils and macrophages [14].

Delayed reactions and cofactors

While IgE-mediated reactions are characteristically rapid, it is important to recognize that the onset of symptoms can be significantly delayed, a phenomenon that can be a diagnostic puzzle for clinicians. When a patient presents with symptoms suggestive of an IgE-mediated reaction but with a delayed onset, clinicians must actively investigate the role of *cofactors*, which can lower a patient's reaction threshold.

Cofactors such as exercise, alcohol, nonsteroidal anti-inflammatory drug (NSAID) use, and concurrent illness can augment the severity of a reaction or may even be required to elicit one, as seen in food-dependent exercise-induced anaphylaxis [3]. A key example of an intrinsically delayed IgE-mediated reaction is *alpha-gal syndrome*, where symptoms characteristically appear 3 to 6 hours after consuming mammalian meat, providing a pathognomonic clue to the diagnosis [15].

Non-IgE-mediated food allergies

These reactions are driven by cellular responses, primarily T-cells, and manifest with delayed, often gastrointestinal, symptoms.

- *Eosinophilic Gastrointestinal Diseases (EGIDs):* EGIDs are a group of disorders defined by pathologic eosinophilic infiltration of specific segments of the gastrointestinal tract, in the absence of other known causes for the eosinophilia [16]. While some patients may have evidence of food-specific IgE, the underlying pathophysiology is considered to be a primarily non-IgE-mediated Th2 inflammatory response.
    - This is powerfully illustrated by *eosinophilic esophagitis (EoE)*, the most common EGID. EoE is notably unresponsive to anti-IgE therapy (omalizumab) but shows significant histologic and symptomatic improvement with *dupilumab*, a biologic that directly targets the core Th2 pathway by blocking the shared receptor for *IL-4 and IL-13* [17]. This differential response confirms that the disease is driven by Th2 cytokines, not by IgE-mediated mechanisms.

Other examples of EGIDs include

- *Eosinophilic Gastritis:* Involves eosinophilic inflammation of the stomach, leading to symptoms like nausea, vomiting, and abdominal pain.
- *Eosinophilic Gastroenteritis:* Affects both the stomach and small intestine, causing a mix of pain, vomiting, and diarrhea.
- *Eosinophilic Enteritis:* Involves the small intestine and is often associated with diarrhea and malabsorption.
- *Eosinophilic Colitis:* Affects the colon (large intestine) and typically presents with bloody diarrhea, particularly in infants.
    - *Food Protein-Induced Enterocolitis Syndrome (FPIES)* is a distinct non-IgE-mediated food allergy and is *not* considered a part of the EGID spectrum, as it is not defined by chronic eosinophilic infiltration [18]. The classic presentation is profuse, delayed vomiting that occurs 1 to 4 hours after ingesting a trigger food, often accompanied by diarrhea, pallor, and lethargy, which can lead to dehydration and shock. FPIES has 2 peak age ranges for onset: it most commonly presents in *early infancy*, triggered by cow's milk, soy, and grains, but it is also increasingly recognized in *adulthood*, where seafood is the most common culprit [19,20]. The diagnosis is entirely clinical, based on a characteristic history, as there are currently *no validated biomarkers* or diagnostic laboratory tests to confirm the condition.
    - Heiner Syndrome: Heiner Syndrome is a rare, non-IgE-mediated hypersensitivity to cow's milk in which IgG-mediated immune complexes are thought to cause alveolar hemorrhage and pulmonary hemosiderosis. It typically presents

in infants with a triad of chronic respiratory symptoms, iron-deficiency anemia, and failure to thrive, with a diagnosis confirmed by the rapid resolution of symptoms upon strict elimination of all cow's milk products [21].

EVALUATION AND DIAGNOSIS

The diagnosis of food allergy is a clinical process integrating a detailed history, evidence of sensitization, and, if necessary, a medically supervised oral food challenge, which remains the gold standard [22].

- Standard IgE-Based Tests: The skin prick test (SPT) and serum-specific IgE (sIgE) are primary tools. It is critical to note that these tests indicate sensitization, not necessarily clinical allergy, and must be interpreted in the context of the patient's history to avoid false positives and overdiagnosis [23].
- Component Resolved Diagnostics (CRD): CRD can significantly improve diagnostic accuracy and risk assessment for several common food allergies. The most clinically useful component tests are as follows:
    - Egg: Ovomucoid (Gal d 1) is a key marker for persistent allergy and risk of reaction to baked egg [24–26].
    - Fish: Parvalbumin is the main marker for fish allergy [26].
    - Milk: Casein (Bos d 8) is associated with persistent allergy and reactions to baked milk [24–26].
    - Peanut: Ara h 2 is the most specific and predictive marker for a true, systemic peanut allergy. Ara h 1 and Ara h 3 are also associated with a higher risk of severe reactions, while Ara h 8 is a marker for cross-reactivity with birch pollen, often associated with milder, oral symptoms [27].
    - Peach: Pru p 7 is a marker associated with severe, systemic reactions [28].
    - Seeds: Ses i 1 (sesame) is the most useful component for sesame allergy diagnosis and risk assessment [26,29].
    - Shrimp: Tropomyosin (Pen m 1) is the most relevant component for diagnosis [24,26].
    - Soy: Gly m 8 is the most relevant component for distinguishing genuine soy allergy from cross-reactivity [26].
    - Tree Nuts: Ana o 3 (cashew), Jug r 1 (walnut), and Cor a 14 (hazelnut) are highly predictive for true allergy and risk of severe reactions [24,26,27].
    - Wheat: Omega-5 gliadin (Tri a 19) is the key component predictive for wheat-dependent exercise-induced anaphylaxis and other severe reactions [24,30].
- *Epitope-Resolved Diagnostics:* Recent head-to-head studies have shown that epitope-resolved IgE diagnostic platforms are superior to both skin prick testing and standard component testing for peanut allergy [31]; however, these platforms have not yet received regulatory approval for routine clinical use.
- *Functional Assays*: The *basophil activation test* measures in vitro degranulation of a patient's basophils in response to an allergen and is more predictive of clinical reactivity than sIgE or CRD, though it is not yet widely available [24].
- *Tests Not Recommended:* Food-specific *IgG4 testing* is a marker of exposure and tolerance, not allergy. Major international guidelines explicitly recommend *against* its use as a diagnostic tool [32]. *Its primary clinical utility is as a biomarker for monitoring the immune response to oral immunotherapy (OIT).*

MANAGEMENT

The cornerstone: avoidance and emergency preparedness

The cornerstone of managing a food allergy is the combination of strict allergen avoidance and a clear, written anaphylaxis action plan. This includes diligent label reading and comprehensive patient and family education.

Treatment of accidental exposures

For the treatment of an acute allergic reaction, it is critical to recognize that *epinephrine is the only first-line, life-saving medication for anaphylaxis*, and its administration should never be delayed. Antihistamines are useful for treating mild, cutaneous symptoms like isolated hives, but they *do not* prevent or treat the severe respiratory or cardiovascular symptoms of anaphylaxis. Therefore, epinephrine should be administered immediately at the first sign of any systemic reaction involving more than just the skin.

- Epinephrine Delivery Systems.
  - *Intramuscular (IM) Epinephrine:* For decades, the standard of care has been the administration of epinephrine via autoinjector into the anterolateral thigh. It remains the gold standard for treating anaphylaxis [4].
  - *Intranasal Epinephrine (A New Delivery System):* Recently, an alternative delivery method has been approved. *Intranasal epinephrine spray (Neffy)* is now also indicated for the emergency treatment of Type I allergic reactions, including anaphylaxis, in patients aged 4 years and older who weigh at least 15 kg [33]. A phase 3 open-label study demonstrated that Neffy was effective in resolving symptoms of moderate (Grade 2) anaphylaxis *triggered by an oral food challenge* in pediatric patients, with a median time to resolution of 16 minutes after a single dose. The most commonly reported immediate local side effects are nasal discomfort, sneezing, rhinorrhea, and nasal congestion. It is important to note that a biphasic reaction requiring a subsequent dose of IM epinephrine has been reported [34].

All patients at risk for anaphylaxis should be prescribed and carry one of these forms of epinephrine at all times.

Allergen immunotherapy

The ultimate goal of treatment is to induce permanent tolerance, a state of nonresponsiveness that persists after therapy is stopped. However, this has proven elusive. The more common and achievable goal of current therapies is desensitization, which is an increase in the reaction threshold while a patient is still on active treatment. A subset of patients may achieve sustained unresponsiveness (SU), which is a temporary state of nonreactivity after discontinuing therapy, but this is distinct from lifelong tolerance [35]. SU has been observed more frequently in younger children, particularly those undergoing early OIT before the age of 4 years, suggesting an age-dependent window of immune plasticity that may facilitate more durable outcomes [36,37]. Mechanistically, SU is associated with persistent immunologic changes such as reduced allergen-specific IgE, increased IgG4/IgA, basophil hyporesponsiveness, and expansion of regulatory T cells, but these changes do not equate to natural tolerance [38].

- *Oral Immunotherapy (OIT):* OIT is highly effective at inducing desensitization. The only FDA-approved product is Palforzia, a standardized peanut allergen powder for patients aged 1 to 17 years [39]. However, the primary limitation of OIT is its safety profile, with a high rate of allergic reactions and a risk of anaphylaxis [40]. Furthermore, achieving long-term SU is less common, as demonstrated in major trials like the POISED study [41].
- *Other Approaches (EPIT, SLIT):* Epicutaneous (EPIT) and sublingual (SLIT) immunotherapies have better safety profiles than OIT but are generally less efficacious [42,43].

Role of adjunctive biologics

A transformative advance is the use of adjunctive biologics. In early 2024, the FDA approved the anti-IgE monoclonal antibody omalizumab to reduce the risk of allergic reactions from accidental exposure to one or more foods in patients aged 1 year and older. Combined treatment with omalizumab and OIT dramatically improves the safety and efficacy of desensitization [44]. In parallel, dupilumab (anti-IL-4Rα) has shown promise as an adjunct to OIT and is revolutionizing the treatment of EoE [45].

Clinical note: atopic dermatitis and food elimination diets

While atopic dermatitis is a major risk factor for developing food allergy, food allergy itself is rarely the primary cause of atopic dermatitis, especially in older children and adults. For this reason, major clinical guidelines strongly recommend against the use of routine or empiric food elimination diets for the management of atopic dermatitis in the absence of a confirmed, specific food trigger [46].

FUTURE CONSIDERATIONS

Future advances are focused on improving the safety of immunotherapy and refining diagnostics. Investigational approaches include modified hypoallergenic proteins and peptide immunotherapy designed to induce T-cell tolerance without activating mast cells [47]. Novel diagnostics such as mast cell activation tests and microbiome analysis offer insights into allergy trajectories, with distinct oral and gut bacterial profiles linked to peanut allergy risk. While not yet sufficiently predictive, microbiome profiling may complement other measures in integrated diagnostic frameworks [48]. Recent advances in diagnostics are also focused on epigenetics. The analysis of DNA methylation signatures has identified patterns in genes crucial for immune regulation (eg, *FOXP3*, *IL4*) and barrier integrity (*FLG*) that are associated with food allergy status and persistence [49,50].

CASE VIGNETTE: IgE-MEDIATED PEANUT ALLERGY

History

A 15 month old male toddler with a history of moderate atopic dermatitis was brought for an allergy evaluation. His parents reported that 15 minutes after his first known ingestion of peanut–a small bite of a peanut butter sandwich–

he developed diffuse urticaria on his chest and face, followed by angioedema of his eyelids and lips. He then began to cough and wheeze. An oral antihistamine administered by the parents provided minimal relief from the urticaria. Due to the persistent respiratory symptoms, he was taken to an emergency department.

Evaluation

In the emergency department, he was diagnosed with anaphylaxis and treated with a single dose of IM epinephrine, which led to the rapid resolution of all symptoms. Subsequent allergy testing revealed a large wheal on skin prick testing to peanut and a markedly elevated serum specific peanut IgE level of 15.8 kU/L. Component testing was primarily positive for Ara h 1, 2, and 6, confirming a high risk for systemic reactions, and the baseline peanut-specific IgG4 was undetectable.

Management and outcome

The patient was diagnosed with a severe IgE-mediated peanut allergy. The family was provided with 2 epinephrine autoinjectors, trained on their use, and given a written Anaphylaxis Action Plan. After a discussion of therapeutic options, the parents opted to proceed with OIT with adjunctive omalizumab.

The treatment protocol was as follows:

- Omalizumab Pretreatment: The patient was pretreated with omalizumab (Xolair) every 4 weeks for 3 doses.
- Accelerated OIT: An accelerated OIT protocol with standardized peanut powder was initiated, and the patient successfully reached the target dose of 2 g of peanut powder over a 2 month period.
- Maintenance and Omalizumab Taper: He was then transitioned to a daily maintenance dose of peanut butter. After 6 months of stable dosing, the omalizumab interval was gradually extended and subsequently discontinued.

As of this writing, the patient has been off omalizumab for 2 months and continues to tolerate his daily maintenance dose of peanut butter without systemic symptoms. Notably, this clinical improvement was accompanied by a significant immunologic shift; his peanut-specific IgG4 level increased from undetectable to 2.4 μg/mL, consistent with the development of blocking antibodies.

CLINICS CARE POINTS

- Sensitization is not a diagnosis: A positive SPT or sIgE only indicates sensitization. A diagnosis of food allergy requires a convincing clinical history and is definitively confirmed by an oral food challenge.
- Component testing refines risk: For certain food allergies, particularly peanut and hazelnut, CRD can help predict the likelihood and potential severity of a clinical reaction, but this predictive value is not as strong for many other foods.

- Epinephrine is the only first-line treatment for anaphylaxis: Antihistamines treat mild, cutaneous symptoms like hives but do not stop the progression of anaphylaxis. Epinephrine should be administered immediately at the first sign of a systemic reaction.
- Do not use food elimination diets for atopic dermatitis: In the absence of a confirmed, specific food trigger, major guidelines strongly recommend against empiric food elimination for atopic dermatitis, as it rarely causes the condition.
- Biologics enhance immunotherapy: Using adjunctive omalizumab with OIT dramatically improves the safety and efficacy of desensitization, making it a viable option for more patients.

DECLARATION OF AI AND AI-ASSISTED TECHNOLOGIES IN THE WRITING PROCESS

During the preparation of this work, the author(s) used AI (open evidence and Gemini) in order to improve readability and language. After using this tool/service, the author(s) reviewed and edited the content as needed and take(s) full responsibility for the content of the publication.

Disclosures

The authors have nothing to disclose.

References

[1] Boyce JA, Assa'ad A, Burks AW, et al. Guidelines for the diagnosis and management of food allergy in the United States: report of the NIAID-sponsored expert panel. J Allergy Clin Immunol 2010;126(6 Suppl):S1–58.
[2] Novembre E, Gelsomino M, Liotti L, et al. Fatal food anaphylaxis in adults and children. Ital J Pediatr 2024;50(1):40.
[3] Iglesia EGA, Kwan M, Virkud YV, et al. Management of food allergies and food-related anaphylaxis. JAMA 2024;331(6):510–21.
[4] Sampson HA, Aceves S, Bock SA, et al. Food allergy: a practice parameter update-2014. J Allergy Clin Immunol 2014;134(5):1016–25.e43.
[5] Warren C, Bartell T, Nimmagadda SR, et al. Socioeconomic determinants of food allergy burden: a clinical introduction. Ann Allergy Asthma Immunol 2022;129(4):407–16.
[6] Commins SP, Satinover SM, Hosen J, et al. Delayed anaphylaxis, angioedema, or urticaria after consumption of red meat in patients with IgE antibodies specific for galactose-alpha-1,3-galactose. J Allergy Clin Immunol 2009;123(2):426–33.
[7] Arnau-Soler A, Tremblay BL, Sun Y, et al. Food allergy genetics and epigenetics: a review of genome-wide association studies. Allergy 2025;80(1):106–31.
[8] Du Toit G, Roberts G, Sayre PH, et al. Randomized trial of peanut consumption in infants at risk for peanut allergy. N Engl J Med 2015;372(9):803–13.
[9] Lu C, Jiang Y, Lan M, et al. Children's food allergy: effects of environmental influences and antibiotic use across critical developmental windows. J Hazard Mater 2024;472:134506.
[10] Carnazza M, Werner R, Tiwari RK, et al. The etiology of IgE-Mediated food allergy: potential therapeutics and challenges. Int J Mol Sci 2025;26(4):1563.
[11] Jutel M, Agache I, Zemelka-Wiacek M, et al. Nomenclature of allergic diseases and hypersensitivity reactions: adapted to modern needs: an EAACI position paper. Allergy 2023;78(11):2851–74.
[12] Gowthaman U, Chen JS, Eisenbarth SC. Regulation of IgE by T follicular helper cells. J Leukoc Biol 2020;107(3):409–18.

[13] Bachtel ND, Cullen JL, Liu M, et al. Intestinal mast cell-derived leukotrienes mediate the anaphylactic response to ingested antigens. Science 2025;389(6760):eadp0246.
[14] Crespo JF, Cabanillas B. Recent advances in cellular and molecular mechanisms of IgE-mediated food allergy. Food Chem 2023;411:135500.
[15] Commins SP, James HR, Kelly LA, et al. The relevance of tick bites to the production of IgE antibodies to the mammalian oligosaccharide Galactose-A-1,3-Galactose. J Allergy Clin Immunol 2011;127(5):1286–93.e6.
[16] Shoda T, Taylor RJ, Sakai N, et al. Common and disparate clinical presentations and mechanisms in different eosinophilic gastrointestinal diseases. J Allergy Clin Immunol 2024;153(6):1472–84.
[17] Dellon ES, Spergel JM. Biologics in eosinophilic gastrointestinal diseases. Ann Allergy Asthma Immunol 2023;130(1):21–7.
[18] Su KW, Shreffler WG, Yuan Q. Gastrointestinal immunopathology of food protein-induced enterocolitis syndrome and other non-immunoglobulin E-mediated food allergic diseases. Ann Allergy Asthma Immunol 2021;126(5):516–23.
[19] Anvari S, Gupta M, Nicolaides R, et al. The evolution of food protein-induced enterocolitis syndrome (FPIES): global trends, emerging triggers, and natural history. Ann Allergy Asthma Immunol 2025;S1081-1206(25):01160-3.
[20] Ahmed M, Poowuttikul P, Chey WD, et al. Adult FPIES: a review of emerging evidence and clinical considerations. Dig Dis 2025;1–12.
[21] Arasi S, Mastrorilli C, Pecoraro L, et al. Heiner syndrome and milk hypersensitivity: an updated overview on the current evidence. Nutrients 2021;13(5):1710.
[22] Sampson HA, Arasi S, Bahnson HT, et al. AAAAI-EAACI practall: standardizing oral food challenges-2024 update. Pediatr Allergy Immunol 2024;35(11):e14276.
[23] Bégin P, Waserman S, Protudjer JLP, et al. Immunoglobulin E (IgE)-mediated food allergy. Allergy Asthma Clin Immunol 2024;20(Suppl 3):75.
[24] Santos A, Al-Ahmed M, Vlieg-Boerstra B, et al. The added value of component-resolved diagnostics to IgE-based food allergy diagnosis. Allergy 2021;76(11):3288–306.
[25] Sicherer SH, Wood RA. Allergy testing in childhood: using allergen-specific IgE tests. Pediatrics 2014;133(5):921–30.
[26] Popescu FD, Ganea E, Batani A, et al. Component-resolved diagnosis of food allergy. World J Methodol 2019;9(2):23–37.
[27] Klemans RJB, van den Holt R, van Os-Medendorp H, et al. The value of specific IgE to peanut and its components for the diagnosis of peanut allergy. Clin Exp Allergy 2015;45(6):1111–9.
[28] Klingel C, Chantran Y, Arif-Lusson R, et al. Pru P 7 sensitization is a predominant cause of severe, cypress pollen-associated peach allergy. Clin Exp Allergy 2019;49(4):526–36, PMID: 30672059.
[29] Kuehn A, Codreanu F, Sahiner UM, et al. The diagnosis of sesame allergy. Curr Allergy Asthma Rep 2010;10(4):261–7.
[30] Ebisawa M, Takahashi K, Takahashi K, et al. Epinephrine nasal spray improves allergic symptoms in patients undergoing oral food challenge, phase 3 trial. J Allergy Clin Immunol Pract 2025 S2213-2198(25)00630-0.
[31] Suárez-Fariñas M, Suprun M, Kearney P, et al. Accurate and reproducible diagnosis of peanut allergy using epitope mapping. Allergy 2021;76(12):3789–97.
[32] Stapel SO, Asero R, Ballmer-Weber BK, et al. Testing for IgG4 against foods is not recommended as a diagnostic tool: EAACI task force report. Allergy 2008;63(7):793–6.
[33] Neffy. FDA drug label. Silver Spring (MD): Food and Drug Administration; 2025.
[34] Ebisawa M, Ito K, Fujisawa T, et al. Japanese guideline for food allergy 2020. Allergol Int 2020;69(3):370–86.
[35] Burks AW, Laubach S, Jones SM. Oral tolerance, food allergy, and immunotherapy: implications for future treatment. J Allergy Clin Immunol 2008;121(6):1344–50.

[36] Barten LJC, Zuurveld M, Faber J, et al. Oral immunotherapy as a curative treatment for food-allergic preschool children: current evidence and potential underlying mechanisms. Pediatr Allergy Immunol 2023;34(11):e14043.
[37] Smeekens JM, Kulis MD, Kim EH, et al. Induction of tolerance to food allergens-younger is better. Pediatr Allergy Immunol 2025;36(10):e70193.
[38] Barshow SM, Kulis MD, Burks AW, et al. Mechanisms of oral immunotherapy. Clin Exp Allergy 2021;51(4):527–35.
[39] PALISADE Group of Clinical Investigators, Vickery BP, Vereda A, Casale TB, et al. AR101 oral immunotherapy for peanut allergy. N Engl J Med 2018;379(21):1991–2001.
[40] Chu DK, Wood RA, French S, et al. Oral immunotherapy for peanut allergy (PACE): a systematic review and meta-analysis of efficacy and safety. Lancet 2019;393(10187):2222–32.
[41] Chinthrajah RS, Purington N, Andorf S, et al. Sustained outcomes in oral immunotherapy for peanut allergy (POISED study): a large, randomised, double-blind, placebo-controlled, phase 2 study. Lancet 2019;394(10207):1437–49.
[42] Fleischer DM, Greenhawt M, Sussman G, et al. Effect of epicutaneous immunotherapy vs placebo on reaction to peanut protein ingestion among children with peanut allergy: the PEPITES randomized clinical trial. JAMA 2019;321(10):946–55.
[43] Fleischer DM, Burks AW, Vickery BP, et al. Sublingual immunotherapy for peanut allergy: a randomized, double-blind, placebo-controlled multicenter trial. J Allergy Clin Immunol 2013;131(1):119–27.
[44] Bird JA, Spergel JM, Jones SM, et al. Efficacy and safety of dupilumab with peanut oral immunotherapy: a phase 2 randomized trial (Dupe-OIT). J Allergy Clin Immunol 2024;153(5):1339–49.
[45] Andorf S, Purington N, Block WM, et al. Anti-IgE treatment with oral immunotherapy in multifood allergic participants: a double-blind, randomised, controlled trial. Lancet Gastroenterol Hepatol 2018;3(2):85–94.
[46] Chu DK, Schneider L, Asiniwasis RN, et al. Atopic dermatitis (eczema) guidelines: 2023 American Academy of Allergy, asthma and Immunology/American College of Allergy, asthma and immunology joint task force on practice parameters GRADE- and Institute of medicine-Based recommendations. Ann Allergy Asthma Immunol 2024;132(3):274–312.
[47] Feuille E, Nowak-Wegrzyn A. Allergen-specific immunotherapies for food allergy. Allergy Asthma Immunol Res 2018;10(3):189–206.
[48] Wong DSH, Santos AF. The future of food allergy diagnosis. Front Allergy 2024;5:1456585.
[49] Safar R, Oussalah A, Mayorga L, et al. Epigenome alterations in food allergy: a systematic review of candidate gene and epigenome-wide association studies. Clin Exp Allergy 2023;53(3):259–75.
[50] Chun Y, Lee JH, Bunyavanich S. Epigenomic and epigenetic investigations of food allergy. Pediatr Allergy Immunol 2024;35(1):e14065.

Advances in Pediatrics 73 (2026) 295–307

ADVANCES IN PEDIATRICS

Hidradenitis in Pediatrics

Soneet Dhillon, MD, MHA[a,1],
Nadine Horneck, MD[b,1], Jan Smogorzewski, MD[c,*]

[a]Department of Internal Medicine, Harbor UCLA, Torrance, CA, USA; [b]Department of Internal Medicine, St Mary Medical Center, Long Beach, CA, USA; [c]Division of Dermatology, Department of Internal Medicine, Harbor UCLA, Torrance, CA, USA

Keywords

• Hidradenitis suppurativa • Intertriginous acne • Pediatrics • Acne inversa
• Verneuil disease

Key points

- Pediatric hidradenitis suppurativa is a chronic inflammatory disease with recurrent painful nodules in flexural sites and a high risk of scarring.
- Diagnosis is done clinically and may be delayed in children.
- Early referral to dermatology and ongoing psychosocial support improves outcomes and quality of life.

INTRODUCTION

Hidradenitis suppurativa (HS) is a chronic, inflammatory skin disease that substantially impacts quality of life. It is traditionally regarded as a postpubertal condition and is therefore infrequently diagnosed in children, with many pediatric cases spanning 15 and 17 years of age [1]. Prepubertal presentation is rare, accounting for approximately 2% of patients with HS [2]. However, true disease prevalence is likely underestimated due to frequent misdiagnosis and delays in care. The diagnosis is made clinically by the recognition of recurrent characteristic inflammatory lesions in intertriginous areas, underscoring the importance of disease awareness and training among pediatric primary care providers. Management of pediatric HS typically combines topical therapies and intralesional steroids with timely escalation to systemic agents and procedures if warranted. Pediatric HS is further complicated by a significant

[1]Contributed equally to the project.

*Corresponding author. *E-mail address:* jsmogorzewski@dhs.lacounty.gov

https://doi.org/10.1016/j.yapd.2025.12.007

Abbreviations

HS	hidradenitis suppurativa
PCOS	polycystic ovary syndrome

comorbidity burden, necessitating ongoing medical and psychosocial support. In this review, we summarize the current understanding of pediatric HS epidemiology, pathogenesis, clinical presentation, and treatment.

PRESENTATION AND DIAGNOSIS DISCUSSION

Clinical features and comorbidities

HS is a clinical diagnosis characterized by tender deep nodules in intertriginous regions that are rich in apocrine glands, such as the axillae, inframammary area, groin, and perianal area. Disease manifestations include cysts, sinus tract formation, purulent drainage, open comedones, and eventually hypertrophic scars. Diagnosis of HS is based on identifying these chronic, characteristic lesions in intertriginous regions. However, the challenge of misdiagnosis and underdiagnosis exists in children, with a reported clinically meaningful diagnostic gap of about 2 years in pediatric HS [3]. Such diagnostic delays may reflect limited access to dermatologic care or insufficient disease recognition among pediatric primary care providers. These delays can ultimately culminate in more advanced presentations with scarring and sinus tract formation .[4].

Clinical manifestations and affected locations of pediatric HS largely resemble those seen in adults [4,5]. However, pediatric patients may present with more subtle findings like comedones, papules, pustules, or isolated abscesses [3]. Thus, the disease has a high potential to be misdiagnosed as acne, folliculitis, or an infection. It is important to recognize, though, that these 3 conditions may also present alongside HS as part of the follicular occlusion tetrad [6]. Given this range of clinical manifestations, the disease is often not suspected, and flares are initially managed in emergency departments with antibiotics or incision and drainage. Recognition of the disease's chronic or recurrent nature and its characteristic location can often guide clinicians toward HS.

Several comorbidities have been identified in pediatric patients with HS, many of which can significantly impact self-esteem and quality of life. In patients aged 12 to 17, a significant association was demonstrated between HS and psychological impacts. About 32% screened positive for depression on the PHQ-9 and disease severity correlated with poorer quality of life on the Skindex-Teen survey [7]. Other studies have reported associations between HS and anxiety, inflammatory bowel disease, Down syndrome, and metabolic syndrome [6,8,9]. Pediatric onset of HS may have a greater association with endocrine comorbidities including acne, premature adrenarche, polycystic ovarian syndrome, hirsutism, diabetes, and adrenal hyperplasia than adult onset [4,6,10]. Clinicians should have a higher level of suspicion for precocious puberty in children with HS and baseline screening can be recommended.

Disease symptoms may also limit physical activity, contributing to higher levels of obesity, mood disorders, and disease progression .[5,10].

Hidradenitis suppurativa severity and staging

The most widely used staging system for HS is the Hurley system, which categorizes patients into 3 stages based on physical findings. Stage I (mild) involves abscess formation without scarring or sinus tract formation; Stage II (moderate) is characterized by recurrent abscesses with sinus tracts and scarring; Stage III (severe) presents with multiple abscesses and interconnected sinus tracts. However, this system has been criticized for not fully capturing the extent of the disease. Other useful scoring tools include the Sartorius scoring system, International Hidradenitis Suppurative Severity Score System, and the Hidradenitis Suppurative Quality of Life system [11]. These scoring tools are largely used for research purposes and the majority of clinically relevant severity assessment does use the Hurley system.

EPIDEMIOLOGY AND RISK FACTORS

The true prevalence of pediatric HS is uncertain because misdiagnosis and diagnostic delay are common. In US population data, prevalence is estimated between 0.017% to 0.03% overall and rises sharply with age [1,2]. A majority of female patients had an average age at onset of 12.5 but diagnosis age of 14.4, with many patients already presenting with scarring at their first dermatology visit, implying the need for earlier recognition in primary care [3].

The 3 risk factors consistently associated with HS in children are female gender, African American race, and elevated body mass index (BMI). A cross-sectional analysis reported a 3.75-fold greater standardized prevalence of HS in girls compared with boys [1]. Research from other countries show regional differences in male-to-female ratios, versus clear female predominance in Europe and North America (~1:3) [12,13]. Racial differences have also been observed, with one study reporting a 3.5-fold greater standardized prevalence in African American children and adolescents compared with Caucasians .[1].

Furthermore, lifestyle and metabolic factors, specifically weight and insulin related comorbidities are consistently implicated and track with disease burden. Similar to adults, obesity has been identified as a key risk factor for pediatric HS [4]. This is potentially related to mechanical friction within skin folds, microbial overgrowth, and systemic inflammation [14]. Obesity has been seen in 40% to 65% of children and type 2 diabetes is seen in 5% of children with HS [3,15]. Height was not found to be a risk factor. These findings suggest that weight loss, nutrition, and healthy lifestyle modifications should be encouraged when managing pediatric HS.

Among adolescent girls, HS also coaggregates with polycystic ovary syndrome (PCOS); pediatric database studies show elevated PCOS prevalence in HS, suggesting that menstrual irregularity, hirsutism, acne, or weight gain should prompt PCOS evaluation alongside HS care [16]. Acne vulgaris was found to be documented in 29% to 51% of patients with HS [3,17].

Beyond weight and androgens, tobacco exposure during adolescence remains a modifiable risk factor. Data in adult patients show that sustained smoking cessation reduces incidences of HS flares over time, supporting strong counseling to avoid cigarettes and e-cigarettes in youth with HS risk or early disease [18]. Specifically, HS onset before the age of 13 was more often associated with nonsmokers and patients under 18 years who smoked were more likely to have gluteal involvement of HS [2,4] Recognizing this regional flare correlation could guide clinicians in identifying pediatric HS patients who could benefit from smoking cessation efforts.

Additionally, genetic predisposition remains a key driver, as 21% to 42% of patients reporting an affected relative, and twin data show high heritability at ~ 77% [3,19]. However, for the majority of patients, HS appears polygenic with a complex inheritance pattern, and variations that cause rare familial forms of HS are the exception and not the rule [13]. Furthermore, there are mixed studies regarding early-onset disease corresponding with a family history or to a higher Hurley stage [2,4]. HS can also co-occur in autoinflammatory syndromes such as pyoderma gangrenosum, acne, and suppurative hidradenitis [20,21].

In summary, pediatric HS is rare but rises sharply through adolescence. There is a disproportionate burden in African American and biracial female patients in European and North American cohorts. The frequent comorbidity, early scarring, and evidence that early intervention improves outcomes underscores the need for earlier recognition and prospective studies to define natural history and optimize care [1,3].

PATHOGENESIS

HS is currently understood as a chronic, immunoinflammatory disorder of the follicular unit with contributions from aberrant keratinization, dysregulated innate and adaptive immune responses, genetic susceptibility, mechanical forces, hormonal milieu, and microbiome [22]. Abnormal infundibular keratinization leads to follicular occlusion resulting in dilation and rupture allowing keratin, hair shafts, and microbes to enter the dermis and trigger an exaggerated cytokine response characterized by IL-1, tumor necrosis factor alpha (TNF-α), and the T helper (Th)17/interleukin (IL)-17 axis to drive neutrophilic infiltration, tissue destruction, sinus tract formation, and scarring [20,22]. In pediatric patients, this biology is further modulated by pubertal changes. Adrenarche and early sex-hormone shifts temporally precede onset, and case–control data link precocious puberty and adolescent PCOS with HS, supporting attention to hyperandrogenic signs in pediatric evaluations [3].

Genetics

Genetic factors play an important role in shaping susceptibility, age at onset, and clinical course of HS. While the majority of pediatric HS appears to follow a polygenic inheritance pattern, rare familial and early-onset cases highlight the contribution of highly penetrant variations. Specifically, loss-of-function variants in the γ-secretase/Notch pathway genes NCSTN, PSENEN, and PSEN1 have been identified in multiplex families [23–25]. These variations disrupt follicular homeostasis, impair keratinocyte differentiation, and amplify innate immune activation, providing a mechanistic explanation for why disease can emerge aggressively at younger ages. Furthermore, the γ-secretase/Notch axis also intersects with androgen-responsive signaling, offering a biologic link to puberty-associated flares frequently seen in adolescents with HS [19].

Together, these findings suggest that HS exists on a genetic spectrum–at one end, rare familial variations drive early and severe disease; at the other, common variants act in concert with environmental factors such as obesity, smoking, and mechanical stress to lower the threshold for disease onset. This framework may explain why pediatric cases often present differently across families, with some showing strong clustering while others emerge sporadically in the context of broader risk factors.

Process to tunneling

Mechanical forces amplify disease in intertriginous, follicle-dense skin, where obesity increases friction, moisture, and hypoxia that promote dysbiosis and microinjury. Stretch marks or scarring can act as templates for new HS lesions, illustrating a *two-hits* model in which local trauma combines with systemic risk to drive lesion development [26]. The HS microbiome further sustains inflammation–epithelialized tunnels harbor polymicrobial, anaerobe-rich communities and biofilms that resist clearance and remain immunologically active, perpetuating cytokine signaling despite surface quiescence [27–29]. Tunnels also show features of an inflamed epidermis, with hyperplasia, neutrophil infiltration, and upregulated cytokines, confirming that they are not passive scars but active drivers of chronic disease [30]. Together, these findings highlight HS tunnels as metabolically and immunologically distinct niches that explain the persistence of lesions and the difficulty of achieving durable remission.

TREATMENTS

Refer to Fig. 1 for disease progression and treatment targets and Fig. 2 for a pediatric-specific treatment algorithm described later.

Current evidence

Across severities, foundational care includes patient and family education on the chronic and relapsing nature of HS, identification of triggers, gentle skin care with antibacterial washes such as benzoyl peroxide or chlorhexidine, and friction reduction through loose clothing [31]. Tracking of menstrual-linked flares in adolescents and cardiometabolic counseling, framed to avoid weight stigma, are important preventive measures [32]. Symptom control should be prioritized: pain, itch, and drainage are addressed with nonopioid analgesics, short courses of topical anesthetics for procedures, and absorbent dressings; integration of psychosocial screening and school accommodations (such as for participation in physical education) supports quality of life [31]. These fundamental treatment guidelines anchor every plan regardless of

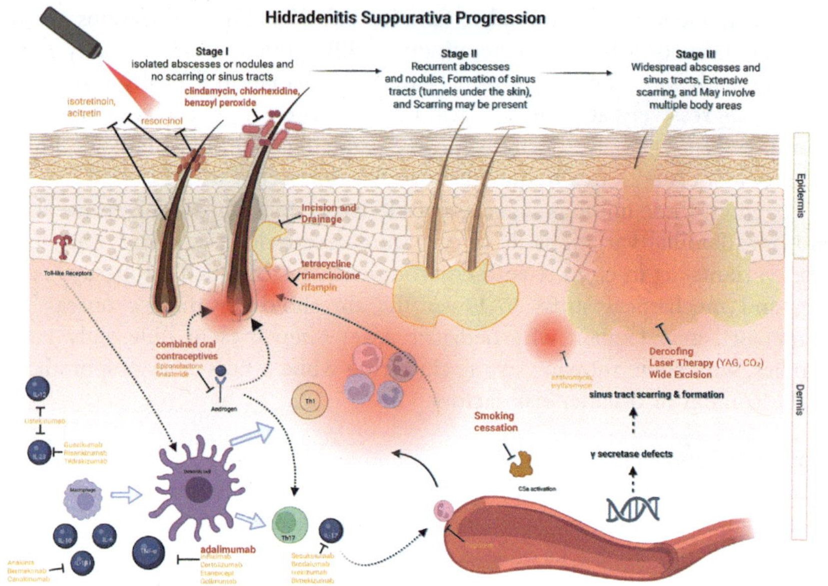

Fig. 1. Progression of HS treatment. Therapies in red text are currently recommended by evidence-based guidelines. Therapies in orange are currently being investigated. (*Created in* BioRender. Dhillon S, et al. (2025) https://BioRender.com/owar4r1.)

severity. Given the progressive nature of HS, it can be useful to initiate the referral process to a dermatologist as soon as HS is suspected.

For mild inflammatory disease, topical clindamycin is considered first-line, often paired with benzoyl peroxide to mitigate bacterial resistance. Intralesional triamcinolone is effective for exquisitely tender nodules. [31,33]. In patients ≥8 years with more active disease, systemic tetracyclines are standard first-line oral agents and may be repeated for flares with antibiotic stewardship and adverse-effect counseling emphasized [31]. For patients with inadequate response, oral clindamycin plus rifampin (300 mg twice daily each) has demonstrated meaningful response rates in prospective studies, though clinicians must monitor for drug–drug interactions and rifampin-associated discoloration [31].

Other antibiotic considerations include a triple regimen of moxifloxacin, metronidazole, and rifampin in older patients [34]. Of note, rifampin will decrease oral contraceptive (OCP) effectiveness [35]. Dapsone may be considered for neutrophilic-predominant disease or antibiotic-intolerant patients, with G6PD testing and hematologic monitoring [35].

Short courses of systemic corticosteroid can help HS flares and be used as a bridge to other systemic therapies, though side effects include sleep disturbance, increased appetite, weight gain, higher postprandial glucose, affected growth, changed moods and energy fluctuations [31].

For moderate-to-severe HS, or earlier in the setting of scarring and tunnel formation, biologic escalation should not be delayed. Adalimumab, an anti–TNF-α

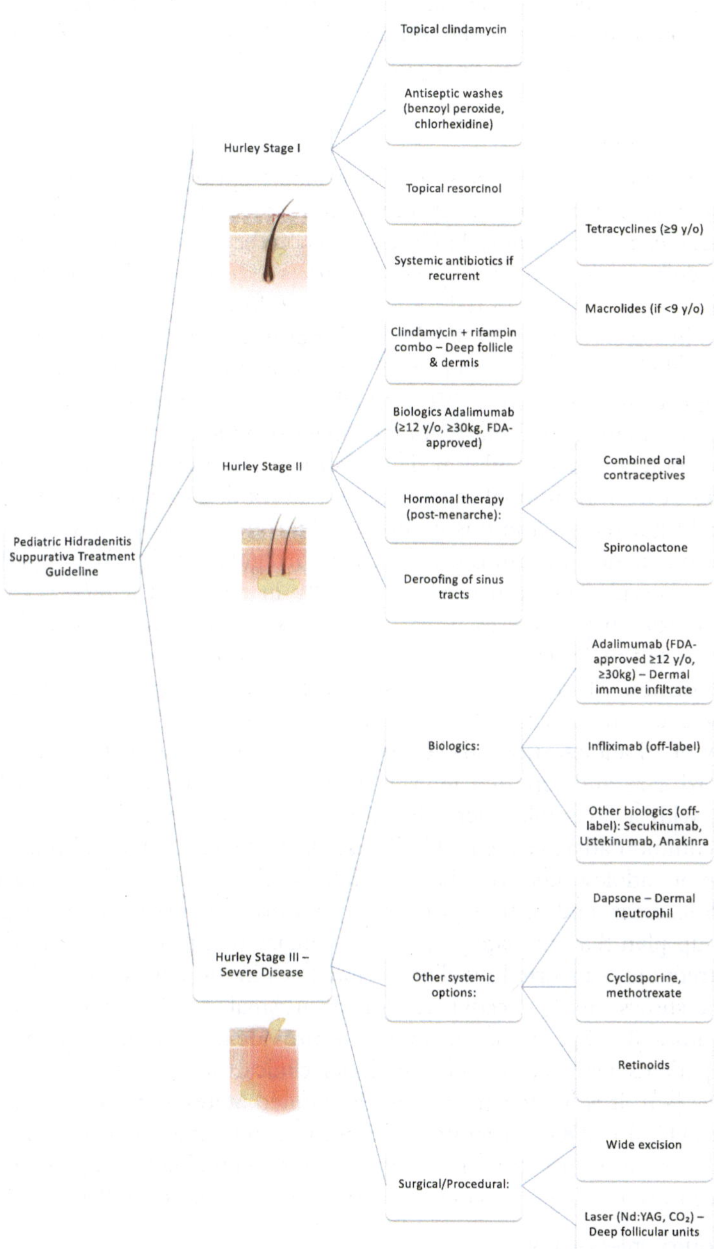

Fig. 2. Support at every stage—antiseptic washes, weight management, pain control, and psychosocial support.

agent, is food and drug adminstration (FDA)-approved for HS in patients ≥12 years with weight-based dosing [36]. IL-17 inhibitors are also FDA-approved in adults and can be upcoming considerations as pediatric data mature [37].

Hormonal strategies

Combined oral contraceptives are a reasonable option for postmenarche adolescents with HS who report cyclical flares, acne, hirsutism, or other signs of androgen excess. The clinical rationale rests on the link between HS and hyperandrogenic states such as polycystic ovary syndrome, and on evidence that hormonal modulation can reduce follicular occlusion and downstream inflammation in select patients [31,35]. Pediatric pathways recommend standard ethinyl estradiol doses paired with third or fourth generation progestins that are less androgenic [35,38]. If OCPs are ineffective or not tolerated, spironolactone can be considered, particularly for its antiandrogenic effect [39,40]. Hyperkalemia is a potential risk in adult patients, but it is uncommon in patients younger than 45 years with normal renal function, so routine electrolyte monitoring is generally not required in this group [41]. Spironolactone is not typically used for male patients and can cause menstrual irregularities in females [40]. Similarly, finasteride has been used successfully in male and female HS patients and has shown promise in pediatric patients but should be used cautiously in adolescent males given that data are sparse [40,42].

Metformin, which targets the insulin metabolic pathways seen in HS, can also be used. In the largest pediatric series to date, a single-center retrospective review of 16 adolescents with Hurley I to II disease used metformin alongside standard care and reported improvement in about half of the evaluable patients, with a favorable tolerability profile and gastrointestinal effects as the most common adverse event [43]. These data support a practical role for metformin in adolescents who have metabolic risk, menstrual irregularity, or PCOS features, and in those who prefer an oral adjunct while moving along a step-up plan that ultimately includes biologics when indicated [35,44].

Isotretinoin, supported by clinical guidelines in the United States but not in Europe shows mixed effectiveness for HS in small retrospective and prospective studies [31]. Specifically, it is noted to provide improvement in younger female patients with facial acne, but lacks clinical benefit for Hurley Stage 3 patients [45]. It is teratogenic and in the United States all patients must enroll in the FDA iPLEDGE program. Acitretin is also teratogenic with a prolonged half-life that warrants extreme caution in those with childbearing potential but has been used in HS with contradictory reports of success [40,45].

Procedural interventions

Procedural interventions are integral to long-term control, typically coordinated with dermatology colleagues. For exquisitely tender inflammatory nodules or early tunnels, acute flares can be managed with corticosteroid injections to reduce pain. Specifically, triamcinolone acetonide intralesional injections can reduce pain within 1 day and decrease erythema and swelling over the first week [46]. For pediatric patients, the lowest effective dose is used to avoid thin skin to limit atrophy or hypopigmentation, while reserving repeat sessions for discrete flares rather than routine maintenance [35]. Comfort can be improved with lidocaine in the injection, topical lidocaine applied before, and age-appropriate distraction techniques [35].

Repeated simple incision and drainage of tunnels is discouraged as it has a recurrence rate of nearly 100% [40]. Rather, tissue-sparing (unroofing of sinus tracts with secondary intention healing), is a well-studied technique in adults that offers durable relief while being tissue-sparing, and is feasible in adolescents [47]. Severe, chronic disease may necessitate wide local excision with grafts or flaps and procedures should be done by pediatric, plastic, or dermatologic surgeons with local or general anesthesia based on age and procedure scope [35].

Many randomized clinical trials have found laser hair removal treatments also effective in improving HS without postprocedure recovery time, but cost is a significant barrier as treatment is often not covered by medical insurance [40,48]. Specifically, long-pulsed 1064-nm Nd:YAG hair-reduction laser reduces inflammatory lesion counts in hair-bearing sites and serves as an adjunct to medical therapy for mature adolescents with coarse terminal hair, proving to be particularly useful in stage I disease.

Adjuvant treatments

Sweating and friction can trigger hidradenitis suppurativa flares, so encourage activities that limit both, and recommend form fitting clothing in skin folds made of moisture wicking fabrics like polyester, spandex, or polypropylene, using antifriction creams or balms. Consideration can also be given to sensitive skin deodorants or botulinum toxin injections for hyperhidrosis [49,50]. To reduce irritation and leakage, suggest high absorbency shorts and undergarments to minimize skin to skin contact, advise against shaving or waxing over lesions, and use tampons or menstrual cups during menses [51].

Dietary modification, such as adopting a Mediterranean diet and reducing high-glycemic foods, has been proposed and studied in adult patients as an adjunctive strategy to reduce insulin resistance–associated inflammation [52–54]. Zinc's immunomodulatory and antioxidant effects make it a plausible adjunct, showing symptomatic improvement in patients who received supplementation alone or combined with other treatments though overall evidence quality remains low and heterogeneous [52,55,56].

Emerging therapies

Biologics now sit at the center of care for HS because many patients progress despite antibiotics, hormones, retinoids, and surgery. Targeted immune modulation can give faster and more durable control of pain, nodules, abscesses, and tunnels with meaningful quality of life improvement [57]. For pediatric patients, approved biologics options are currently limited to the tumor necrosis factor alpha inhibitor, adalimumab. Several additional mechanistic targets under active investigation may expand options for refractory pediatric cases in coming years, which include IL-17 inhibitors, janus kinase (Jak) inhibitors, bruton tyrosine kinase (BTK) inhibitors, and biologics that target the Il-36, IL-1 $\propto$ and IL-β pathways [57].

These biological agents, when approved, may expand options, which are relevant for pediatricians who coordinate care with dermatology and need to plan vaccination review, pregnancy prevention counseling for patients with childbearing potential, and infection risk screening before immunomodulator therapy.

SUMMARY

Pediatric patients with HS often first present to pediatricians, family physicians, or emergency department clinicians, where the disease is frequently misclassified as folliculitis or acne rather than HS [17]. Early recognition shortens the median delay to diagnosis–consider HS in tweens and teens with recurrent, painful *boils* that relapse in the same intertriginous sites and leave scars, and connect with dermatology early [58]. Counsel on medication-specific cautions, embed mental-health support, sleep counseling, and school participation plans into routine follow-up [31]. Before biological initiation, screen for tuberculosis and hepatitis B and update nonlive immunizations; coordinate timing of live vaccines with pediatric infectious diseases when potent immunosuppression is planned [35]. A multidisciplinary partnership between pediatrics and dermatology improves outcomes and adherence, particularly when procedural and systemic therapies are combined.

CLINICS CARE POINTS

Pearls

- Suspect HS in children and adolescents with recurrent painful nodules, abscesses, or draining tracts in flexural areas.
- Connect to a dermatologist early.
- Screen systematically for comorbidities and triggers. Assess weight, menstrual irregularity or PCOS features, mood symptoms, and tobacco exposure, and provide counseling, school accommodations, and clear plans for pain and drainage.

Pitfalls

- Misinterpreting lesions as *simple boils* or acne delays referral and risks scarring and sinus tract formation.
- Overreliance on antibiotics without addressing HS pathophysiology.
- Overlooking HS in male patients, who may be underrepresented in pediatric cohorts, can delay diagnosis and care.

Disclosure

The authors have nothing to disclose.

References

[1] Garg A, Wertenteil S, Baltz R, et al. Prevalence estimates for hidradenitis suppurativa among children and adolescents in the United States: a Gender- and age-adjusted population analysis. J Invest Dermatol 2018;138(10):2152–6.
[2] Deckers IE, van der Zee HH, Boer J, et al. Correlation of early-onset hidradenitis suppurativa with stronger genetic susceptibility and more widespread involvement. J Am Acad Dermatol 2015;72(3):485–8.
[3] Liy-Wong C, Kim M, Kirkorian AY, et al. Hidradenitis suppurativa in the pediatric population: an international, multicenter, retrospective, cross-sectional study of 481 pediatric patients. JAMA Dermatol 2021;157(4):385–91.
[4] Garcovich S, Fania L, Caposiena D, et al. Pediatric hidradenitis suppurativa: a cross-sectional study on clinical features and treatment approaches. J Cutan Med Surg 2022;26(2):127–34.
[5] Górecka A, Barańska-Rybak W, Lewandowski M, et al. Pediatric-onset hidradenitis suppurativa: a case series of 42 patients. Advances in Dermatology and Allergology/Postępy Dermatologii i Alergologii 2024;41(5):525–9.
[6] Kimball AB, Sundaram M, Gauthier G, et al. The comorbidity burden of hidradenitis suppurativa in the United States: a claims data analysis. Dermatol Therapy 2018;8(4):557–69.
[7] McAndrew R, Lopes FC, Sebastian K, et al. Quality of life in hidradenitis suppurativa: a cross-sectional study of a pediatric population. J Am Acad Dermatol 2021;84(3): 829–30.
[8] Garg A, Malviya N, Strunk A, et al. Comorbidity screening in hidradenitis suppurativa: evidence-based recommendations from the US and Canadian hidradenitis suppurativa foundations. J Am Acad Dermatol 2022;86(5):1092–101.
[9] Tiri H, Jokelainen J, Timonen M, et al. Somatic and psychiatric comorbidities of hidradenitis suppurativa in children and adolescents. J Am Acad Dermatol 2018;79(3):514–9.
[10] Liy-Wong C, Pope E, Lara-Corrales I. Hidradenitis suppurativa in the pediatric population. J Am Acad Dermatol 2015;73(5):S36–41.
[11] Zouboulis CC, Prens EP, Sayed CJ, et al. International hidradenitis suppurativa severity scoring system (IHS4) as a holistic measure of hidradenitis suppurativa disease severity compared with Hurley staging: a post hoc analysis of the SUNRISE and SUNSHINE phase 3 trials of secukinumab. J Eur Acad Dermatol Venereol 2024;38(6).
[12] Ingram JR. The epidemiology of hidradenitis suppurativa. Br J Dermatol 2020;183(6): 990–8.
[13] Kaya G, Özgen FP, Kelahmetoğlu O, et al. Demographic features, clinical characteristics, and comorbid relation in hidradenitis suppurativa: a population-based study. Original Research. Front Med 2025;11–2024; https://doi.org/10.3389/fmed.2024.1499509.
[14] Balgobind A, Finelt N, Strunk A, et al. Association between obesity and hidradenitis suppurativa among children and adolescents: a population-based analysis in the United States. J Am Acad Dermatol 2020;82(2):502–4.
[15] Mehta S, Metko D, Lam JM. Obesity in pediatric hidradenitis suppurativa: a scoping review. Pediatr Dermatol 2025;42(1):91–4.
[16] Garg A, Neuren E, Strunk A. Hidradenitis Suppurativa is associated with polycystic ovary syndrome: a population-based analysis in the United States. J Invest Dermatol 2018;138(6): 1288–92; https://doi.org/10.1016/j.jid.2018.01.009.
[17] Hallock KK, Mizerak MR, Dempsey A, et al. Differences between children and adults with hidradenitis suppurativa. JAMA Dermatol 2021;157(9):1095–101.
[18] Kim SR, Choi YG, Jo SJ. Smoking cessation and risk of hidradenitis suppurativa development. JAMA Dermatol 2024;160(10):1056–65.
[19] van Straalen KR, Prens EP, Willemsen G, et al. Contribution of genetics to the susceptibility to hidradenitis suppurativa in a large, cross-sectional Dutch twin cohort. JAMA Dermatol 2020;156(12):1359–62.
[20] Ingram JR. The genetics of hidradenitis suppurativa. Dermatol Clin 2016;34(1):23–8.

[21] Braun-Falco M, Kovnerystyy O, Lohse P, et al. Pyoderma gangrenosum, acne, and suppurative hidradenitis (PASH)–a new autoinflammatory syndrome distinct from PAPA syndrome. J Am Acad Dermatol 2012;66(3):409–15.
[22] Frew JW. Intrinsic factors in the pathogenesis of hidradenitis suppurativa: genetics, hormones, and the microbiome. J Am Acad Dermatol 2024;91(6):S12–6.
[23] Nomura Y, Nomura T, Sakai K, et al. A novel splice site mutation in NCSTN underlies a Japanese family with hidradenitis suppurativa. Br J Dermatol 2013;168(1):206–9.
[24] Pink AE, Simpson MA, Desai N, et al. γ-Secretase variations in hidradenitis suppurativa: new insights into disease pathogenesis. J Invest Dermatol 2013;133(3):601–7.
[25] Sun Q, Broadaway KA, Edmiston SN, et al. Genetic variants associated with hidradenitis suppurativa. JAMA Dermatol 2023;159(9):930–8.
[26] Boer J, Jemec GBE. Mechanical forces and Hidradenitis Suppurativa. Exp Dermatol 2021;30(2):212–5.
[27] Ring HC, Sigsgaard V, Thorsen J, et al. The microbiome of tunnels in hidradenitis suppurativa patients. J Eur Acad Dermatol Venereol 2019;33(9):1775–80.
[28] Soto-Moreno A, Haselgruber-de Francisco S, León-Pérez J, et al. The microbiome in Hidradenitis Suppurativa tunnels: a systematic review. Int J Dermatol 2025;64(10):1802–12.
[29] Guet-Revillet H, Jais JP, Ungeheuer MN, et al. The microbiological landscape of anaerobic infections in Hidradenitis Suppurativa: a prospective metagenomic study. Clin Infect Dis 2017;65(2):282–91.
[30] Byrd AS, Carmona-Rivera C, O'Neil LJ, et al. Neutrophil extracellular traps, B cells, and type I interferons contribute to immune dysregulation in hidradenitis suppurativa. Sci Transl Med 2019;11(508); https://doi.org/10.1126/scitranslmed.aav5908.
[31] Alikhan A, Sayed C, Alavi A, et al. North American clinical management guidelines for hidradenitis suppurativa: a publication from the United States and Canadian Hidradenitis Suppurativa Foundations: part I: diagnosis, evaluation, and the use of complementary and procedural management. J Am Acad Dermatol 2019;81(1):76–90.
[32] Shalom G, Freud T, Harman-Boehm I, et al. Hidradenitis suppurativa and metabolic syndrome: a comparative cross-sectional study of 3207 patients. Br J Dermatol 2015;173(2): 464–70.
[33] Molinelli E, Brisigotti V, Simonetti O, et al. Efficacy and safety of topical resorcinol 15% versus topical clindamycin 1% in the management of mild-to-moderate hidradenitis suppurativa: a retrospective study. Dermatol Ther 2022;35(6):e15439; https://doi.org/10.1111/dth.15439.
[34] Delage M, Jais J-P, Lam T, et al. Rifampin-moxifloxacin-metronidazole combination therapy for severe Hurley stage 1 hidradenitis suppurativa: prospective short-term trial and 1-year follow-up in 28 consecutive patients. J Am Acad Dermatol 2023;88(1):94–100.
[35] Cotton CH, Chen SX, Hussain SH, et al. Hidradenitis suppurativa in pediatric patients. Pediatrics 2023;151(5); https://doi.org/10.1542/peds.2022-061049.
[36] Kimball AB, Okun MM, Williams DA, et al. Two phase 3 trials of adalimumab for Hidradenitis Suppurativa. N Engl J Med 2016;375(5):422–34.
[37] Kimball AB, Jemec GBE, Alavi A, et al. Secukinumab in moderate-to-severe hidradenitis suppurativa (SUNSHINE and SUNRISE): week 16 and week 52 results of two identical, multicentre, randomised, placebo-controlled, double-blind phase 3 trials. Lancet 2023;401 (10378):747–61.
[38] Svoboda RM, Nawaz N, Zaenglein AL. Hormonal treatment of acne and hidradenitis suppurativa in adolescent patients. Dermatol Clin 2022;40(2):167–78.
[39] Lee A, Fischer G. A case series of 20 women with hidradenitis suppurativa treated with spironolactone. Australas J Dermatol 2015;56(3):192–6.
[40] Johnston LA, Alhusayen R, Bourcier M, et al. Practical guidelines for managing patients with Hidradenitis Suppurativa: an update. J Cutan Med Surg 2022;26(2_suppl):2S–24S.
[41] Layton AM, Eady EA, Whitehouse H, et al. Oral spironolactone for acne vulgaris in adult females: a hybrid systematic review. Am J Clin Dermatol 2017;18(2):169–91.

[42] Khandalavala BN, Do MV. Finasteride in Hidradenitis Suppurativa: a "Male" Therapy for a Predominantly "Female" disease. J Clin Aesthet Dermatol 2016;9(6):44–50.
[43] Moussa C, Wadowski L, Price H, et al. Metformin as adjunctive therapy for pediatric patients with Hidradenitis Suppurativa. J Drugs Dermatol JDD 2020;19(12):1231–4.
[44] Chung CS, Park SE, Hsiao JL, et al. A review of Hidradenitis Suppurativa in special populations: considerations in children, pregnant and breastfeeding women, and the elderly. Dermatol Ther 2024;14(9):2407–25.
[45] Frew JW, Hawkes JE, Krueger JG. Topical, systemic and biologic therapies in hidradenitis suppurativa: pathogenic insights by examining therapeutic mechanisms. Therapeutic Advances in Chronic Disease 2019;10:2040622319830646; https://doi.org/10.1177/2040622319830646.
[46] Riis PT, Boer J, Prens EP, et al. Intralesional triamcinolone for flares of hidradenitis suppurativa (HS): a case series. J Am Acad Dermatol 2016;75(6):1151–5.
[47] Leszczynska M, Diaz LZ, Peña-Robichaux V. Surgical deroofing in pediatric patients with hidradenitis suppurativa. Pediatr Dermatol 2022;39(3):502–5.
[48] Naouri M, Maruani A, Lagrange S, et al. Treatment of hidradenitis suppurativa using a long-pulsed hair removal neodymium:yttrium-aluminium-garnet laser: a multicenter, prospective, randomized, intraindividual, comparative trial. J Am Acad Dermatol 2021;84(1):203–5.
[49] Von der Werth J, Williams H. The natural history of hidradenitis suppurativa. J Eur Acad Dermatol Venereol 2000;14(5):389–92.
[50] Thompson A, Fernandez J, Rick J, et al. Identifying triggers for hidradenitis suppurativa flare: a patient survey. Br J Dermatol 2021;185(1):225–6.
[51] Collier E, Shi VY, Parvataneni RK, et al. Special considerations for women with hidradenitis suppurativa. Int J Women's Dermatol 2020/03/01/2020;6(2):85–8.
[52] Vural S, Baskurt D, Yldrc Ş, et al. Evaluating dietary considerations in hidradenitis suppurativa: a critical examination of existing knowledge. Int J Dermatol 2024;63(8):987–98.
[53] Barrea L, Fabbrocini G, Annunziata G, et al. Role of nutrition and adherence to the mediterranean diet in the multidisciplinary approach of hidradenitis suppurativa: evaluation of nutritional status and its association with severity of disease. Nutrients 2018;11(1):57.
[54] Lorite-Fuentes I, Montero-Vilchez T, Arias-Santiago S, et al. Potential benefits of the mediterranean diet and physical activity in patients with hidradenitis suppurativa: a cross-sectional study in a Spanish population. Nutrients 2022;14(3):551.
[55] Poveda I, Vilarrasa E, Martorell A, et al. Serum zinc levels in hidradenitis suppurativa: a case–control study. Am J Clin Dermatol 2018;19(5):771–7.
[56] Hessam S, Sand M, Meier NM, et al. Combination of oral zinc gluconate and topical triclosan: an anti-inflammatory treatment modality for initial hidradenitis suppurativa. J Dermatol Sci 2016;84(2):197–202.
[57] Garg A, Hsiao J, Porter ML, et al. Current treatments and future directions for Hidradenitis Suppurativa: a narrative review of completed and ongoing phase 3 clinical trials of biologic therapies. Dermatol Ther 2025/09/01 2025;15(9):2361–77.
[58] Kokolakis G, Wolk K, Schneider-Burrus S, et al. Delayed diagnosis of hidradenitis suppurativa and its effect on patients and healthcare system. Dermatology 2020;236(5):421–30.

Advances in Pediatrics 73 (2026) 309–322

ADVANCES IN PEDIATRICS

Sleep Disturbances in Pediatric Craniofacial Syndromes

Katie Tribuls, DO[a], Carolyn Madden, APRN[b], Sagarika Nallu, MD[c,*]

[a]Department of Pulmonary, Critical Care and Sleep Medicine, University of South Florida Morsani School of Medicine, Tampa, FL, USA; [b]Department of Pediatrics, University of South Florida Morsani College of Medicine, Tampa, FL, USA; [c]University of South Florida Morsani College of Medicine, Tampa, FL, USA

Keywords

- Craniofacial • Craniofacial syndromes • Craniofacial abnormalities
- Sleep disturbances • Pediatric sleep-disordered breathing
- Pediatric obstructive sleep apnea

Key points

- Children with craniofacial abnormalities are at high risk for developing sleep disturbances.
- Sleep-disordered breathing in children with craniofacial abnormalities is often multifactorial.
- Screening for sleep disorders in children with craniofacial abnormalities is an important part in the care of these children.
- A multidisciplinary approach is often required for management of sleep disorders in these children.
- Early management of sleep disorders can improve quality of life and reduce cardiovascular risk in children with craniofacial abnormalities.

INTRODUCTION

Sleep disturbances are a problem in childhood, and they can have a profound influence on overall health. Restorative sleep is critical for proper neurocognitive development during this critical period of growth. Sleep deprivation contributes to deficits in mental and behavioral health, including emotional and

*Corresponding author. University of South Florida, Mosani College of Medicine, 13101 Bruce B Downs Boulevard, Tampa, FL 33612. *E-mail address:* snallu@usf.edu

https://doi.org/10.1016/j.yapd.2025.12.008
0065-3101/26/

Abbreviations

BP	blood pressure
CBC	complete blood count
CPAP	continuous positive airway pressure
CSA	central sleep apnea
HNS	hypoglossal nerve stimulation
OSA	obstructive sleep apnea
PAP	positive airway pressure
PSG	polysomnography
SDB	sleep-disordered breathing

mood dysregulation, increased anxiety and depression, and decreased concentration. Sufficient sleep is necessary for the regulation of growth and metabolic hormones, whereas insufficient sleep can contribute to impaired glucose tolerance and reduced insulin sensitivity. Regular sleep has been shown to strengthen immune system function with reduced susceptibility to infection [1]. In addition to consequences for the child, disrupted sleep and insufficient sleep in children can have detrimental psychological effects on parents, contributing to strife within the family unit [2].

This article seeks to fill knowledge gaps in screening for and identifying common sleep disorders in the pediatric population. Sleep disturbances in this population require a different treatment approach compared with the adult population, and pediatricians play a crucial role in identifying potential sleep disorders [3]. Many sleep disorders often go unrecognized or are mislabeled as behavioral problems. Children with craniofacial abnormalities are at particular risk for sleep disturbances. The authors have divided common pediatric sleep diagnoses into sleep-related respiratory disorders and nonrespiratory disorders.

RESPIRATORY DISORDERS

Children with craniofacial abnormalities experience a continuum of sleep-disordered breathing (SDB), which ranges from primary snoring, upper airway resistance syndrome, obstructive sleep apnea (OSA), and, less frequently, hypoventilation. The mildest form of SDB is primary snoring, which is common and can be the first sign of increased upper airway resistance. Upper airway resistance syndrome involves increased airway collapsibility with narrowing of the airway. Its presentation can be similar to that of impaired sleep, with accompanying daytime complaints. However, it is usually not accompanied by hypoxemia and does not meet the full criteria for OSA. OSA is characterized by repetitive partial or complete collapse of the upper airway associated with intermittent episodes of associated hypoxemia and nighttime arousals. The pathophysiology of pediatric OSA can be complex and is often multifactorial, especially in patients with craniofacial abnormalities. Both anatomic factors, like craniofacial abnormalities, which can lead to a reduced upper airway size, and nonanatomic factors can predispose a child to SDB [4].

Nonanatomic features include hypotonia and neuromuscular dysfunctions that can impair upper airway muscle tone and stability, leading to increased upper airway collapsibility during sleep, even in the absence of significant airway narrowing. Hypoventilation syndromes can present as a more severe form of SDB, associated with sustained hypoventilation and hypercapnia with or without apneas. These syndromes can be seen in children with severe craniofacial abnormalities as well as children with neuromuscular involvement.

The prevalence of sleep disorders in pediatric patients with craniofacial abnormalities approaches 25%, with patients with syndromic conditions being at particular risk [5]. There are many pediatric genetic or congenital syndromes associated with OSA, including Pierre Robin sequence, Down syndrome, Crouzon syndrome, Treacher Collins syndrome, Muenke syndrome, and Apert syndrome (Table 1) [6]. These syndromes are characterized by distinct craniofacial abnormalities, and patients often have systemic involvement affecting multiple organ systems. They frequently have multiple anomalies that contribute to a markedly higher prevalence of OSA owing to complex, multilevel obstruction and structural abnormalities. Nonsyndromic craniofacial abnormalities occur in isolation, often in otherwise healthy children, but even isolated features may predispose the child to OSA.

Central sleep apnea (CSA) is a less common condition that has been reported in children with craniofacial abnormalities. It is characterized by episodes of cessation of airflow with associated lack of respiratory effort. Usually, CSA in children is benign and related to arousal and transitions from wake to sleep. However, frequent CSAs while asleep can be associated with developmental disorders and can indicate a more serious pathologic condition that should prompt further evaluation by a sleep specialist. Pathologic CSA is typically found in the context of associated structural neurologic conditions, genetic conditions affecting respiratory control, or cardiac abnormalities [7]. Children with syndromic craniosynostosis and Chiari malformations are at increased risk, and central events may present alongside obstructive events. Typically, if

Table 1
Craniofacial abnormalities that increase the risk for sleep-disordered breathing

Chromosomal disorders	Syndromic craniosynostosis conditions	Syndromic craniofacial microsomia conditions	Isolated conditions
Trisomy 21	Apert syndrome	Treacher Collins syndrome	Cleft lip
Trisomy 18	Crouzon syndrome	Pierre Robin syndrome	Cleft palate
Prader Willi syndrome	Pfeiffer syndrome	22q11.2 deletion syndrome	Micrognathia/retro
Smith-Magenis syndrome	Muenke syndrome		Craniosynostosis
	Saethre-Chotzen syndrome		High arched palate
	Carpenter syndrome		

CSA is identified, further investigation into neurologic and cardiac issues is warranted with an echocardiogram and a brain MRI, with management directed at addressing the underlying cause.

SDB can have profound consequences. It can lead to poor sleep quality and has also been associated with a poorer quality of life, especially in children with syndromic craniosynostosis [8]. Children with SDB, including OSA, also exhibit a significantly increased risk for elevated blood pressure (BP), not only during nocturnal sleep but also during daytime resting periods [9]. This elevation in BP has been attributed to repeated arousals, intermittent hypoxemia, and activation of the sympathetic nervous system, all of which contribute to persistent alterations in autonomic cardiovascular regulation. Notably, even habitual snoring in children who do not meet diagnostic criteria for SDB has been independently associated with higher daytime resting BP, suggesting that upper airway resistance and sleep fragmentation, irrespective of apneic events, may influence cardiovascular risk profiles in pediatric populations [10]. In addition, childhood OSA has been associated with deficits of IQ as well as abnormal neuronal metabolism, which could impair cognitive potential [11].

Medical history

A detailed history can reveal significant clues when evaluating patients with sleep disturbances. Although some children may present with daytime fatigue and sleepiness, children with SDB more often present with disrupted sleep or neurobehavioral issues. Nocturnal symptoms can include snoring, labored breathing, diaphoresis, paradoxic chest and abdominal movement, or "belly breathing," and frequent movements during sleep. Daytime symptoms may include poor school performance, mood issues including depression, aggressive behavior, morning headaches, inappropriate napping, and difficulty arousing from sleep. Some children may initially present with concerns for attention-deficit/hyperactivity disorder with inattentiveness, hyperactivity, and lack of impulse control. Nocturnal enuresis, particularly in children who have already obtained bladder control, can be a sign of sleep disturbance. Failure to thrive is another critical sign that can be seen in SDB.

In children with craniofacial abnormalities, a thorough understanding of their facial anomalies is imperative. Although some craniofacial anomalies may present as isolated malformations, others may present as part of a syndromic condition, which can have multisystem involvement. If the craniofacial abnormality is part of a syndromic condition in children with suspected SDB, further characterization of the genetic or chromosomal disorder, as well as the specific anatomic site affected, can help guide risk assessment and management strategies. Children with craniofacial abnormalities are more likely to have neurocognitive and developmental delays. They can also have vision or hearing deficits, which can further predispose them to behavioral issues. Concomitant medical conditions can also provide insight regarding the risk of SDB. A history of allergic rhinitis should raise concern because of the strong correlation between chronic allergies and adenotonsillar hypertrophy, and subsequent SDB. Chiari malformations and other conditions associated with increased intracranial pressure have been associated with OSA, and to some degree, CSA. Cardiac abnormalities and restrictive lung diseases can also contribute to central sleep disorders in the pediatric population.

In pediatric patients with craniofacial abnormalities, a thorough surgical history is essential when evaluating sleep disturbances, particularly SDB. Surgical interventions significantly alter upper airway anatomy and dynamics, often influencing both the severity and the presentation of SDB. Key procedures to document include adenotonsillectomy, mandibular distraction osteogenesis, midface advancement, cleft palate repair, tongue-lip adhesion, and tracheostomy, noting the timing, staging, and clinical outcomes of each [12,13]. In addition, orthodontic interventions, including rapid maxillary expansion and mandibular advancement, may impact airway patency and should be considered in sleep evaluations [7]. History of tracheostomy, decannulation, or use of temporary airway support devices provides insight into the severity of previous airway compromise. In addition, surgeries for other system comorbidities, including cardiac or neurologic, may also affect sleep physiology.

It is important to review medications and consider their potential impact on sleep, specifically, medications that can cause decreased respiratory drive. Children with Prader-Willi syndrome who are on human growth hormone should be monitored for signs of SDB. Antiepileptics, in particular gabapentin and valproic acid, have been associated with an increased risk of OSA [14].

Several environmental factors may increase the risk of developing OSA in children. Maternal smoking during pregnancy and exposure to smoke after birth are both associated with high rates of OSA. Air pollution has been associated with an increased risk of snoring and OSA.

Neonatal and birth history can provide useful information when evaluating the risk for SDB in children. Prematurity is associated with central apnea of prematurity, fragmented sleep, and increased rates of OSA later in childhood [15]. A history of mechanical ventilation, low birth weight, or neonatal airway interventions may indicate underlying airway instability or structural compromise, underscoring the need for early sleep evaluation in this high-risk group [16].

Physical examination

A careful physical examination can provide great insight when treating children with craniofacial malformation. Children may present with isolated craniofacial abnormalities or with several, as in the case of many syndromic conditions. Special attention should be paid to the mouth, jaw, oropharynx, and nose, as these areas largely affect the risk of SDB.

Adenotonsillar hypertrophy is the most common cause of OSA in children with and without craniofacial abnormalities. Because of naturally narrow airways in children, enlargement of these soft tissues predisposes them to airway obstruction, especially in children with craniofacial abnormalities. In the general pediatric population, adenoidal and tonsillar hypertrophy are positively associated with OSA, with an even greater risk if both adenoid and tonsillar hypertrophy occur together [17,18]. In children with other craniofacial abnormalities, adenotonsillar hypertrophy may further compromise an already narrowed airway. The Modified Mallampati score is a useful tool that clinicians should use when assessing airway risk for SDB. Higher scores, class III or IV, are strongly associated with an increased risk and severity of OSA in children and may indicate limited response to adenotonsillectomy [19,20].

Mandibular size and position should be closely evaluated as mandibular hypoplasia, micrognathia, and retrognathia can lead to posterior displacement of the tongue and subsequent airway obstruction. The Jaw Index is a tool clinicians can use in neonates and infants to identify the severity of micrognathia and can be particularly useful in identifying future risks of airway obstruction, especially in cases of Pierre Robin sequence [21,22].

When evaluating the palate, findings of a high arched palate, narrow palatal width, and cleft palate can contribute to an overall smaller airway. Cleft palate is a common birth defect, affecting approximately 1 in 1000 live births in the United States, according to the National Institutes of Health [23,24]. Cleft palate may be unilateral or bilateral and may or may not accompany a cleft lip. It has been associated with reduced upper airway size, even after surgical repair. Palatal surgeries are one of the many surgical interventions that can contribute to the development of velopharyngeal insufficiency or dysfunction, which can further contribute to SDB [25].

Macroglossia can be commonly found in syndromic craniofacial syndromes, causing narrowing of the airway. Glossoptosis, backward and downward displacement of the tongue, may be seen alone or in conjunction with macroglossia, leading to obstruction of the retroglossal airway [26]. Dental features and malocclusions associated with increased risk of SDB in children with craniofacial abnormalities include mandibular retrognathia, increased overjet, anterior open bite, posterior crossbite, narrow and high-arched palate, and convex facial profile.

Nasal abnormalities may be common in patients with syndromic abnormalities. Low nasal arch, nasal stenosis, and other deformities, including deviated septum, hypoplastic nasal bones, or narrow nasal vault, decrease the cross-sectional area of the nasal airway. Evaluating the nasal turbinates may reveal hypertrophy or pallor, which can be seen in chronic allergic rhinitis and can contribute to snoring and upper airway resistance. In addition, a deviated septum may also contribute to nasal obstruction. Nasal obstruction in general leads to increased airflow resistance and a greater tendency for mouth breathing. Mouth breathing is a risk factor for SDB, and it can further alter craniofacial growth, thereby perpetuating airway compromise.

Additional physical examination findings unrelated to the oral airway can also provide insight. Infraorbital darkening can be seen in children with allergies, which, as previously mentioned, is associated with SDB. In certain craniosynostosis syndromes, fundoscopic examinations can reveal signs of elevated intracranial pressure, which is positively associated with OSA. Chest wall examination evaluating for pectus excavatum or carinatum should be done. Chest wall abnormalities can contribute to restrictive lung and hypoventilation with resultant nocturnal hypoxemia or hypercapnia. Cardiac findings of a prominent S3 on auscultation should raise concern about potential heart failure, which can be seen in severe cases of SDB, both as a contributing factor and as a side effect. Evidence of clubbing should also be noted and can indicate chronic hypoxemia.

Abnormal vital signs, specifically hypertension and an elevated body mass index, should raise concern when screening for SDB. Obesity in the pediatric population is a growing concern and is an independent risk factor for OSA in healthy children. However, in children with craniofacial malformations, obesity may play a smaller role (Table 2) [27].

Screening

Screening for proper sleep should be as essential as screening for proper diet, exercise, and safety at every well-child visit. Current recommendations from the American Academy of Pediatrics include screening all pediatric patients for snoring [28]. In children with craniofacial abnormalities, however, both the American Heart Association and the American Academy of Pediatrics recommend a low threshold for screening and polysomnography (PSG) owing to the high risk and potential for severe disease [28,29]. Fig. 1 presents an algorithm for screening these children. The gold standard for screening and

Table 2
Examination findings in children at risk for sleep-disordered breathing

Treacher Collins syndrome	Mandibular hypoplasia, zygomatic arch hypoplasia
Pierre Robin sequence	Micrognathia, glossoptosis
Apert syndrome	Maxillary hypoplasia, highly arched palate, cleft palate, V-shaped maxillary dental arch, class 3 malocclusion
Crouzon syndrome	Beaked nose, midface hypoplasia
Pfeiffer syndrome	Midface hypoplasia, craniosynostosis (cloverleaf skull)
Muenke syndrome	Brachycephaly, midface hypoplasia, high arched palate, cleft palate
Saethre-Chotzen syndrome	Facial asymmetry, deviated septum
Carpenter syndrome	Brachycephaly, flat nasal bridge, narrow high-arched palate, hypoplastic mandible and/or maxilla, obesity
Nager syndrome	Micrognathia, maxillary hypoplasia, choanal atresia
Stickler syndrome	Micrognathia, maxillary hypoplasia, short genioglossus, soft tracheal cartilage
Trisomy 21	Flat facial profile, flat nasal bridge, protruding tongue, short neck, narrow palate, hypotonia, obesity
Prader-Willi syndrome	Brachycephaly, hypotonia, obesity secondary to hyperphagia, growth hormone deficiency
22q11.2 deletion syndrome	Retrognathia, micrognathia, palatal abnormalities (cleft, velopharyngeal insufficiency), facial hypoplasia, craniosynostosis
Smith-Magenis syndrome	Midface hypoplasia, brachycephaly, mandibular prognathism

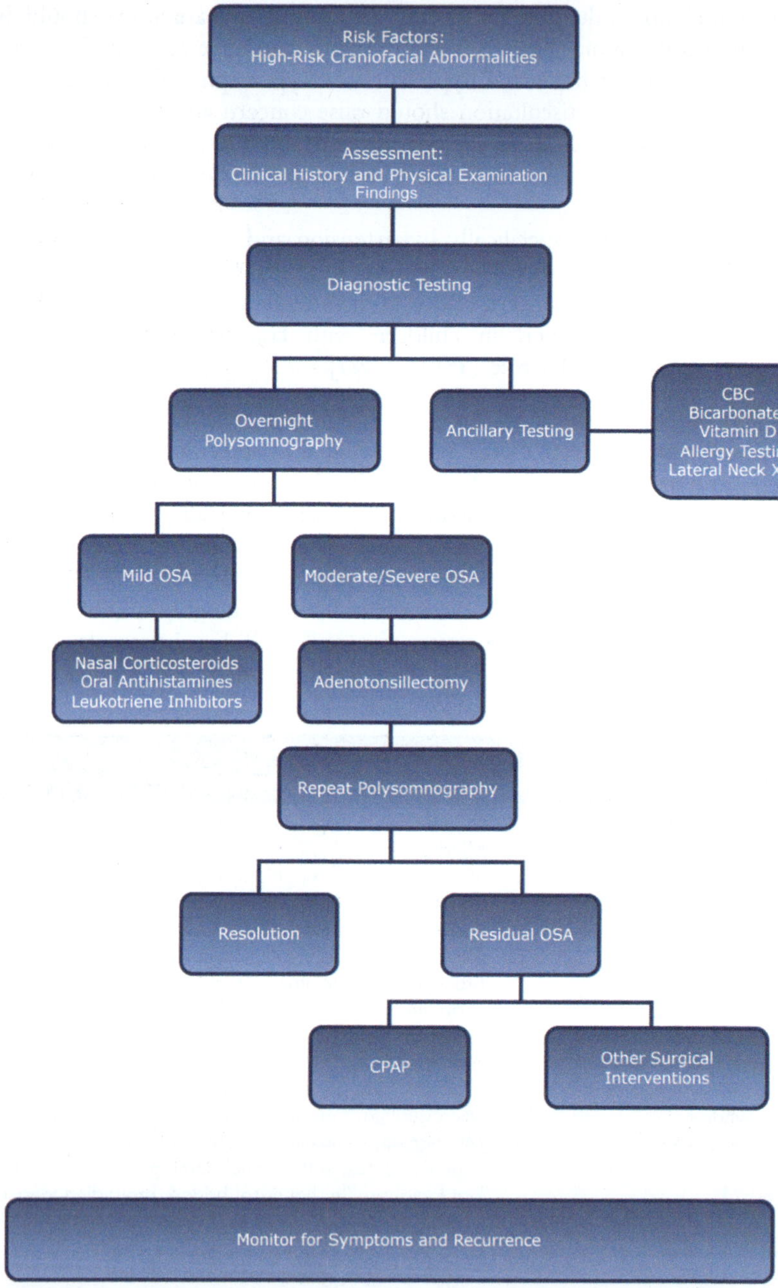

Fig. 1. Screening algorithm for SDB in children with craniofacial abnormalities.

diagnosis for pediatric SDB in all ages is an overnight, attended in-laboratory PSG. Severity is determined by the number of respiratory events that occur per hour, which are further categorized as either obstructive events, central events, or mixed. Other parameters monitored during PSGs include oximetry, carbon dioxide levels, limb movements, and electroencephalogram to characterize sleep staging.

In cases of mild OSA without significant symptoms, the use of nasal corticosteroids, oral antihistamines, and leukotriene inhibitors can be effective. If there is persistence of symptoms or PSG reveals moderate or severe OSA, surgical intervention is indicated, with adenotonsillectomy generally considered first-line treatment. Unfortunately, the cure rate with adenotonsillectomy is lower in children with craniofacial abnormalities, usually owing to multilevel sites of obstruction. After surgical intervention, a repeat PSG 3 months postprocedure is recommended to ensure resolution of the SDB. If residual sleep apnea is identified on repeat PSG, referral to a sleep specialist can help guide the next intervention. In this situation, a multidisciplinary team is often required [30]. The American Academy of Otolaryngology–Head and Neck Surgery recommends that children with craniofacial abnormalities and persistent OSA after tonsillectomy and adenoidectomy should be managed with a combination of medical and surgical options tailored to the site and severity of obstruction [31]. In cases where the baseline PSG shows complex sleep disorders, including a combination of OSA or severe OSA, early referral to a sleep specialist can be useful. Other surgical options may be warranted at this time, depending on the level of obstruction. A drug-induced sleep endoscopy may be useful in this case to help identify the site of obstruction and help dictate further management. Successful treatment of complex SDB may require collaborations with dentists and orthodontists, otolaryngologists, oral and maxillofacial specialists, and plastic and reconstructive surgeons.

If surgical options fail to correct the OSA or if a nonsurgical option is desired, continuous positive airway pressure (CPAP) can be considered. It is effective in severe OSA and with multilevel obstruction. Before the initiation of positive airway pressure (PAP) therapy in children, a PAP titration PSG is required during which PAP is titrated throughout the night to achieve resolution of sleep-related breathing disorder. AutoPAP therapy is not typically used in pediatric patients, except in the rare case of older adolescents who have already physically matured. Adequate CPAP usage may be challenging to use in certain pediatric patients, especially in children with neurodevelopmental delays. When there is trouble tolerating CPAP, a sleep specialist can often provide guidance to both parents and physicians on techniques to improve compliance.

Hypoglossal nerve stimulation (HNS) is an emerging therapy that is effective in adolescents with trisomy 21. Multiple prospective studies, case series, and systematic reviews demonstrate that HNS produces a 50% to 85% reduction in the apneic-hypopneic index in most pediatric patients with Down syndrome, with many achieving values in the normal or mild OSA range after device titration [32,33]. Currently, HNS is approved for adolescents older than 13 years old, with prospective studies also showing initial safety and efficacy in younger children [34]. Although there have been a few case reports of HNS in other genetic and craniofacial disorders, such as Treacher Collins syndrome, HNS has only been robustly studied in the trisomy 21 population; further research is needed [35].

In certain scenarios, ancillary testing may be pertinent for investigating the cause of SDB. Evaluating adenoid size on sagittal radiographs can provide information if there is concern for snoring or OSA. Laboratory work can be particularly useful in revealing underlying SDB sequelae. Chronic intermittent hypoxia may lead to polycythemia. Chronic hypoventilation may result in elevated serum bicarbonate levels. Vitamin D deficiency has also been correlated with an increased risk of OSA [36]. For children with snoring and chronic allergies, allergy testing may be warranted.

NONRESPIRATORY SLEEP DISORDERS

Although children with craniofacial anomalies are particularly prone to SDB, other sleep disturbances may also be present. Nonrespiratory sleep disorders encompass a variety of conditions, including circadian rhythm disorders, insomnias, hypersomnia, parasomnias, and sleep-related movement disorders. Although poor sleep hygiene, insomnia, and restless leg syndrome can be common, parasomnias and central disorders of hypersomnolence are less commonly seen in the general pediatric population. Parasomnias, including sleepwalking/sleep talking, can be associated with SDB and should be ruled out as a potential cause first.

History and physical examination

Similar to SDB, nonrespiratory sleep disturbances can present as behavioral problems and poor school performance. Many of the symptoms of nonrespiratory sleep disturbances can overlap; thus, a detailed history can be useful. A detailed evaluation, including the sleep-wake schedule, meals, caffeine, medications, napping, activities, bedroom environment, and the bedtime routine, is vital information when determining the cause of the sleep disturbance. Bedtime resistance and frequent and prolonged awakenings can be seen in insomnia, circadian rhythm disorders, and restless leg syndrome. Extensive bedtime routines to help the child fall asleep are frequently seen in sleep association–type insomnia, which is contrasted to limit-setting insomnia, which may manifest as resistance to bedtime, stalling, or frequent "curtain calls." Restlessness or frequent repositioning may indicate restless leg syndrome. Excessive daytime sleepiness with frequent napping can be seen in the setting of nearly all sleep disturbances; however, episodes of sudden temporary loss of muscle tone associated with cataplexy should raise concern for narcolepsy.

A history of neurodevelopment delay or autism should be noted, as these children are at risk for insomnia, poor sleep hygiene, and circadian rhythm disorders [37]. Gastrointestinal or malabsorption issues can lead to vitamin and iron deficiencies, which can contribute to restless leg syndrome. Children with Smith-Magenis syndrome, in particular, are at significant risk for circadian mismatch owing to the inverted melatonin secretion, which can cause severely irregular sleep patterns and be quite challenging to manage [38].

All medications should be noted. Certain stimulants can be associated with insomnia if taken late in the day. Certain medications used for mood can also contribute to increased daytime sleepiness and should be reviewed in children with concern for hypersomnia. In addition, several medications, including antihistamines, anxiolytics, or mood stabilizers, can alter the natural architecture of sleep. Antihistamines have also been associated with an increased risk of restless leg syndrome.

Most nonrespiratory disorders do not have specific physical examination findings. Findings of pallor of the inner eyelids and nails may be the most evident finding in iron-deficiency anemia, which may have the strongest correlation with restless leg syndrome. Pagophagia can be associated with iron-deficiency anemia.

Screening

In children with craniofacial abnormalities who experience sleep disturbances, screening for nonrespiratory disorders is important if SDB has been ruled out. If there is no evidence of SDB breathing on PSG or if there are persistent sleep disturbances after the SDB has been appropriately treated, further evaluation may be required. Ensuring adequate sleep time and good sleep hygiene is of utmost importance. A sleep diary, completed over the course of 2 weeks by the caregiver, can reveal irregular patterns in the circadian rhythm and identify behavioral factors that can contribute to poor sleep.

Recognition and diagnosis of sleep-related movement disorders in children with craniofacial abnormalities require a high index of suspicion and often necessitate overnight PSG with limb EMG channels, as well as clinical screening for restless leg syndrome symptoms and periodic limb movements. Evaluation for restlessness during sleep should include evaluation for restless leg syndrome as well as ruling out sleep-related breathing disorders. Given the strong correlation of iron deficiency and restless leg syndrome, laboratory tests should be ordered to check for iron deficiency and should include complete blood count (CBC) with differential, total serum iron, ferritin, and transferrin levels. To properly interpret the ferritin level, a CBC should be ordered at the same time to rule out an infection or active inflammation that can lead to falsely elevated levels of ferritin, given its acute phase reactant property. Vitamin D and B12 deficiencies should be considered for evaluation of daytime fatigue [39].

If there are concerns of excessive daytime sleepiness in children with craniofacial abnormalities, further testing may be required. If no identified organic cause is identified, such as sleep-related breathing disorders, movement disorders, poor sleep hygiene, and/or medications that contribute to excessive daytime sleepiness, then further evaluation with a multiple sleep latency test can be considered to evaluate for central disorders of hypersomnolence, for example, narcolepsy.

SUMMARY

Although now more widely recognized, sleep disturbances in the general pediatric population are still largely undiagnosed. This underdiagnosis is of particular concern in children with craniofacial abnormalities. Sleep disorders and disturbances in children with craniofacial abnormalities are associated with a higher burden of cardiovascular and adverse respiratory consequences. They are also at higher risk for CSA. Many genetic syndromes associated with craniofacial abnormalities are associated with neurocognitive delays, motor deficits, and abnormal muscle tone, which affects their respiratory clearance, secretions, and so forth. This significantly impacts the quality of breathing and ventilation during sleep and leads to multiple awakenings throughout the night, leading to poor quality of sleep in the children as well as their caregivers. Early intervention not only improves their sleep quality but also lessens the burden on their cardiovascular system and overall well-being.

CLINICS CARE POINTS

- Evidence shows that patients with craniofacial syndromes or abnormalities are at higher risk for sleep disturbances and also can have more than one concomitant sleep disorder.
- Children with craniofacial abnormalities pose higher risk for nocturnal hypoxemia due to sleep disordered breathing and are thus, predispose to sleep disruption, irregular sleep/wake cycle and behavioral changes due to sleep deprivation.
- Due to the complexity of craniofacial abnormalities and genetic syndromes, these children's sleep issues are often overlooked and require need more clinical and thorough evaluation than the pediatric general population.
- Compared to the general pediatric population, in these children evaluation of sleep disorders requires a comprehensive, multidisciplinary workup incorparating sleep medicine, surgery, pulmonology, neurology, otolargynology and behavioral medicine.

Acknowledgments

The authors wish to acknowledge the help of Sanvi Soma, who provided administrative assistance and literature review for this article.

References

[1] Garbarino S, Lanteri P, Bragazzi NL, et al. Role of sleep deprivation in immune-related disease risk and outcomes. Commun Biol 2021;4(1):1304, PMID: 34795404; PMCID: PMC8602722.

[2] Morgenthaler TI, Owens J, Alessi C, et al, American Academy of Sleep Medicine. Practice parameters for behavioral treatment of bedtime problems and night wakings in infants and young children. Sleep 2006;29(10):1277–81, PMID: 17068980.

[3] Meltzer LJ, Williamson AA, Mindell JA. Pediatric sleep health: it matters, and so does how we define it. Sleep Med Rev 2021;57:101425; https://doi.org/10.1016/j.smrv.2021.101425:PMID: 33601324; PMCID: PMC9067252.
[4] Kim KA, Kim SJ, Yoon A. Craniofacial anatomical determinants of pediatric sleep-disordered breathing: a comprehensive review. J Prosthodont 2025;34(S1):26–34, PMID: 39557815; PMCID: PMC12000634.
[5] Moraleda-Cibrián M, Edwards S, Kasten S, et al. Sleep-related movement disorders and growing pains: differences in daytime and bedtime behavior in 2-6 year old children with cleft palate. Sleep Med 2021;85:303–8, PMID: 34391005.
[6] Kruszka P, Rolle M, Kahle KT, et al. Muenke syndrome. In: Adam MP, Feldman J, Mirzaa GM, et al, editors. GeneReviews® [internet]. Seattle (WA): University of Washington, Seattle; 2006. p. 1993–2025. Available at: https://www.ncbi.nlm.nih.gov/books/NBK1415/.
[7] Sivaram G, Jawad K, El-Kersh K, et al. Sleep-disordered breathing in children with craniofacial syndromes. Cleft Palate Craniofac J 2025;17:10556656251378588; https://doi.org/10.1177/10556656251378588:PMID: 40961264.
[8] Bannink N, Maliepaard M, Raat H, et al. Obstructive sleep apnea-specific quality of life and behavioral problems in children with syndromic craniosynostosis. J Dev Behav Pediatr 2011;32(3):233–8, PMID: 21297497.
[9] Bhattacharjee R, Kheirandish-Gozal L, Pillar G, et al. Cardiovascular complications of obstructive sleep apnea syndrome: evidence from children. Prog Cardiovasc Dis 2009;51(5):416–33, PMID: 19249448.
[10] Li S, Jin X, Yan C, et al. Habitual snoring in school-aged children: environmental and biological predictors. Respir Res 2010;11(1):144.
[11] Halbower AC, Degaonkar M, Barker PB, et al. Childhood obstructive sleep apnea associates with neuropsychological deficits and neuronal brain injury. PLoS Med 2006;3(8):e301; https://doi.org/10.1371/journal.pmed.0030301:PMID: 16933960; PMCID: PMC1551912.
[12] Ma LK, Zhang ZY, Tang XJ, et al. Respiratory outcome of mandibular distraction osteogenesis on obstructive sleep apnea in craniofacial microsomia: a retrospective study. J Craniomaxillofac Surg 2023;51(6):355–9.
[13] Garg RK, Afifi AM, Garland CB, et al. Pediatric obstructive sleep apnea: consensus, controversy, and craniofacial considerations. Plast Reconstr Surg 2017;140(5):987–97, PMID: 29068938.
[14] Jullian-Desayes I, Revol B, Chareyre E, et al. Impact of concomitant medications on obstructive sleep apnoea. Br J Clin Pharmacol 2017;83(4):688–708, PMID: 27735059; PMCID: PMC5346880.
[15] Sadras I, Reiter J, Fuchs N, et al. Prematurity as a risk factor of sleep-disordered breathing in children younger than two years: a retrospective case-control study. J Clin Sleep Med 2019;15(12):1731–6, PMID: 31855158; PMCID: PMC7099182.
[16] Cristea AI, Ren CL, Amin R, et al. Outpatient respiratory management of infants, children, and adolescents with post-prematurity respiratory disease: an official American thoracic society clinical practice guideline. Am J Respir Crit Care Med 2021;204(12):e115–33.
[17] Kang KT, Chou CH, Weng WC, et al. Associations between adenotonsillar hypertrophy, age, and obesity in children with obstructive sleep apnea. PLoS One 2013;8(10):e78666; https://doi.org/10.1371/journal.pone.0078666:PMID: 24205291; PMCID: PMC3808373.
[18] Ferreira VHDC, Miura CS, Lupoli BAC, et al. Adenoid hypertrophy is directly associated with the severity of OSA in obese children: a pilot study. Braz J Otorhinolaryngol 2025;91(6):101694; https://doi.org/10.1016/j.bjorl.2025.101694:PMID: 40753942.
[19] Suri JC, Sen MK, Venkatachalam VP, et al. Outcome of adenotonsillectomy for children with sleep apnea. Sleep Med 2015;16(10):1181–6.

[20] Kumar HV, Schroeder JW, Gang Z, et al. Mallampati score and pediatric obstructive sleep apnea. J Clin Sleep Med 2014;10(9):985–90.
[21] van der Haven I, Mulder JW, van der Wal KG, et al. The jaw index: new guide defining micrognathia in newborns. Cleft Palate Craniofac J 1997;34(3):240–1.
[22] Breugem CC, Evans KN, Poets CF, et al. Best practices for the diagnosis and evaluation of infants with robin sequence: a clinical consensus report. JAMA Pediatr 2016;170(9):894–902.
[23] Mai CT, Isenburg JL, Canfield MA, et al. National population-based estimates for major birth defects, 2010–2014. Birth Defects Research 2019;111:1420–35.
[24] National Institute of Dental and Craniofacial Research. Prevalence of cleft lip & cleft palate I data & statistics. 2022. Available at: https://www.nidcr.nih.gov/research/data-statistics/craniofacial-birth-defects/prevalence. Accessed October 27, 2025.
[25] Hirschberg J. Results and complications of 1104 surgeries for velopharyngeal insufficiency. ISRN Otolaryngol 2012;2012:181202; https://doi.org/10.5402/2012/181202: PMID: 23724266; PMCID: PMC3658639.
[26] Schweiger C, Manica D, Kuhl G. Glossoptosis. Semin Pediatr Surg 2016;25(3):123–7, PMID: 27301596.
[27] Moraleda-Cibrián M, Edwards SP, Kasten SJ, et al. Symptoms of sleep disordered breathing in children with craniofacial malformations. J Clin Sleep Med 2014;10(3):307–12, PMID: 24634629; PMCID: PMC3927437.
[28] Baker-Smith CM, Isaiah A, Melendres MC, et al. Sleep-disordered breathing and cardiovascular disease in children and adolescents: a scientific statement from the American heart association. J Am Heart Assoc 2021;10(18):e022427; https://doi.org/10.1161/JAHA.121.022427.
[29] Marcus CL, Brooks LJ, Draper KA, et al. Diagnosis and management of childhood obstructive sleep apnea syndrome. Pediatrics 2012;130(3):e714–55.
[30] Moraleda-Cibrián M, Edwards SP, Kasten SJ, et al. Obstructive sleep apnea pretreatment and posttreatment in symptomatic children with congenital craniofacial malformations. J Clin Sleep Med 2015;11(1):37–43, PMID: 25515281; PMCID: PMC4265656.
[31] Ishman SL, Maturo S, Schwartz S, et al. Expert consensus statement: management of pediatric persistent obstructive sleep apnea after adenotonsillectomy. Otolaryngol Head Neck Surg 2023;168(2):115–30.
[32] Larrow DR, Marcus KS, Gipson K, et al. Upper airway stimulation for children and adolescents with Down syndrome: long-term Follow-Up. Laryngoscope 2025;135(3):1218–22, PMID: 39381939.
[33] Diercks GR, Wentland C, Keamy D, et al. Hypoglossal nerve stimulation in adolescents with Down syndrome and obstructive sleep apnea. JAMA Otolaryngol Head Neck Surg 2018;144(1):37–42.
[34] Kim M, Xu LJ, Shih E, et al. Hypoglossal nerve stimulator for obstructive sleep apnea in children with Down syndrome younger than 13. Int J Pediatr Otorhinolaryngol 2025;196:112497; https://doi.org/10.1016/j.ijporl.2025.112497:PMID: 40714532.
[35] Wong ACL, Jones A, Stone A, et al. Combination CPAP and bilateral hypoglossal nerve stimulation for obstructive sleep apnea in Treacher Collins syndrome: first case report. J Clin Sleep Med 2023;19(1):197–9, PMID: 36038987; PMCID: PMC9806783.
[36] Kheirandish-Gozal L, Peris E, Gozal D. Vitamin D levels and obstructive sleep apnoea in children. Sleep Med 2014;15(4):459–63.
[37] Rana M, Kothare S, DeBassio W. The assessment and treatment of sleep abnormalities in children and adolescents with autism spectrum disorder: a review. J Can Acad Child Adolesc Psychiatry 2021;30(1):25–35.
[38] Potocki L, Glaze D, Tan DX, et al. Circadian rhythm abnormalities of melatonin in smith-magenis syndrome. J Med Genet 2000;37(6):428–33.
[39] Al-Shawwa B, Ehsan Z, Ingram DG. Vitamin D and sleep in children. J Clin Sleep Med 2020;16(7):1119–23.

Advances in Pediatrics 73 (2026) 323–334

ADVANCES IN PEDIATRICS

Approach to a Child with Gait Disturbances

Chaithanya Reddy Bandi V, MD[a], Sagarika Nallu, MD[b,*]

[a]Division of Pediatric Neurology, Department of Pediatrics, University of South Florida Morsani School of Medicine, Tampa, FL, USA; [b]University of South Florida Morsani School of Medicine, Tampa, FL, USA

Keywords

• Gait disturbances • Balance issues • Childhood • Ataxia • Spasticity • Dystonia • Myopathy • Functional

Key points

- A focused and structured gait assessment may have significant implications for both diagnosis and treatment of underlying neurologic disorders.
- Understanding the normal variations in gait related to different ages is essential to prevent unnecessary investigations and alleviate parents' concerns.
- Neurologic disorders are a common cause of gait disturbances in pediatric patients.
- The step-by-step approach to gait assessment presented in the article facilitates the prompt diagnosis of underlying neurologic disorders in a clinical setting.
- Positive clinical signs, such as inconsistency, incongruence, variability, and distractibility, help establish an early diagnosis of functional gait disorders, rather than waiting to exclude organic causes, to expedite multidisciplinary rehabilitation care.

INTRODUCTION

The prevalence of gait disorders in pediatric patients varies depending on the definitions used and the populations studied. In a large, nationally representative sample from the United States, it was found that 5.3% of children aged 3 to 17 years experienced dizziness and balance problems. The rates were higher

*Corresponding author. Department of Pediatric Neurology, University of Florida, Morsani College of Medicine, 13101 Bruce B Downs Boulevard, Tampa, FL 33612. *E-mail address:* snallu@usf.edu

https://doi.org/10.1016/j.yapd.2025.12.014
0065-3101/26/

Abbreviations

AT	ataxia telangiectasia
FA	Friedreich ataxia

among older children and showed some variation by sex and ethnicity [1]. The prevalence of childhood ataxias and pediatric cerebellar disorders, which are a subset of gait disorders, is estimated to be 26 cases per 100,000 children in Europe and 21.9 cases per 100,000 in a Finnish cohort [2,3]. However, these figures may underestimate the true global burden of these conditions.

Notably, almost 90% of children with gait disorders are being labeled with "unspecified dizziness," indicating the need for improvement of diagnostic methods used by physicians to evaluate children's balance issues. A focused assessment could help identify specific underlying causes and lead to effective treatment strategies [4].

In this review, the authors briefly discuss normal gait development and then outline the approach to addressing gait abnormalities, with a particular focus on neurologic gait disorders. A special note on functional gait disorders is also provided, along with a summary.

NORMAL GAIT

A gait cycle is typically composed of the following 2 phases: stance (foot is in contact with the ground) and swing (foot is off the ground). The cycle begins when one heel strikes the ground. As the body weight shifts forward, it is supported by the stance leg on the same side, while the opposite leg swings forward. Eventually, the foot of the opposite leg strikes the ground, completing the cycle and initiating a new one. It is important to understand several key terms that are essential for defining gait (Table 1).

The normal development of gait in children follows a predictable sequence of advancements, beginning with independent walking, which typically occurs around 12 to 15 months of age [5]. In the early stages of walking, children display a wide base of support, short step lengths, increased cadence, and excessive double support time (percentage of time, while walking, when both feet are on the ground). As children grow older, improvements in neuromuscular control and balance lead to increased walking speed and stride length, as well as decreased cadence and double support time [6–8].

Table 1
Terminology

Term	Definition
Velocity	Distance covered in a given time
Cadence	Steps per minute
Stride length	Distance covered by the gait cycle
Step length	Distance covered during the swing phase of a single leg
Step width or base	Distance between the left and right feet while walking

Children typically adopt a mature heel-to-strike pattern by the age of 2 to 3 years, with improved consistency of spatiotemporal gait characteristics. Stride-to-stride variability continues to be higher in this age group compared with older children [6,7,9]. Between the ages of 3 and 6, further improvements occur, including increased walking speed and stride length, along with a decreased base of support and intraindividual gait variability. Nonetheless, stride width continues to show variability in this population [6,10,11].

Most children aged 7 to 8 years exhibit gait patterns that resemble those of adults, including aspects such as velocity, stride length, and support phases. Some features related to stride dynamics and lower-extremity growth may continue to develop into adolescence [9,12,13]. By age 7, children's ability to walk in a straight line with enhanced stability approaches adult levels [14]. Throughout children's development, gait remains symmetric, although differences related to sex and pelvic movement may become apparent during later childhood [10,11].

It is important to understand the normal variations in gait that often prompt parents to seek consultation (Table 2). If these variations persist beyond the typical age of resolution or continue to progress and cause pain, further evaluation is necessary.

NEUROLOGIC GAIT DISORDERS

Gait is a complex motor behavior that is coordinated by the nervous system and requires the harmonious functioning of networks involving muscles, the spinal cord, the brainstem, the cerebellum, the basal ganglia, and the cerebral cortex. The brainstem, especially the mesencephalic locomotor region, plays a crucial role in integrating signals from higher brain centers to initiate and regulate gait and postural tone [15]. Sensory inputs, including proprioceptive, vestibular, visual, and cutaneous signals, are essential for coordinating smooth gait by providing continuous feedback to the higher centers, which helps to allow real-time adjustments to posture, limb movement, and balance during walking. Gait disorders can thus arise from disruption at various levels, with clinical phenotypes specific to the underlying neurologic impairment. The

Table 2
Gait variation

Normal gait variation	Expected age of resolution
Toe walking	3 y
In-toeing (walking with patella and feet facing inward)	8 y
Internal tibial version (walking with patella facing forward and feet pointing inward)	3 y
Metatarsus adductus (flexible C-shaped lateral border of feet)	6 y
Bowlegs (genu varum)	18 mo
Knock knees (genu valgum)	7 y
Flat feet	6 y

associated compensatory strategies, such as altered walking patterns, often follow to maintain stability [16,17].

Gait assessment should commence with an observation of the patient's walking style as they enter the examination room. An effective approach is to have the patient walk down a long, free hallway that allows them to reach their maximum walking speed. During this time, observe various aspects of their gait, starting with symmetry and then noting stride length, step length, velocity, cadence, and step base. Pay special attention to key findings, such as posture, arm swing, leg stiffness, knee lift, and pelvic lurching, as these can provide valuable insights. A neurologic examination focusing on muscle bulk, muscle tone, sensory perception, and reflexes may reveal potential underlying causes of gait abnormalities. In addition, certain clinical maneuvers can help uncover clinically relevant information. The Grower sign (asking the patient to rise from a sitting or supine position on the floor without using arms to push off) as well as heel or toe walking reveal subtle proximal and distal muscle weakness, respectively [18]. The Romberg test (asking the patient to stand with feet together, eyes open, and then with eyes closed) and tandem walking (heel-to-toe) are well-established sequential maneuvers for evaluating sensory ataxia and dynamic gait balance. The authors discuss the common neurologic causes of abnormal gait in detail in later discussion.

Spasticity

Spasticity is characterized by stiffness caused by velocity-dependent hypertonia, resulting from dysfunction of the central motor pathways in the brain or spinal cord. It typically involves the co-contraction of antagonist muscles and is often accompanied by varying degrees of weakness and reduced joint mobility. This stiffness, combined with the associated weakness, leads to distinct and recognizable patterns in gait.

In patients with spasticity involving bilateral lower extremities (such as spastic paraparesis), excessive stiffness of the thigh adductors, along with weakness in the typical distribution involving bilateral hip flexors, hip abductors, knee flexors, and foot dorsiflexors, contributes to a characteristic scissoring gait pattern. Equinus posture, which causes forefoot contact, results in abnormal scraping against the ground while walking. Weakness in the bilateral hip flexors and abductors limits the ability to swing the leg outward at the hip (circumduction), reducing foot clearance in these patients [19,20]. In contrast, the unaffected limb helps by moving the pelvis to compensate when the affected limb swings outward, improving forefoot clearance and leading to a characteristic circumduction gait in patients with unilateral spasticity (hemiparesis). In addition, ipsilateral arm posturing may be seen, including forearm pronation and elbow flexion. In cases of subclinical spasticity, signs of these gait patterns can be observed when the patient is asked to walk more quickly. During clinical examination in these patients, hyperreflexia and an extensor plantar response are commonly noted, along with increased muscle tone and weakness [19,20].

Brain and spinal cord imaging precedes the other steps in the evaluation process. Metabolic and genetic studies will follow if imaging is a normal study to rule out cerebral palsy mimickers [21]. Physical therapy outperforms other medical interventions, such as baclofen administration, Botox injections, and selective dorsal rhizotomy, in benefiting these patients. Remember, management should focus on targeting specific functional goals rather than just treating spasticity, as the latter alone may cause detrimental effects if weakness and instability coexist.

Dystonia

Dystonia refers to stiffness that is hypothesized to be secondary to poor gaiting by the basal ganglia, leading to abnormal, excessive motor cortical activity that manifests as intermittent or sustained contractions of antagonistic muscle groups, resulting in abnormal postures or twisting movements. It is not a velocity-dependent phenomenon. Dystonia syndromes are often initially focal and episodic in nature, particularly in the lower extremities. Some may remain focal, and others may progress to generalization. The clinical presentation fluctuates, as the tone can vary with action (task-specific) and improve dramatically with sensory stimulation (sensory trick). The clinical presentation of task-specific dystonia, for example, dystonia limited to forward walking, can be confused with a functional neurologic disorder.

The effect of dystonia on gait is predominantly owing to overriding extensor muscle activity and twisting movements. Leg extension, ankle inversion, toe walking, and in-toeing, which are either episodic or persistent, are common gait abnormalities. In addition, specific gait patterns have been described in various clinical contexts, such as the "dragging leg," the "hobby horse gait," the "high-stepping cock-walk gait" [22,23]. Diurnal fluctuation, milder in the morning after waking up, then progressively worsening as the day goes on, reaching its peak in severity in the evening, is typically seen in classic dopa-responsive dystonia, particularly Segawa disease, and is attributed to circadian changes in dopamine synthesis and neurotransmission in the nigrostriatal pathways [24]. The clinical examination should focus on other associated movement disorders, such as spasticity and myoclonus, which can provide clues whether the dystonia is combined or syndromic.

Paroxysmal dystonias are another critical group. These conditions are often genetic and differ from others in that they are predominantly episodic and associated with specific triggers. Triggers include sudden change in movement (kinesogenic), caffeine or alcohol, but have no relation to movement (nonkinesogenic), or prolonged exercise (lance-type). The characteristic feature is the absence of clinical symptoms between episodes. Treatment usually focuses on specific therapies, such as carbamazepine (kinesogenic) or avoidance of triggers (eg, lance-type, which are induced by prolonged exercise) [25].

MRI of the brain is often the initial diagnostic investigation. The clinical context and imaging findings may dictate other subsequent investigations, including thyroid profile, serum urate for Lesch-Nyhan syndrome, blood film for acanthocystosis, copper and ceruloplasmin levels for Wilson disease, paired blood and cerebrospinal fluid (CSF) glucose for GLUT-1 defects, CSF neurotransmitters, and so forth. Genetic evaluation is particularly relevant if the clinical picture suggests monogenic dystonia, such as DYT1, DYT11, or PANK2/PLA2G6. Intrathecal baclofen, Botox injections, gabapentin, clonidine, and trihexyphenidyl are the established therapeutic options in these patients. Levodopa should be considered as initial treatment for patients with a clinical picture suggestive of dopa-responsive dystonia, as well as for dystonia of undetermined cause [26]. The patients with GLUT-1 defects respond best to the ketogenic diet. Deep brain stimulation is worth considering in patients with primary dystonia whose families have exhausted other options [27].

Chorea and athetosis

Chorea and athetosis are involuntary, purposeless movements that reflect dysfunction at different levels of basal ganglia circuits [28]. Chorea is characterized by dancing-like or fidgety gestures, notable for random, irregular, and discrete movements that flow from one body part to another. In contrast, athetosis is continuous, slow, writhing in nature, similar to the movements of a cat's tail. It predominantly involves the distal extremities. The term "choreoathetosis" is commonly used in the literature, as both movement types are concurrent in several clinical conditions, such as dyskinetic cerebral palsy and Sydenham chorea [29].

Gait in patients with chorea is affected by unpredictable, brief movements that cause unwanted deviations of the legs or trunk, breaking down the planned movement, resulting in instability, difficulty maintaining a steady pace, and a higher risk of falls. The child may seem restless, and the step-to-step variation can be seen. Athetosis, which causes continuous unwanted movements in the distal extremities, leads to persistent instability and an undulating or snakelike gait, with difficulty maintaining the step-to-step rhythm. Importantly, hypotonia, weakness, and additional movement disorders should be assessed during the clinical examination as they further compound gait difficulties [29].

Postinfectious syndromes, dyskinetic cerebral palsy, and autoimmune conditions, such as *N*-methyl-D-aspartate encephalitis, are common causes. Specific genetic associations have been recently identified. Benign hereditary chorea results from a mutation in the NKX2-1 gene. ADCY-5 mutation is associated with early-onset generalized chorea, which characteristically affects perioral and facial muscles. Levetiracetam, tetrabenazine, and valproate help control chorea symptoms. Nonetheless, treating the underlying disorder is the best approach for these patients. Deep brain stimulation is successfully used to prevent life-threatening fluctuations in patients with GNAO-1 mutations [30].

Myoclonus

Myoclonus is a movement disorder characterized by rapid, involuntary, brief jerky movements lasting between 10 and 50 milliseconds, resulting from the sharp contraction or relaxation of one or more muscle groups. The abrupt and brief nature differentiates myoclonus from chorea and athetosis. Pathophysiology is heterogeneous. It can be secondary to lesions within the cortical or subcortical regions, basal ganglia, brainstem, or spinal cord. The underlying mechanism is abnormal neuronal excitability and a deficit in inhibitory control, culminating in abrupt synchronized muscle activation [31].

The effect of this movement disorder on gait is largely due to the disruption of smooth, coordinated movement; the jerks can be focal, segmental, or generalized. Their occurrence at different phases of the walking cycle causes marked instability and significant risk of falls, resulting in a wide-based, irregular gait. Clinical history taking and examination should aim to document whether jerks occur at rest, are action-triggered or stimulus-driven (cortical nonepileptic), irregular (subcortical), or rhythmic (cortical epileptic) [32]. Progressive forms are frequently genetic and associated with neurodegeneration [33]. An understanding of other associated defects, such as ataxia (progressive myoclonus epilepsies) and dystonia (*SGCE* myoclonic-dystonia [SGCE-M-D]), enables the clinician to better understand gait manifestations, particularly in patients with progressive courses.

Video electroencephalogram differentiates epileptic from nonepileptic myoclonus [32]. Epileptic myoclonus can be a part of epilepsy syndromes as well as progressive myoclonic epilepsies. Antiepileptic medications are used to control epileptic myoclonus. Nonepileptic myoclonus, for example, opsoclonus-myoclonus, is usually treatment-resistant. Therapeutic options targeting the underlying disorder may help in these cases.

Ataxia

Ataxia refers to the impaired ability to execute voluntary movements as planned, owing to poor balance and coordination, rather than secondary to weakness or involuntary muscle contractions. One form is sensory ataxia, where the defective position sensations (proprioception) result in compromised sensory information and motor control abnormalities. Another group is cerebellar ataxia, which is primarily due to dysfunction of the cerebellum and its connections within the cerebellothalamocortical network [34].

A high-stepping and stamping gait is characteristic of sensory ataxia. The defective proprioception hampers the ability to appreciate the position of legs and joints in space during the normal step cycle. Therefore, compensatory leg lifting higher than usual, followed by heel striking the ground as a slap, helps the patient receive increased sensory feedback through other sensory routes and auditory prompts [35]. In addition, a slightly wide-based gait with or without reduced stride length can also be seen. All these features may worsen when the patients walk in the darkness or close their eyes. Positive Romberg sign and decreased or absent deep tendon reflexes are the supportive examination findings in these patients [34].

Cerebellar ataxic gait, particularly owing to midline vermis dysfunction, is typically associated with slow, wide-based gait with reduced stride length. As these patients have difficulty accelerating and stopping movements, their gait patterns have been described as stumbling, lurching, or drunken. Clinical examination may reveal other cerebellar signs, such as scanning speech, dysmetria, and dysdiadochokinesia. During the Romberg test, the patient exhibits excessive unsteady stance regardless of whether their eyes are open or closed [34].

Ataxias can be secondary to acute conditions or chronic progressive disorders. Acute cerebellitis, postinfectious acute cerebellar ataxias, and the Miller Fisher variant of Guillain-Barré syndrome are prime examples of acute associations. Ataxia is usually reversible with or without treatment in these conditions. Ataxia telangiectasia (AT) and Friedreich ataxia (FA) are chronic progressive disorders. Elevated serum alpha-fetoprotein levels aid in the early diagnosis of AT in young children with unexplained ataxia, as ocular telangiectasia becomes evident in late childhood [36]. This helps prevent unnecessary radiation exposure to children with AT. FA is a multisystem disease characterized by ataxia, cardiomyopathy, diabetes, axonal neuropathy, areflexia, and extensor plantar response. As there is no curative treatment, these patients require lifelong multidisciplinary treatment. Abetalipoproteinemia, ataxia with vitamin E deficiency, and Hashimoto encephalopathy are examples of disorders that respond to treatment. Multiple episodic ataxias have been recently identified, with the evolution of genetic technology, each with distinct characteristic features. The differentiation among them is beneficial, as some have treatment options, such as acetazolamide, for episodic ataxia type-2.

Neuropathy

Neuropathic (lower motor neuron) gait refers to gait disturbances that are secondary to lesions or pathologic condition involving anterior motor neurons, nerve routes, or peripheral nerves. Depending on the extent of involvement, the weakness is nonetheless mainly focal and asymmetric.

Gait is typically described as high stepping (steppage) in patients with weakness in the ankle dorsiflexors, as they flex excessively at the hip and knee during the swing phase to compensate and allow foot clearance [37]. An audible slap may be noted as the foot touches the ground. Patients with weakness in the knee extensors often fail to lock their knees during the stance phase, which can result in knee buckling and falls [38].

Observing the different stages of the patient's walk helps to better understand and identify clues to neuropathic gait abnormalities. Preservation of deep tendon reflexes (except in the distribution of neuropathy) and low to normal tone, along with sparing of some muscle groups, such as the iliopsoas, favors neuropathic weakness. In addition, bladder dysfunction is not typically seen in these patients (except with cauda equina lesions), compared with those with upper motor neuron weakness.

Hereditary neuropathies are a vital differential in pediatric cases. Nerve conduction studies and electromyography are helpful for a better understanding, and specific genetic tests are used for confirmation. Acquired causes, such as mononeuritis multiplex secondary to chronic inflammatory demyelinating polyradiculoneuropathy, vasculitis, and infectious causes, as well as deficiencies of vitamins, such as B12, are essential to identify, as they are treatable.

Myopathy

Symmetric and proximal weakness in the lower extremities is characteristically seen in patients with myopathies.

Gait abnormalities, ranging from slow step speed and reduced stride length to increased step base and a characteristic waddling pattern, can be observed. In addition to proximal weakness, compensatory pelvic tilt and lordosis contribute to the evolution of a typical waddling gait. The transition from a typical plantigrade to toe walking may also be observed as the disease advances and weakness progresses. The natural history of Duchenne muscular dystrophy provides the best example for understanding these gait dynamics [39].

At times, it can be challenging to differentiate between neuropathic and myopathic presentations. The symmetric and proximal nature, with relative preservation of reflexes and lack of sensory involvement, suggests myopathic weakness. Tone is relatively preserved on clinical examination. The Trendelenburg test (asking the patient to bear weight on one leg to assess drooping on the opposite side) and the Gower maneuver help detect proximal weakness at the bedside.

Detailed clinical examination, followed by genetic studies and muscle biopsies, aids in the diagnosis of developmental muscle disorders. Nerve conduction studies, particularly repetitive stimulations, identify myasthenia gravis as well as congenital myasthenia syndromes. In addition, it is essential to consider the reversible causes of myopathies, such as thyroid and parathyroid abnormalities, as well as vitamin E deficiency, when evaluating these patients.

FUNCTIONAL GAIT DISORDERS

Functional gait disorders are becoming an essential group of gait disorders, characterized by variable and inconsistent gait patterns that are incongruent to any established neurologic disorders, given the lack of a plausible neuroanatomic basis. Knowledge of gait patterns aids in the early diagnosis of functional gait abnormalities. Bizarre gait patterns do not confirm a functional nature. For instance, patients with dystonia can present with bizarre and twisted gait. Conversely, dystonic gaits are consistent in that the same patterns superimpose repeatedly at identical time points during the gait cycle [40]. Patients with lower limb dystonia can add an exception to this consistency: forward walking triggers task-specific dystonia and foot drop, whereas backward walking or running transiently resolves the dystonia. Similarly, a cautious gait is not always a functional phenomenon. Apart from reasonable psychological adjustment, a cautious gait can be seen in patients with higher-level (frontal) disorders, such as apraxia [41].

Functional gait disorder can be present in isolation or in combination with other functional movement disorders, such as chorea and dystonia. Positive clinical signs include excessive slowness, dragging one lower extremity, ataxia (inability to stand), and abasia (inability to walk), excessive demonstration of effort (huffing and puffing), knee buckling, falling toward support, and noneconomic posture, among others, suggestive of a functional gait disorder [41]. In addition, children may show improvements when distracted, dramatic changes in gait patterns, and sometimes revert to usual activities in different contexts, such as playing or running, which are not typical for causes with an organic basis [41]. History taking should aim to determine whether there are accompanying recent psychosocial stressors, physical illness, or trauma. Absence of definite neurologic deficits on examination, along with the inconsistency between the stated disability and observed function, favors functional cause.

Overall, positive clinical signs, such as inconsistency, incongruence, variability, and distractibility, help establish an early diagnosis, rather than waiting to exclude organic causes. However, basic investigations are reasonable to be conducted as they help reassure families. Importantly, it is vital to be open and honest with parents when discussing clinical details for which no organic explanation is expected. This approach helps prevent unnecessary detailed investigations and expedite multidisciplinary rehabilitation care, to which many young children respond positively [42].

SUMMARY

Gait disorders are common in the pediatric age group and are often labeled as unspecified dizziness. This review discusses normal gait variation expected at various stages of development and then provides a comprehensive, step-by-step approach to gait assessment from a neurology perspective. Common neurologic causes are discussed, focusing on their effects on gait, history, and examination findings to elucidate pathophysiology, and to guide diagnostic investigations and management. This understanding helps the clinician to promptly recognize the underlying neurologic cause and initiate effective interventions. Recognition of functional gait disorders requires experience. An attempt is made to provide a brief overview of this topic to help readers understand their nature and the importance of considering them in differentials.

CLINICS CARE POINTS

- Gait disorders in Pediatric population requires a comprehensive history and physical examination to differentiate normal variations from pathological etiologies.
- A thorough understanding of motor developmental stages in children can minimize misdiagnosis and further aid in accurate diagnostic testing.
- Identifying functional gait disorders from neurological gait disorders requires clinical expertise.

Acknowledgments

The authors wish to acknowledge the help of Sanvi Soma, who provided administrative assistance and literature review for this paper.

References

[1] Li CM, Hoffman HJ, Ward BK, et al. Epidemiology of dizziness and balance problems in children in the United States: a population-based study. J Pediatr 2016;171:240–7.e73.
[2] Musselman KE, Stoyanov CT, Marasigan R, et al. Prevalence of ataxia in children: a systematic review. Neurology 2014;82(1):80–9.
[3] Granath K, Huhtaniska S, Ellonen J, et al. Phenotypic heterogeneity in genetic and acquired pediatric cerebellar disorders. Mov Disord 2025;40(9):1851–62.
[4] O'Reilly RC, Morlet T, Nicholas BD, et al. Prevalence of vestibular and balance disorders in children. Otol Neurotol 2010;31(9):1441–4.
[5] Størvold GV, Aarethun K, Bratberg GH. Age for onset of walking and prewalking strategies. Early Hum Dev 2013;89(9):655–9.
[6] Rygelová M, Uchytil J, Torres IE, et al. Comparison of spatiotemporal gait parameters and their variability in typically developing children aged 2, 3, and 6 years. PLoS One 2023;18(5):e0285558.
[7] Preis S, Klemms A, Müller K. Gait analysis by measuring ground reaction forces in children: changes to an adaptive gait pattern between the ages of one and five years. Dev Med Child Neurol 1997;39(4):228–33.
[8] Tsuyuki C, Hiraga H, Sudo M, et al. Estimability study on the age of toddlers' gait development based on gait parameters. Sci Rep 2023;13(1):2958.
[9] Hausdorff JM, Zemany L, Peng C, et al. Maturation of gait dynamics: stride-to-stride variability and its temporal organization in children. J Appl Physiol 1999;86(3):1040–7.
[10] Gieysztor E, Kowal M, Paprocka-Borowicz M. Gait parameters in healthy preschool and school children assessed using wireless inertial sensor. Sensors (Basel) 2021;21(19):6423.
[11] Wang S, Cui H, Tang T, et al. Key points of development of motor skills in childhood embodied in gait parameters. Gait Posture 2023;104:51–7.
[12] Froehle AW, Nahhas RW, Sherwood RJ, et al. Age-related changes in spatiotemporal characteristics of gait accompany ongoing lower limb linear growth in late childhood and early adolescence. Gait Posture 2013;38(1):14–9.
[13] Ito T, Noritake K, Ito Y, et al. Three-dimensional gait analysis of lower extremity gait parameters in Japanese children aged 6 to 12 years. Sci Rep 2022;12(1):7822.
[14] Miyagishima S, Mani H, Sato Y, et al. Developmental changes in straight gait in childhood. PLoS One 2023;18(2):e0281037.
[15] Takakusaki K. Neurophysiology of gait: from the spinal cord to the frontal lobe. Mov Disord 2013;28(11):1483–91.
[16] Felicetti G, Thoumie P, Do MC, et al. Cutaneous and muscular afferents from the foot and sensory fusion processing: physiology and pathology in neuropathies. J Peripher Nerv Syst 2021;26(1):17–34.
[17] Wuehr M, Schniepp R, Schlick C, et al. Sensory loss and walking speed related factors for gait alterations in patients with peripheral neuropathy. Gait Posture 2014;39(3):852–8.
[18] Chang RF, Mubarak SJ. Pathomechanics of Gowers' sign: a video analysis of a spectrum of Gowers' maneuvers. Clin Orthop Relat Res 2012;470(7):1987–91.
[19] Clewes K, Hammond C, Dong Y, et al. Neuromuscular impairments of cerebral palsy: contributions to gait abnormalities and implications for treatment. Front Hum Neurosci 2024;18:1445793.
[20] Papageorgiou E, Simon-Martinez C, Molenaers G, et al. Are spasticity, weakness, selectivity, and passive range of motion related to gait deviations in children with spastic cerebral palsy? A statistical parametric mapping study. PLoS One 2019;14(10):e0223363.
[21] Pearson TS, Pons R, Ghaoui R, et al. Genetic mimics of cerebral palsy. Mov Disord 2019;34(5):625–36.

[22] Schuberth K, Ramani PK, Beemarajan E, et al. Child neurology: *KMT2B*-related dystonia in a young child with worsening gait abnormality. Neurology 2023;101(7):328–32.
[23] Correa-Vela M, Carvalho J, Ferrero-Turrion J, et al. Early recognition of SGCE-myoclonus-dystonia in children. Dev Med Child Neurol 2023;65(2):207–14.
[24] Segawa M. Hereditary progressive dystonia with marked diurnal fluctuation. Brain Dev 2011;33(3):195–201.
[25] Erro R, Bhatia KP. Unravelling of the paroxysmal dyskinesias. J Neurol Neurosurg Psychiatry 2019;90(2):227–34.
[26] Trau SP, Gallentine WB, Mikati MA. Child neurology: a young child with an undiagnosed case of dystonia responsive to l-dopa. Neurology 2020;94(7):326–8.
[27] Duga V, Giossi R, Romito LM, et al. Long-term globus pallidus internus deep brain stimulation in pediatric non-degenerative dystonia: a cohort study and a meta-analysis. Mov Disord 2024;39(7):1131–44.
[28] Robottom BJ, Factor SA, Weiner WJ. Movement disorders emergencies part 2: hyperkinetic disorders. Arch Neurol 2011;68(6):719–24.
[29] Zomorrodi A, Wald ER. Sydenham's chorea in Western Pennsylvania. Pediatrics 2006;117 (4):e675–9.
[30] Decraene B, Smeets S, Remans D, et al. Deep brain stimulation for GNAO1-associated dystonia: a systematic review and meta-analysis. Neuromodulation 2024;27(3):440–6.
[31] Sanger TD, Chen D, Fehlings DL, et al. Definition and classification of hyperkinetic movements in childhood. Mov Disord 2010;25(11):1538–49.
[32] Dijk JM, Tijssen MA. Management of patients with myoclonus: available therapies and the need for an evidence-based approach. Lancet Neurol 2010;9(10):1028–36.
[33] Christensen CK, Walsh L. Movement disorders and neurometabolic diseases. Semin Pediatr Neurol 2018;25:82–91.
[34] Expert Panel on Neurological Imaging, Wang LL, Thompson TA, Shih RY, et al. ACR appropriateness criteria® dizziness and ataxia: 2023 update. J Am Coll Radiol 2024;21(6S): S100–25.
[35] Macefield VG, Norcliffe-Kaufmann LJ, Axelrod FB, et al. Relationship between proprioception at the knee joint and gait ataxia in HSAN III. Mov Disord 2013;28(6):823–7.
[36] Amirifar P, Ranjouri MR, Lavin M, et al. Ataxia-telangiectasia: epidemiology, pathogenesis, clinical phenotype, diagnosis, prognosis and management. Expert Rev Clin Immunol. 2020;16(9):859–71.
[37] Wojciechowski E, Sman A, Cornett K, et al. Gait patterns of children and adolescents with Charcot-Marie-Tooth disease. Gait Posture 2017;56:89–94.
[38] Poage C, Roth C, Scott B. Peroneal nerve palsy: evaluation and management. J Am Acad Orthop Surg 2016;24(1):1–10.
[39] Kennedy RA, de Valle K, Adams J, et al. Characterising gait in paediatric neuromuscular disorders: an observational study of spatio-temporal gait in a clinical cohort. Disabil Rehabil 2022;44(23):7023–9.
[40] Lidstone SC, Araújo R, Stone J, et al. Ten myths about functional neurological disorder. Eur J Neurol 2020;27(11):e62–4.
[41] West E, Shah U. Diagnosis of functional weakness and functional gait disorders in children and adolescents. Semin Pediatr Neurol 2022;41:100955.
[42] Chouksey A, Pandey S. Functional movement disorders in children. Front Neurol 2020;11:570151.

Advances in Pediatrics 73 (2026) 335–351

ADVANCES IN PEDIATRICS

Management of Foreign Bodies

Beads, Coins, and Magnets

Bindi Naik-Mathuria, MD, MPH[a,*], Fereshteh Salimi Jazi, MD[b]

[a]University of Texas Medical Branch, Galveston, TX, USA; [b]University of California San Diego, Rady Children's Hospital, San Diego, CA, USA

Keywords

• Magnet • Button battery • Coin • Water bead • Sharp objects

Key points

- Pediatric foreign body ingestion is a frequent emergency; coins, magnets, button batteries, and water beads pose the highest risks requiring prompt diagnosis and object-specific management strategies.
- Multiple magnet ingestion can rapidly cause bowel necrosis and fistulas; urgent removal or surgery is required when magnets attract across intestinal loops or symptoms develop.
- Button batteries cause liquefactive necrosis within minutes; esophageal impaction requires removal within 2 hours, with honey or sucralfate used as preendoscopic protective measures.
- Water bead ingestion presents diagnostic challenges owing to radiolucency; polyethylene glycol or Gastrografin may help passage, but most symptomatic cases require surgical intervention.
- Prevention relies on parental education, safe product design, and updated regulations targeting magnets, batteries, and expanding polymers like water beads to minimize pediatric ingestion injuries.

INTRODUCTION

Foreign body ingestion remains one of the most common and potentially serious emergencies in the pediatric population. Children under the age of 5 are especially vulnerable because of their natural oral exploratory behaviors and limited ability to distinguish between edible and hazardous objects [1,2].

*Corresponding author. Department of surgery, University of Texas Medical Branch, 301 University Boulevard, Galveston, TX 77555. *E-mail address:* B.naikmathuria@gmail.com

https://doi.org/10.1016/j.yapd.2025.12.001

Abbreviations

CPSC	Consumer Product Safety Commission
CT	computed tomography
GI	gastrointestinal
NASPGHAN	North American Society for Pediatric Gastroenterology, Hepatology and Nutrition
PEG	polyethylene glycol

Each year, tens of thousands of ingestions are reported to US poison control centers, with coins, magnets, button batteries, and small toy parts being the most frequently implicated objects [3,4].

Although many ingested foreign bodies pass spontaneously, certain types pose serious risks and require urgent medical or surgical intervention. High-risk objects, such as button batteries, multiple magnets, water beads, and sharp-pointed items, can lead to complications, including mucosal erosion, pressure necrosis, perforation, fistula formation, and bowel obstruction [1,5].

Diagnosis typically begins with a detailed history and physical examination, although in many cases, the ingestion is unwitnessed. Plain radiographs remain the mainstay of evaluation; however, some foreign bodies–such as water beads and plastic items–are radiolucent and may require high clinical suspicion and additional imaging modalities like ultrasound or computed tomography (CT) for diagnosis [3,6–8].

The evolution of pediatric foreign body ingestion has paralleled changes in toy manufacturing and consumer product trends. Over the past decade, a significant increase in morbidity has been attributed to ingestion of multiple high-powered magnets and button batteries, particularly in younger children [1,9]. Meanwhile, the increase of superabsorbent polymer water beads has introduced a new radiolucent hazard, often diagnosed only after symptoms of obstruction appear [8,10].

This article reviews the diagnosis and management of pediatric foreign body ingestion, with a focus on object-specific risks and treatment strategies.

MAGNETS

Prevalence and risk

Magnet ingestion, particularly those involving high-powered neodymium magnets, has become an increasingly recognized cause of serious gastrointestinal (GI) injury in children over the past 2 decades [1,5,11]. Although a single magnet may pass uneventfully through the GI tract, the ingestion of multiple magnets can result in severe complications owing to the attractive forces between them across layers of bowel [5,12]. Children between the ages of 6 months and 6 years are most affected, although ingestion in older children and adolescents–sometimes linked to imitation of tongue piercings–has also been reported [3,12].

Multiple magnet ingestion can lead to pressure necrosis, bowel wall erosion, fistula formation, bowel obstruction, volvulus, and perforation. These complications often develop rapidly and may occur even in asymptomatic children [9,12–14]. A multicenter retrospective review reported a significant increase in surgical interventions and complication rates following the reintroduction of high-powered magnet sets to the US market after a temporary regulatory ban was lifted [15].

Diagnosis

Diagnosis begins with a thorough history, although ingestion is often unwitnessed. Children may present with nonspecific symptoms, such as vomiting, abdominal pain, or irritability, or may be entirely asymptomatic early in the course [5,7,9,13]. Plain abdominal radiographs are the first-line imaging modality. When multiple magnets are stacked or attract across intestinal walls, they may appear as a single radiopaque object on imaging, obscuring the true risk [12,13]. Certain radiographic clues–such as separation of magnets by air-filled loops, unusual object shapes, or multiple beads aligned along a curved path–should raise suspicion for multiple magnet ingestion [3,16]. In unclear cases, additional imaging (eg, lateral views, serial films, or CT scan) may help differentiate between benign and high-risk scenarios (Fig. 1A, B) [3,12,17].

Management

Management depends on the number of magnets, their location, the time since ingestion, time interval between the ingested magnets, and whether the child is symptomatic [13,18]. The key concern is whether the magnets are in different loops of bowel and exerting force across them, increasing the risk of pressure necrosis, fistula, or perforation [13].

An evidence-based algorithm adopted from Hussain and colleagues [19], proposed by North American Society for Pediatric Gastroenterology, Hepatology and Nutrition (NASPGHAN), stratifies patients based on clinical presentation

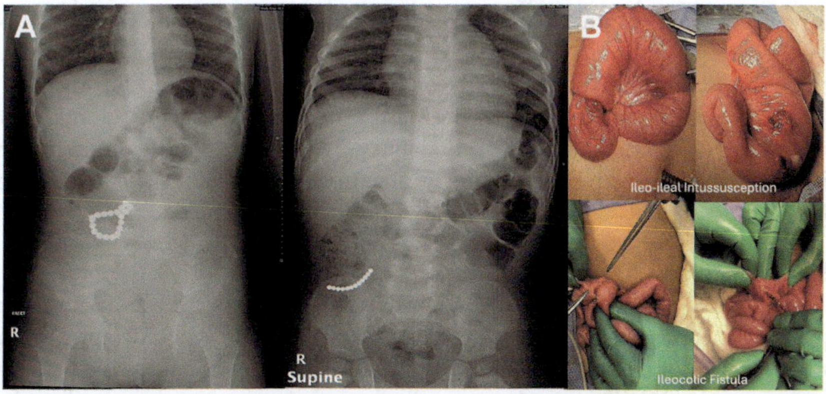

Fig. 1. (*A*) Radiographic view and (*B*) operative complications of magnets. (Altokhais T (2021) Magnet Ingestion in Children Management Guidelines and Prevention. Front. Pediatr. 9:727988. https://doi.org/10.3389/fped.2021.727988.)

and imaging findings [3,19]. This algorithm has been incorporated in multiple literatures and recommend following management (Fig. 2):

- Single asymptomatic magnet: Often managed conservatively with observation and serial radiographs.
- Multiple magnets:
  - All magnets visualized in the stomach:
    - Urgent endoscopic removal is generally indicated. However, in the authors' practice, if the magnets are clearly attached to each other on imaging and small enough to pass through the pylorus, then observation with serial imaging is feasible. If no movement within 12 to 24 hours, then they should be removed by endoscopy.
  - Magnets beyond the pylorus:
    - Asymptomatic child with movement: Continue observation until complete passage.
    - Asymptomatic child, no interval movement in 12 to 24 hours: Surgical exploration should be considered given the assumption that the magnets are attached through the intestinal wall.
    - Symptomatic or radiologic signs of perforation/obstruction: Proceed directly to laparoscopy or laparotomy.

Early surgical intervention is often favored, particularly when symptoms develop or magnets fail to progress [13,19,20]. Delayed surgery has been associated with increased rates of bowel injury and resection. When operating, surgeons may encounter multiple enteroenteric fistulas, transmural necrosis, or magnets embedded in adjacent intestinal loops [21,22]. Laparoscopic exploration might be challenging owing to the magnets adhering to the instruments.

BUTTON BATTERIES

Prevalence and risk

Button battery ingestion represents one of the most life-threatening pediatric foreign body ingestions, particularly in children under 5 years of age [1,6]. With widespread use in household electronics and toys, these small, shiny batteries are often mistaken for candy or coins by young children [6]. Incidence has increased significantly over the past 2 decades, with corresponding increases in major complications and fatalities [3,23]. The 20-mm lithium battery is most associated with severe esophageal injuries because of its size and voltage [6,24].

Pathophysiology

Tissue injury occurs rapidly following mucosal contact with the battery. The primary mechanism is generation of an external electrolytic current, leading to hydrolysis of tissue fluids and production of hydroxide ions at the battery's negative pole [25]. This results in an alkaline environment and causes liquefactive necrosis, which can begin within 15 minutes of contact [6,25]. Prolonged impaction may result in perforation, tracheoesophageal fistula, strictures, vocal cord paralysis, and even fatal hemorrhage from aortoesophageal fistulas [26].

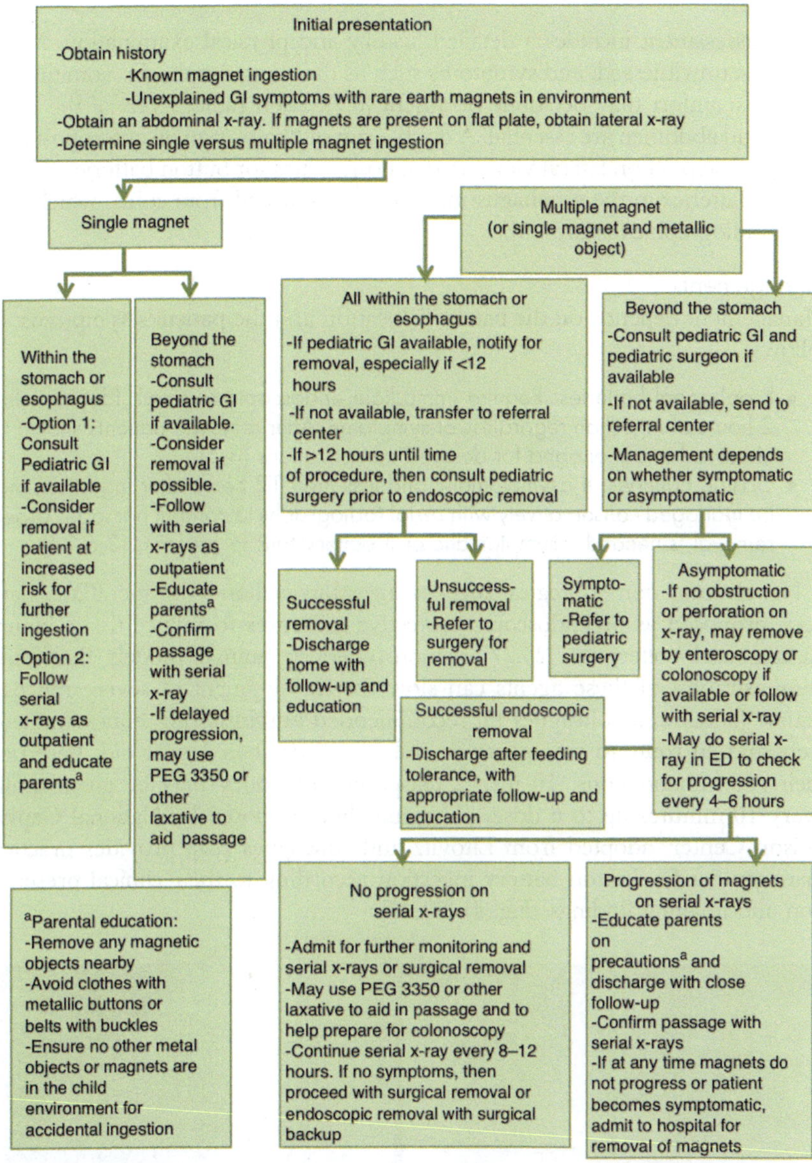

Fig. 2. Proposed management algorithm by NASPGHAN for magnet ingestion in children. ED, emergency department. (Hussain, S.Z., Bousvaros, A., Gilger, M., Mamula, P., Gupta, S., Kramer, R. and Noel, R.A. (2012), Management of Ingested Magnets in Children. Journal of Pediatric Gastroenterology and Nutrition, 55: 239-242. https://doi.org/10.1097/MPG.0b013e3182687be0.)

Diagnosis

Initial assessment includes a detailed history and physical examination. Many cases are unwitnessed, and symptoms such as drooling, dysphagia, vomiting, or chest discomfort may be subtle or absent [6,7]. Plain radiographs of the neck, chest, and abdomen are essential. A double-rim or "halo" sign on anteroposterior view and step-off on lateral view are diagnostic clues for button batteries (Fig. 3) [6,23]. Batteries in the esophagus must be distinguished from coins, which lack these radiographic features [3].

Management

Management depends on the battery's location and the patient's symptoms, as follows:

- Esophageal batteries: Require immediate endoscopic removal, ideally within 2 hours of ingestion regardless of symptoms. After removal, patients should be observed and managed for delayed complications [3,6].
- Gastric batteries: If asymptomatic and less than 12 hours after ingestion, may be managed conservatively with serial radiographs to confirm passage. Urgent removal is needed if symptomatic or if battery fails to progress [3,6,24].

Novel mitigation strategies, such as ingestion of honey or sucralfate, have been proposed as preendoscopic protective measures to reduce tissue injury. Anfang and colleagues [25,27] demonstrated in animal models that early administration of these agents can slow the development of severe mucosal injury. Jatana and colleagues [6] recommended administering honey immediately and en route to emergency in children older than 1 year old. Based on their recommendations, 10 mL (2 teaspoons) of honey may be given orally every 10 minutes up to 6 doses. The guideline proposed by National Capital Poison Center, adopted from Litovitz and colleagues [23], provides practical management for button battery ingestion according to their clinical presentation and imaging findings (Fig. 4) [23,28].

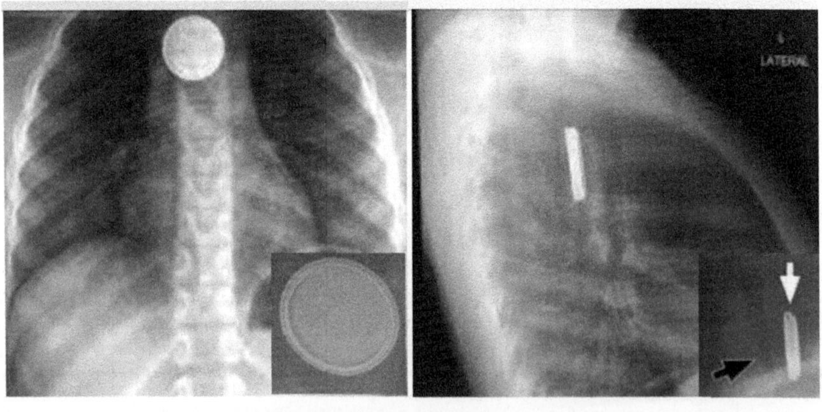

Fig. 3. Anteroposterior (Halo sign) and lateral (Step-off sign) radiographic views of a button battery.

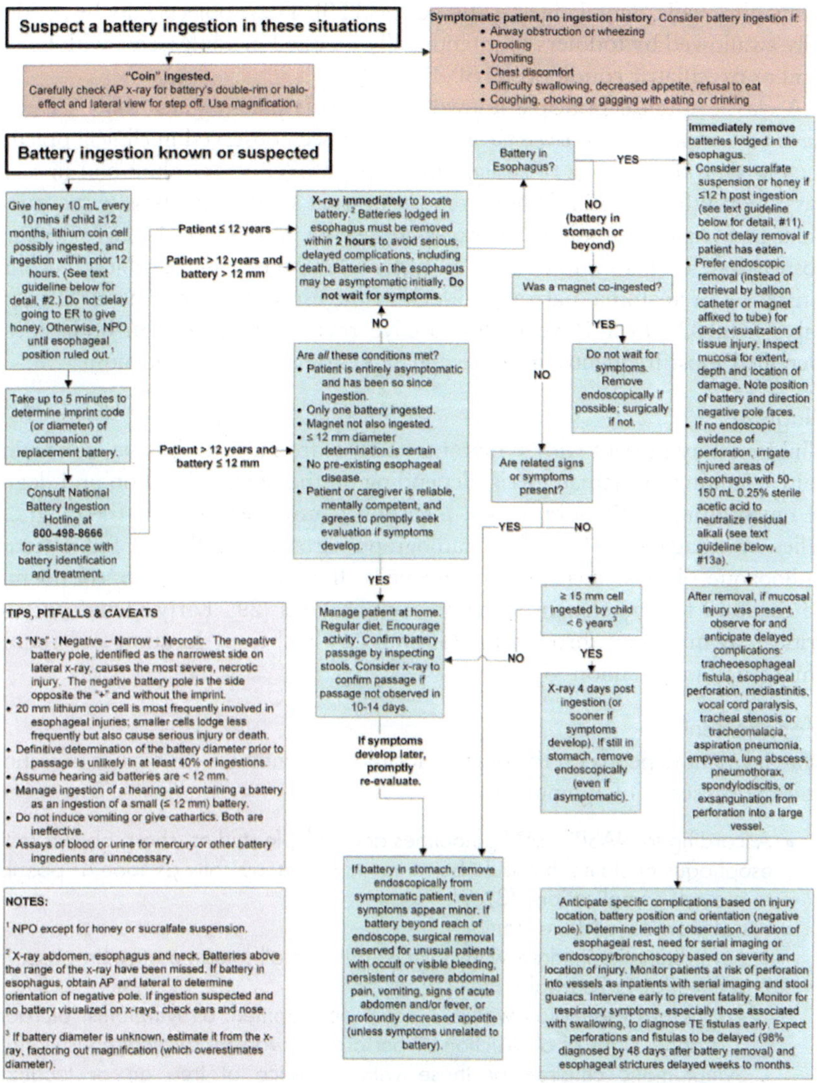

Fig. 4. Proposed management algorithm by National Capital Poison Center for button battery ingestion. (National Capital Poison Center. Battery ingestion triage and treatment guideline. Washington (DC): National Capital Poison Center; 2018 [updated June 2018. Available from: https://www.poison.org/battery/guideline.)

SHARP OBJECTS

Prevalence and risk

Ingestion of sharp-pointed objects in children, although less frequent than coins or batteries, poses a higher risk of morbidity owing to the potential for perforation or penetration of the GI tract. Common sharp foreign bodies include needles, safety pins, nails, dental objects, and bones [3,29]. These objects may be accidentally swallowed by toddlers or intentionally ingested in adolescents with behavioral or psychiatric conditions [5,30,31].

A classic surgical principle known as Jackson's axiom states that *"advancing points perforate and trailing points do not."* This has been observed in clinical practice, such as with the passage of straight pins, which often travel blunt end first and pass uneventfully [3,32]. Although most ingested sharp items pass without incident, their rigid and pointed nature increases the likelihood of mucosal injury, obstruction, or perforation. Risk is further heightened if the object becomes lodged in an anatomic narrowing, such as the esophagus, pylorus, or ileocecal valve [3,32,33]. In a 10-year retrospective review, sharp foreign bodies were identified most frequently in the esophagus, stomach, and duodenum [29].

Diagnosis

Children may present with symptoms such as drooling, dysphagia, abdominal pain, vomiting, or hematemesis, depending on the object's location and degree of mucosal injury. In some cases, ingestion is unwitnessed, and the diagnosis relies on imaging [29,32]. Plain radiographs are often sufficient for detecting radiopaque objects, such as pins and nails; however, CT or ultrasound may be required for radiolucent items or complications [29]. Early identification is critical, as migration through the GI wall can lead to perforation and require emergency intervention [3].

Management

Management depends on the object's location, orientation, time since ingestion, and the presence of symptoms.

- According to NASPGHAN guidelines and multiple studies, sharp objects in the esophagus or stomach should be removed endoscopically as soon as possible to prevent complications [3,29].
- For objects beyond the stomach:
  - Asymptomatic children with objects in the small intestine may be observed with serial radiographs.
    - Lack of progression within 3 days, development of symptoms, or radiographic signs of obstruction or perforation warrant surgical consultation.
  - Symptomatic children or those with evidence of free air or localized tenderness require prompt surgical intervention (Fig. 5) [3].

NONSHARP OBJECTS

Prevalence and risk

Nonsharp object ingestion accounts for most pediatric foreign body cases, especially in children under 5 years of age, who explore their environment orally [34]. Commonly ingested items include coins, small toy parts, jewelry, buttons, and beads [35]. Although most of these pass through the GI tract without incident, certain characteristics–such as size, shape, and composition–can increase the risk of impaction, obstruction, or mucosal injury [3,36].

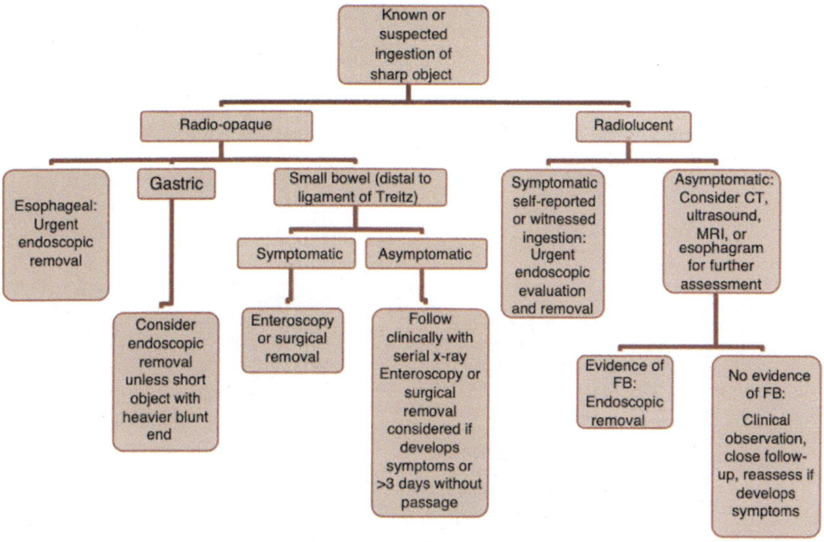

Fig. 5. Proposed management algorithm by NASPGHAN for sharp object ingestion. (*From* Hussain SZ, Bousvaros A, Gilger M, et al. Management of ingested magnets in children. J Pediatr Gastroenterol Nutr. 2012;55(3):239–42.)

Coins are the most frequently ingested foreign body in children, particularly among toddlers. Most coins pass spontaneously, but complications can occur if they lodge in the esophagus or airway, especially if the child is symptomatic [37]. Beads and other small, rounded objects pose a lower risk of injury but may still cause obstruction depending on their size and the anatomy of the GI tract [3,36].

Diagnosis

Diagnosis begins with a careful history and physical examination, but many ingestions are unwitnessed. Plain radiographs are typically sufficient to detect radiopaque items, such as coins, jewelry, and some beads [36]. However, radiolucent items (eg, some plastics or wooden toys) may require advanced imaging, such as ultrasound or CT, if symptoms develop [1,3].

Key radiographic indicators of esophageal foreign bodies include a circular object in the coronal plane on anteroposterior views (coin), and the "double rim" sign, which helps differentiate button batteries from coins [38]. Evaluation should include chest and abdominal films to assess location and identify signs of obstruction or perforation.

Management

Most nonsharp objects that have passed beyond the esophagus can be managed conservatively with observation, especially if the child is asymptomatic (Fig. 6)

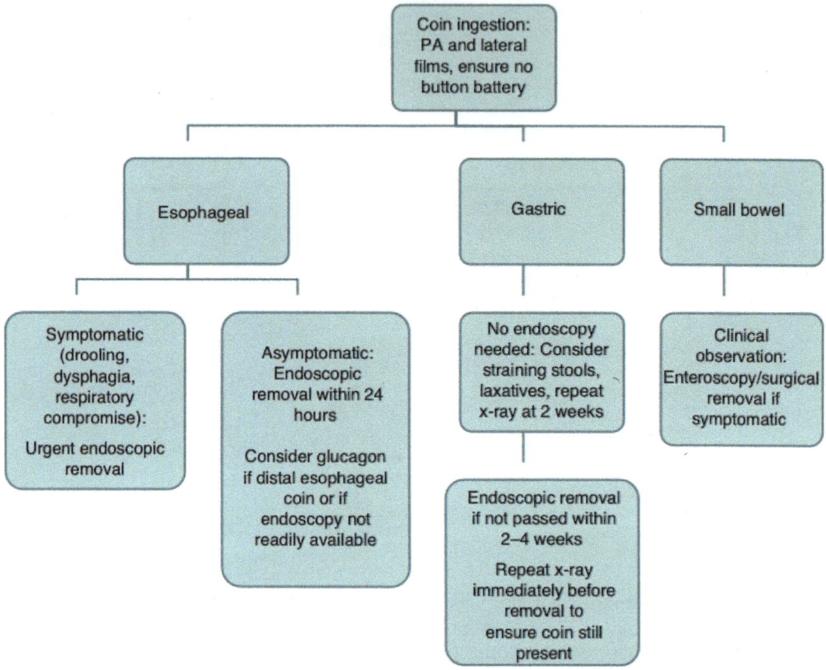

Fig. 6. Proposed algorithm by NASPGHAN for management of coin ingestion. (*From* Hussain SZ, Bousvaros A, Gilger M, et al. Management of ingested magnets in children. J Pediatr Gastroenterol Nutr. 2012;55(3):239–42.)

[1,3,36]. Key considerations, which include object location, size, and time since ingestion, are as follows.

- Esophageal objects:
  - Symptomatic: Require urgent removal owing to risk of airway compromise or esophageal injury.
  - Asymptomatic and present less than 24 hours: May be observed briefly with serial radiographs, but removal is generally preferred.

Several techniques have been described for esophageal retrieval that are summarized in Table 1 [2,39–41].

- Gastric and beyond:
  - Small, blunt objects (eg, coins, marbles) may be managed conservatively in asymptomatic patients with serial radiographs.
  - In general, objects with a diameter more than 2.5 cm or longer than 6 cm are less likely to pass through the gastric pylorus or the duodenum C-loop. When feasible, these objects should be removed upon presentation to prevent potential obstruction [1,3].
  - If the object fails to progress within 3 to 4 days, or if symptoms develop (vomiting, pain), endoscopic or surgical intervention is warranted.
  - Children with prior GI surgery, strictures, or multiple ingestions require more cautious evaluation and possibly earlier intervention [1,3,36].

Table 1
Techniques for removal of coins in the esophagus [42]

Method	Description	Advantages	Risks/limitations
Rigid esophagoscopy	Direct visualization and removal under general anesthesia	Safe, controlled, effective	Requires operating room and anesthesia
Bougienage	Manual advancement into stomach	Can be done without anesthesia	Risk of pushing against obstruction/ perforation
Foley catheter removal	Blind retrieval using balloon catheter	Quick in trained hands	Aspiration risk, no visualization
Glucagon	Smooth muscle relaxant, aids in passage	Noninvasive, adjunctive	Limited data, not always effective

Salazar JH. Foreign body ingestion American College of Surgeon Clinical Congress; October 2024; San Francisco, CA2024.

WATER BEADS

Prevalence and risk

Water beads–also known as hydrogel beads or superabsorbent polymers–are small, colorful toys marketed for play, decoration, and sensory therapy [43]. When dry, they are tiny and easy to ingest; however, once exposed to moisture, they can expand more than 400 times their original size [8,44]. This property poses a significant risk of bowel obstruction when ingested by children, especially toddlers who may mistake them for candy [8,43,44].

Although ingestion of water beads is less common than coins or batteries, the incidence of water bead–related emergency visits has been increasing [8,43]. A recent US study reported an estimated 7800 water bead–related pediatric emergency department visits between 2016 and 2023, with nearly half involving ingestion [43]. Most cases involve children under 5 years old, with ingestion occurring most frequently in children aged 1 to 2 years [43]. In some reports, children have ingested large quantities–up to 1200 unexpanded beads, which was approximately one tablespoon, in a case report [43]. The beads can expand variably when in contact with GI fluids, and their size has been shown to increase in higher pH environments, such as the small intestine [45]. As a result, the beads may pass the pylorus but become lodged in the small intestine [44,45]. Because of their radiolucency, water beads often go undetected on standard imaging, leading to delays in diagnosis and management [43] (Fig. 7A–C).

Diagnosis

Diagnosis of water bead ingestion is often challenging. Many cases are unwitnessed, and the beads may not appear on plain radiographs because of their radiolucent nature [8,43]. Children may present with nonspecific symptoms, such as vomiting, abdominal distension, or irritability, mimicking viral gastroenteritis or constipation [43].

Ultrasound may reveal bowel dilatation or intraluminal masses, and CT imaging can help identify obstructing masses or signs of perforation, but diagnosis

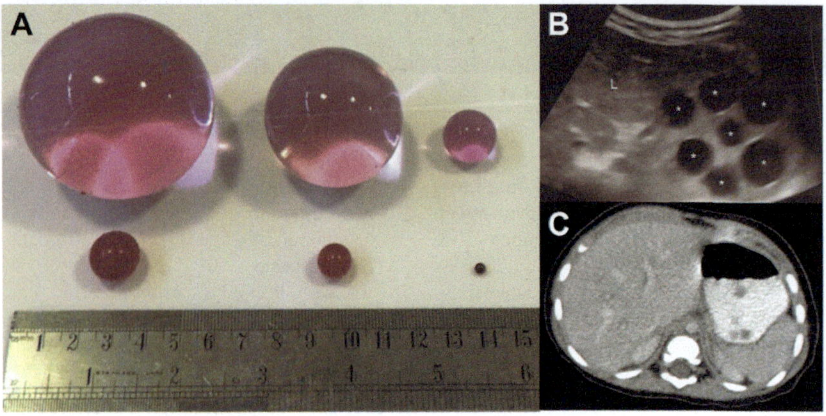

Fig. 7. Water beads expansion potential (*A*), Ultrasound view (*B*), and CT view (*C*) [10,43,44].

often relies on clinical suspicion and parental reporting [8,43]. In several published cases, diagnosis was only made after exploratory laparotomy revealed distended bowel loops obstructed by water beads [8,43]. Although endoscopy can be useful to diagnose and remove beads located in the stomach or duodenum, it cannot rule out the presence of distally located beads [8].

Management

Management, as follows, depends on the time since ingestion, size and location of the beads, and the presence of symptoms:

- Asymptomatic ingestion: Observation may be appropriate if ingestion was recent and the beads have not yet expanded. However, because of their radiolucent nature, standard imaging may appear normal even when beads are present. If suspicion remains high despite negative imaging, advanced imaging, such as CT or ultrasound, or diagnostic endoscopy/laparoscopy, may be necessary to evaluate for retained beads. Asymptomatic patients should be monitored closely, especially if the quantity ingested is unknown or if the child is under 2 years of age [8,44,45].
    - *Polyethylene glycol (PEG):* In select stable, asymptomatic patients without signs of perforation, PEG-based whole bowel irrigation has been used as a noninvasive strategy to promote bead transit and avoid surgery [45].
    - *Gastrografin:* Oral Gastrografin has also been proposed as a potential therapy to promote passage of ingested water beads by creating an osmotic gradient that may shrink the beads and stimulate peristalsis. A case report documented successful passage of a water bead after Gastrografin administration without surgical intervention. Although promising, this approach lacks high-level evidence and should be considered cautiously, ideally in consultation with surgery and radiology [10].
- Symptomatic children: Those presenting with signs of obstruction (eg, vomiting, abdominal distension) require urgent imaging and surgical evaluation. A

retrospective study reported that 95% of symptomatic patients ultimately required surgical intervention, including bowel resection in severe cases [8,44].
- Endoscopic removal: May be considered if the beads are visualized in the stomach or proximal duodenum. However, endoscopy cannot rule out the presence of distally located beads, and its utility is limited if the beads have already passed into the small bowel [8].
- Surgical intervention: Indicated in cases of bowel obstruction or evidence of perforation. Repeat laparotomy may be necessary if beads are missed on initial exploration [8,43].

Hachem and colleagues [45] proposed an algorithm for water bead injection in children according to patient's clinical presentation and size of the beads (Fig. 8).

Prevention and public health

Pediatric foreign body ingestion remains a significant public health concern, particularly in children under 5 years of age. The ubiquity of small household items, evolving toy designs, and inconsistent regulatory standards have contributed to a steady rate of emergency department visits and hospitalizations despite awareness campaigns and clinical guidelines [1,3,34,36].

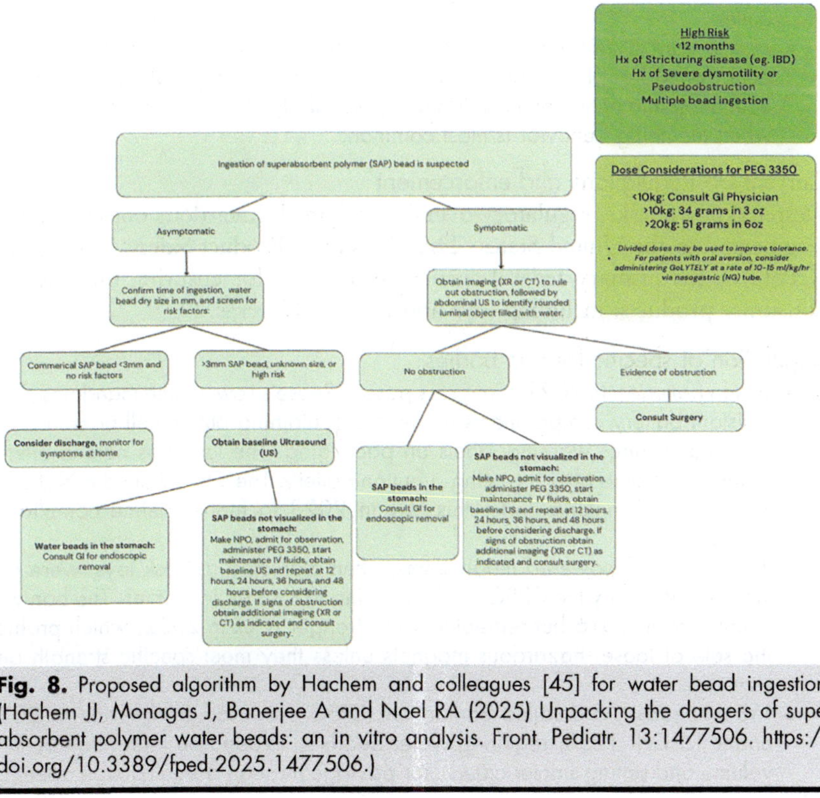

Fig. 8. Proposed algorithm by Hachem and colleagues [45] for water bead ingestion. (Hachem JJ, Monagas J, Banerjee A and Noel RA (2025) Unpacking the dangers of super absorbent polymer water beads: an in vitro analysis. Front. Pediatr. 13:1477506. https://doi.org/10.3389/fped.2025.1477506.)

Primary prevention strategies

Preventing foreign body ingestion requires a multifaceted approach involving caregivers, health care providers, manufacturers, and policymakers. Effective strategies include the following:

- *Parental education:* Educating caregivers about common household hazards—such as button batteries, magnets, water beads, and small toy components—is crucial. Visual reminders (eg, packaging labels, toy warnings) and anticipatory guidance during well-child visits have been shown to increase awareness and reduce risky exposures.
- *Age-appropriate product labeling:* Many ingestions occur when children access toys or objects not designed for their age group. Clear and standardized warning labels are essential to guide safe product use.
- *Safe storage practices:* Storing hazardous objects like batteries, magnets, and small electronics out of reach and sight of young children is a simple yet underutilized preventive measure. Lockable storage containers and child-proofing measures are particularly important for households with toddlers [13,15,43].

Community and provider involvement

- *Public awareness campaigns:* National initiatives, such as those sponsored by the American Academy of Pediatrics or Safe Kids Worldwide, have disseminated educational materials through pediatric clinics, schools, and media outlets.
- *Health care provider counseling:* Pediatricians, family physicians, and emergency providers play a critical role in prevention by incorporating ingestion risk education into anticipatory guidance, particularly at developmental milestones when mouthing behavior is most common.

Current US Regulations and enforcement

Despite known risks, regulatory oversight of small, hazardous objects remains fragmented in the United States. The Consumer Product Safety Commission (CPSC) is the primary federal agency responsible for ensuring the safety of consumer products, including toys and household items.

Regulation of specific foreign bodies

- *Button batteries:* In 2022, Congress passed Reese's Law, which mandates child-resistant battery compartments in devices containing button cell or coin batteries and requires warning labels on packaging. The law was named after a toddler who died after ingesting a button battery. The CPSC issued a Notice of Proposed Rulemaking under this law in 2023 to further define compliance testing.
- *Magnets:* High-powered magnet sets, often marketed as desk toys, were previously banned by the CPSC in 2012 owing to a surge in injuries. The ban was overturned in 2016 but reinstated with stronger rules in 2022, which prohibit the sale of loose, hazardous magnets unless they meet specific strength and size criteria.
- *Water beads:* As detailed earlier, the CPSC proposed a new rule in 2024 under 16 CFR 1250, requiring water beads to expand no more than 50% in volume and setting stricter criteria for passage through a small-gauge opening.

This followed a dramatic increase in ingestion-related injuries and retailer-driven market withdrawal.

Challenges in enforcement

- *Scope gaps:* Many regulations apply only to toys marketed to children under age 3, leaving products intended for older children or adults—such as decorative beads, gel blasters, or adult desk toys—less stringently controlled.
- *Inconsistent compliance:* Enforcement depends on manufacturer reporting and third-party testing, which may be inconsistently implemented. Some products, particularly from international sellers, may not meet US safety standards or include adequate warnings.

FUTURE DIRECTIONS

Calls for more comprehensive legislation and international harmonization of safety standards follow:

- Expanding mandatory product testing to cover items marketed for older children and teens.
- Creating centralized injury registries to better monitor trends and guide policy.
- Enhancing cooperation with online retailers to remove unsafe listings.

CLINICS CARE POINTS

- Button battery ingestion is a surgical emergency; esophageal batteries require immediate removal, regardless of symptoms or fasting status.
- Asymptomatic presentation does not exclude severe injury, particularly with button batteries or multiple magnet ingestions.
- Multiple magnet ingestion carries a high risk of pressure necrosis and perforation, even when objects appear distal on imaging.
- Honey or sucralfate may reduce esophageal injury from button batteries, but should never delay endoscopic removal.
- Plain radiographs may underestimate injury severity; clinical suspicion should guide escalation of care.
- Failure to identify magnet number and timing of ingestion is a common pitfall that leads to delayed intervention.
- Caregiver education at discharge is essential, as delayed complications may occur even after apparent object passage.

DECLARATION

During the preparation of this work, the authors used ChatGPT in order to improve readability and language. After using this tool/service, the authors reviewed and edited the content as needed and take full responsibility for the content of the publication.

Disclosure

The authors do not have anything else to disclose.

References

[1] Lee JH. Foreign body ingestion in children. Clin Endosc 2018;51(2):129–36.
[2] Choe JY, Choe BH. Foreign body removal in children using foley catheter or magnet tube from gastrointestinal tract. Pediatr Gastroenterol Hepatol Nutr 2019;22(2):132–41.
[3] Kramer RE, Lerner DG, Lin T, et al, North American Society for Pediatric Gastroenterology, Hepatology, and Nutrition Endoscopy Committee. Management of ingested foreign bodies in children: a clinical report of the NASPGHAN endoscopy committee. J Pediatr Gastroenterol Nutr 2015;60(4):562–74.
[4] Fergusson JA, Malecky G, Simpson E. Lead foreign body ingestion in children. J Paediatr Child Health 1997;33(6):542–4.
[5] Khorana J, Tantivit Y, Phiuphong C, et al. Foreign body ingestion in pediatrics: distribution, management and complications. Medicina (Kaunas) 2019;55(10).
[6] Jatana KR, Rhoades K, Milkovich S, et al. Basic mechanism of button battery ingestion injuries and novel mitigation strategies after diagnosis and removal. Laryngoscope 2017;127(6): 1276–82.
[7] Quitadamo P, Anselmi F, Caldore M, et al. Foreign body ingestion in children: beware of disk batteries and multiple magnets. Acta Paediatr 2021;110(10):2862–4.
[8] Bollettini T, Mogiatti M, Benigna A, et al. Water beads: expanding toy and 'new' problem for paediatric surgeons and community. J Paediatr Child Health 2025;61(2):204–8.
[9] Strickland M, Rosenfield D, Fecteau A. Magnetic foreign body injuries: a large pediatric hospital experience. J Pediatr 2014;165(2):332–5.
[10] Williams J, Pumiglia L, Zhang B, et al. The Itsy-Bitsy water bead went Down the baby's Mmuth. Will Ddinking Ggstrografin Hhlp to Ffush Ii Oot?". J Surg Res 2024;304:273–9.
[11] Chen QJ, Wang LY, Chen Y, et al. Management of foreign bodies ingestion in children. World J Pediatr 2022;18(12):854–60.
[12] Chen Y, Chen Q, Qian Y, et al. Individualized treatment of multiple magnetic foreign body ingestion in children. J Laparoendosc Adv Surg Tech 2025;35(1):94–100.
[13] Altokhais T. Magnet ingestion in children management guidelines and prevention. Front Pediatr 2021;9:727988.
[14] Luo Y, Cui X, Zhou J, et al. Development and validation of a clinical nomogram for predicting complications from pediatric multiple magnet ingestion: a large retrospective study. Am J Gastroenterol 2025;120(3):642–9.
[15] Flaherty MR, Buchmiller T, Vangel M, et al. Pediatric magnet ingestions after federal rule changes, 2009-2019. JAMA 2020;324(20):2102–4.
[16] Blevrakis E, Raissaki M, Xenaki S, et al. Multiple magnet ingestion causing instestinal obstruction and entero-enteric fistula: which imaging modality besides radiographs? A case report. Ann Med Surg 2018;31:29–33.
[17] Guelfguat M, Kaplinskiy V, Reddy SH, et al. Clinical guidelines for imaging and reporting ingested foreign bodies. AJR Am J Roentgenol 2014;203(1):37–53.
[18] Nugud AA, Tzivinikos C, Assa A, et al, Gastrointestinal Committee of ESPGHAN. Pediatric magnet ingestion, diagnosis, management, and prevention: a european society for paediatric gastroenterology hepatology and nutrition (ESPGHAN) position paper. J Pediatr Gastroenterol Nutr 2023;76(4):523–32.
[19] Hussain SZ, Bousvaros A, Gilger M, et al. Management of ingested magnets in children. J Pediatr Gastroenterol Nutr 2012;55(3):239–42.
[20] Li XL, Zhang QM, Lu SY, et al. Accidental ingestion of multiple magnetic beads by children and their impact on the gastrointestinal tract: a single-center study. BMC Pediatr 2024;24(1):5.
[21] Alareefy A, Barnawi E, Alrashed R, et al. Pediatric magnet ingestion with delayed presentation: case series from tertiary center in Saudi Arabia. Pediatr Health Med Therapeut 2023;14:231–6.

[22] Alansari AN, Baykuziyev T, Soyer T, et al. Magnet ingestion in growing children: a multi-center observational study on single and multiple magnet incidents. Sci Rep 2024;14(1):4575.
[23] Litovitz T, Whitaker N, Clark L, et al. Emerging battery-ingestion hazard: clinical implications. Pediatrics 2010;125(6):1168–77.
[24] Leinwand K, Brumbaugh DE, Kramer RE. Button battery ingestion in children: a paradigm for management of severe pediatric foreign body ingestions. Gastrointest Endosc Clin N Am 2016;26(1):99–118.
[25] Anfang RR, Jatana KR, Linn RL, et al. pH-neutralizing esophageal irrigations as a novel mitigation strategy for button battery injury. Laryngoscope 2019;129(1):49–57.
[26] Karnecki K, Pieśniak D, Jankowski Z, et al. Fatal haemorrhage from an aortoesophageal fistula secondary to button battery ingestion in a 15-month-old child. Case report and literature review. Leg Med 2020;45:101707.
[27] Silva Júnior DSD, Markus JR, Lopes AB, et al. Protocol of care for foreign-body ingestion in children: a qualitative study. Rev Assoc Med Bras 2022;68(9):1270–5.
[28] Center NCP. Battery ingestion triage and treatment guideline Washington (DC): National capital poison center; 2018. 2018. Available at: https://www.poison.org/battery/guideline.
[29] Quitadamo P, Battagliere I, Del Bene M, et al. Sharp-pointed foreign body ingestion in pediatric age. J Pediatr Gastroenterol Nutr 2023;76(2):213–7.
[30] McMahon K, Conners GP, Mohseni M. Pediatric foreign body ingestion. StatPearls: StatPearls Publishing Copyright © 2025. StatPearls Publishing LLC; 2025.
[31] Wu W, Lv Z, Xu W, et al. An analysis of foreign body ingestion treatment below the pylorus in children. Medicine 2017;96(38):e8095.
[32] Karthikeyan VS, Ansari MG, Suresh R, et al. Spontaneous passage of long, sharp gastrointestinal foreign body in a child. BMJ Case Rep 2015;2015.
[33] Emeka CK, Chukwuebuka NO, Tochukwu EJ. Foreign body in the gastrointestinal tract in children: a tertiary hospital experience. Afr J Paediatr Surg 2023;20(3):224–8.
[34] Salman H, Gürsoy Koca T, Dereci S, et al. Foreign body ingestion and management in children. Pediatr Emerg Care 2022;38(11):617–20.
[35] Oliva S, Romano C, De Angelis P, et al, Italian Society of Pediatric Gastroenterology Hepatology and Nutrition SIGENP, and The Italian Association of Hospital Gastroenterologists and Endoscopists AIGO. Foreign body and caustic ingestions in children: a clinical practice guideline. Dig Liver Dis 2020;52(11):1266–81.
[36] Uyemura MC. Foreign body ingestion in children. Am Fam Physician 2005;72(2):287–91.
[37] Gurevich Y, Sahn B, Weinstein T. Foreign body ingestion in pediatric patients. Curr Opin Pediatr 2018;30(5):677–82.
[38] Poddar U, Samanta A. Foreign body ingestion in children: the menace continues. Indian Pediatr 2022;59(9):716–7.
[39] Erginel B, Kaba M, Karadag CA, et al. Foley catheter technique for the extraction of coins lodged in the upper esophagus of children. BMC Pediatr 2023;23(1):605.
[40] Heinzerling NP, Christensen MA, Swedler R, et al. Safe and effective management of esophageal coins in children with bougienage. Surgery 2015;158(4):1065–70 [discussion: 71-2].
[41] Mantegazza C, Ferraro S, Biganzoli D, et al, SIGENP Endoscopy Working Group. Foreign body ingestion in children: definition of a nomogram to predict surgical or endoscopic intervention. Dig Liver Dis 2024;56(2):312–21.
[42] Salazar JH. Foreign body ingestion American College of Surgeon Clinical Congress; October 2024; San Francisco, CA2024.
[43] Joynes HJ, Kistamgari S, Casavant MJ, et al. Pediatric water bead-related visits to United States emergency departments. Am J Emerg Med 2024;84:81–6.
[44] Cairns R, Brown JA, Buckley NA. Dangerous toys: the expanding problem of water-absorbing beads. Med J Aust 2016;205(11):528.
[45] Hachem JJ, Monagas J, Banerjee A, et al. Unpacking the dangers of super absorbent polymer water beads: an in vitro analysis. Front Pediatr 2025;13:1477506.

Advances in Pediatrics 73 (2026) 353–370

ADVANCES IN PEDIATRICS

Climate Stewardship in the Clinical Setting

McKenna F. Parnes, PhD, MSEd[a,b,*], Elliott M. Weiss, MD, MSME[a,b], H. Mollie Grow, MD, MPH[a]

[a]Department of Pediatrics, University of Washington School of Medicine, Seattle, WA, USA; [b]Treuman Katz Center for Pediatric Bioethics & Palliative Care, Seattle Children's Research Institute, Seattle, WA, USA

Keywords

• Health care sustainability • Climate change • Environmental health • Climate stewardship

Key points

- Given the disproportionate impact of climate change on children and their health, pediatricians and other pediatric health clinicians have a critical role in mitigating and adapting to climate change and ensuring sustainability of the health care system that serves children.
- Health care systems contribute to climate change through all aspects of clinical care, and sustainability should be embedded into all dimensions.
- Pediatric clinicians are needed at individual levels to inform patients and families about climate and health, at community level to change institutions through climate stewardship, and at the larger system level to help transform health care policies and practices into sustainable approaches.

INTRODUCTION

What is climate change and how does it affect health and health care?

Climate change is one of the most pressing issues of our time, affecting not just our physical environment, but also the health and well-being of people globally. Definitions of *climate change* refer to the long-term changes in weather patterns and the related effects on the Earth's climate system [1] (see Table 1 for

*Corresponding author. Treuman Katz Center for Pediatric Bioethics and Palliative Care, Seattle Children's Research Institute, 1900 9th Avenue, M/S JMB-6, Seattle, WA 98101. *E-mail address:* mckenna.parnes@seattlechildrens.org

https://doi.org/10.1016/j.yapd.2026.02.003

Abbreviation

PPE Personal protective equipment

definitions of terms). Greenhouse gases such as carbon dioxide, methane, and nitrous oxide, trap heat in the atmosphere and increase Earth's surface temperature. Human activities including burning of fossil fuels, deforestation and land use practices, waste management, and overconsumption and industrialization, account for the majority of greenhouse gas emissions [2].

In 2024, global surface temperatures surpassed 1.5° Celsius (~1.55° Celsius) above pre-industrial levels, breaching the Paris Agreement, an international climate change treaty, limit set in 2015. While a single year above 1.5° Celsius is not catastrophic, if current trends continue, the threats to both people and the planet will become more severe and potentially irreversible. Without the bold multi-national cooperation necessary to drastically reduce emissions, the World Economic Forum estimates that by 2050, climate change could lead to an additional 14.5 million deaths, nearly $13 trillion in global economic losses, and over $1 trillion in added costs to health care systems [3]. The World Bank estimates that as early as 2030, an additional 100 million people could be pushed

Table 1
Climate change and health terms and definitions

Term	Definition
Climate change [1]	Long-term changes in weather patterns and the related effects on the Earth's climate system
Climate stewardship in health care [80]	The involvement of health care professionals and systems to help implement and deliver evidence-based responses to climate change health challenges
Climate justice [81]	Recognizing and addressing the inequitable impacts of climate change and prioritizing the health and safety of individuals and communities who face the greatest risk
Health care sustainability [47]	The implementation of cost-efficient, environmentally friendly practices to support healthy and resilient environments and communities over time
Health care decarbonization [82]	The act of reducing greenhouse gas emissions resulting from human activity in the health care sector
Adaptation [83]	Actions taken to minimize the potential impacts of climate change and to reduce, with the least cost, the adverse effects on health
Mitigation [84]	Efforts aimed at reducing or preventing greenhouse gas emissions or enhancing their removal from Earth's atmosphere
One Health [31]	An integrated approach that recognizes the inextricable link among human health, animal health, and environmental health and calls for collaborative, interdisciplinary work to obtain optimal health
Circularity [85]	Minimizing waste and maximizing resource efficiency through practices like maintenance, repair, reuse, remanufacturing, and recycling

below the poverty line due to climate change impacts [4]. Delays in the adoption of clean energy solutions and lack of regulation or enforcement of laws for major industry contributors has prevented meaningful change [5].

Increased temperatures lead to greater frequency and severity of extreme weather events, including excessive heat, droughts, wildfires, and more severe storms. In turn, extreme weather events worsen environmental exposures such as air pollution, contaminants in water and soil, disease vectors and allergens by disrupting ecosystems [6]. For example, droughts and heatwaves led to more frequent and intense wildfires, releasing smoke and particulate matter, and threaten agriculture, impacting food security and nutrition. Higher temperatures and stagnant conditions from heatwaves also increase ground-level ozone, while warmer, longer seasons increase pollen and allergens, exacerbating asthma. Heavy rains and floods overwhelm sewage systems, contaminating water sources and recreational water. Increased temperatures and flooding also create new breading grounds for vectors like mosquitos and ticks, increasing disease risk and spread. Extreme weather events also worse displacement by destroying homes and infrastructure, eliminating livelihoods (eg, farming, fishing) and forcing people to flee their homes and communities as climate migrants. These events and exposures have significant impacts on human health, increasing rates of morbidity and mortality through direct impacts (eg, injury, death, or trauma exposure due to extreme weather events) as well as indirect impacts (eg, air pollution, spread of vector-borne diseases, food and water insecurity, displacement, exacerbation of pre-existing conditions) [7].

Health care systems are also having to respond to the effects of extreme weather events on supply chains. Disruptions to supply chains have direct effects on patient care. When Hurricane Helene hit North Caroline in September 2024, a primary supplier of US hospital IV fluids incurred damages that led to a pause in production for almost 4 months, resulting in the cancellation and postponement of surgeries and procedures nationally [8]. These extreme weather events cost billions of dollars and have grown substantially over a 40 year period, increasing from an average of about 9 events per year in the 1980s to 27 events documented in 2024 [9].

Pediatric vulnerability to climate change

Pediatric patients are among the most vulnerable to the adverse health effects of climate change and environmental exposures given their immature physical and cognitive systems [10]. Many children also engage in outdoor play or sports, resulting in high rates of exposure to air pollution and heat [11]. As compared to adults, children breathe in more air and consume more food and water per pound of body weight thus potentially exposing them to relatively more contaminants. Because their organs are still developing, they are more susceptible to damage from poor air quality and extreme heat [12].

According to the United Nations Children's Fund Children's Climate Risk Index, which measures risk based on exposure to climate and environmental hazards and children's vulnerability to these hazards, nearly one billion children live in extremely high-risk countries based on their exposure to adverse impacts of climate change [13]. Moreover, the health effects of climate change and environmental exposures are not experienced equally across all pediatric populations–for example, children who are racial and ethnic minorities are 8 times more likely to suffer from pediatric asthma and have a 1.3 times higher risk of premature death due to pollutant exposure [14]. Given the disproportionate impact of climate change on children and their health, pediatricians and other pediatric health clinicians have a critical role in mitigating the impact of climate change on the health of their patients and communities and advocating for *climate justice*.

Organizations around the world, including the United Nations [15], the World Health Organization [16,17], the American Academy of Pediatrics [18], and Health Care Without Harm [19]–a global advocacy organization whose mission is transform health care so that it reduces its environmental impact, promotes sustainability, and leads in environmental and health justice–have issued calls to action to address the effects of climate change on children's health. These organizations urge pediatric clinicians and the health care sector to incorporate climate change considerations and advocacy into clinical practice, training and continuing education curricula, health care operations, and local, national, and international policy recommendations. From this urgent call, we advocate for action at the level of health care providers and health care systems.

The role of pediatric clinicians

Pediatric clinicians are considered one of the most trusted sources of information for families on how to support their children's physical and mental health [20]. As trusted communicators and champions of children's health, pediatric clinicians must be fully aware of climate-related health risks, capitalize on opportunities to integrate discussions about risks into patient care. While the evidence for the adverse impact of climate change on children's health is well established, there is a critical need to educate families on how to prepare and protect their children from climate change's health risks. Leveraging the trust and impact of children's hospitals and providers when developing and disseminating educational interventions about climate change is one way to increase the reach and uptake of this message.

Pediatric clinicians' roles in sustainable health care are multifold. We present opportunities at each level of the socio-ecological framework, as others have used [21], from individual impact behavior change in patients up to system level policies (Fig. 1). Several pediatric specialties recommend consideration for and incorporation of climate and health discussions into clinical practice, and clinical tools have emerged to empower clinicians in climate stewardship so they are better able to integrate climate change awareness into patient care [22]. Table 2 offers guidance summarized from these specialties on how to discuss climate change in pediatric care settings [22–25]. It is important that these conversations occur both in primary care and specialty clinical

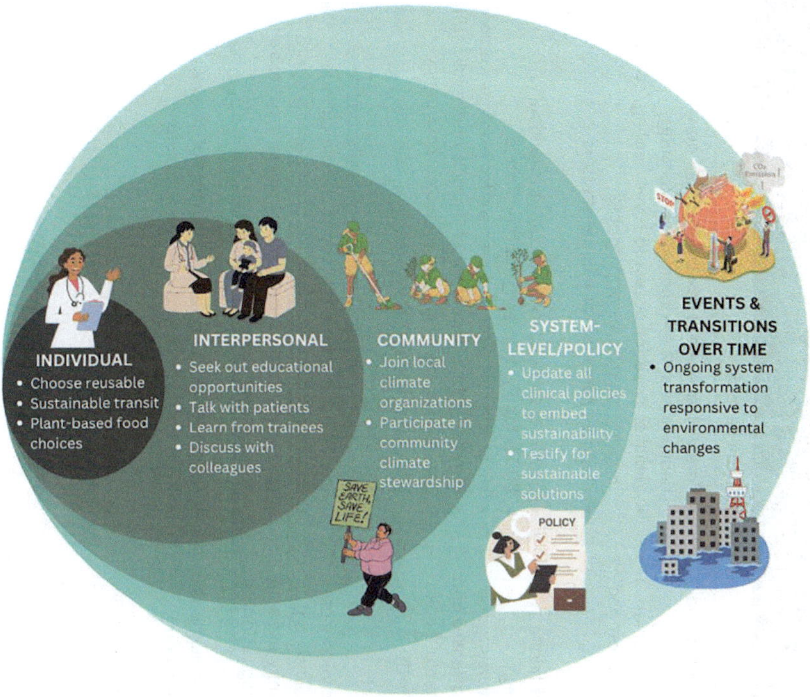

Fig. 1. Socioecological framework of pediatric clinician roles to address climate change in health care.

encounters; depending on the specific condition, specialty medical providers may be able to provide more nuanced and specific recommendations for addressing health impacts of climate change based on a child's needs. This may include providing brief one-pagers virtually or in clinic before an upcoming season (eg, spring allergies, summer heat) that discuss local climate risks (eg, air pollution, extreme heat, disease vectors), health-specific anticipatory guidance (eg, air quality monitoring, weather-informed decision making, recognizing symptoms of heat illness). Pediatric clinicians can also share actionable advice to support climate change mitigation and adaptation. For example, discussing a plant-forward diet and reducing consumption of red and processed meats, which has benefits for both cardiovascular health benefits and emissions reductions; encouraging walking, biking, or public transit to promote physical activity and reduce local air pollution; creating a summer wildfire smoke action plan to map out engaging indoor activities that can replace outdoor play when air quality health risk is high.

Increasing pediatric provider knowledge and education about climate change and health impacts is also critical. Pediatric clinicians have a great opportunity to engage in bidirectional learning with residents and trainees. Understanding

Table 2
Examples of climate-related actions available to pediatric clinicians

Setting	Sample activity	Why these matter
Neonatology and newborn nursery [24]	• Discharge counseling on impact of heat illness and wildfire smoke for babies • Offer counseling on vulnerability to environmental exposures (eg, forever chemicals, microplastics) and at-home solutions to reduce risks • Track heat-related birth outcomes	• Parents leave with knowledge about how to reduce health harms of environmental exposures • Identifies need for access to home heating/cooling support, referrals as appropriate • Prepares nurseries for climate stressors
Primary care [22,86]	• Screen for environmental determinants of health • Provide counseling on healthy active living	• Supports early intervention and prevention • Builds family awareness and resilience
Emergency medicine/ Urgent care [76,87,88]	• Inform caregivers on how rising temperatures, poor air quality, and changes in vector-borne diseases and allergens affect pediatric physical and mental health • Share solutions for mitigating extreme effects of extreme weather events	• Helps families plan and prepare for extreme weather • Greater public awareness of impacts and solutions can reduce extreme weather-related emergency department/urgent care visits
Psychiatry/Psychology [10,89,90]	• Screen for climate distress • Integrate climate-informed practice into clinical care (eg, therapeutic treatment, medication counseling) • Add mental health to school and community extreme weather emergency preparedness plans (eg, establish peer support programs)	• Equips children and families with skills to reduce mental health consequences of climate change • Ensures children and families are receiving appropriate care and intervention to recover from extreme weather exposure
Gastroenterology [78,79]	• Inform families of environmental impacts on gut health (eg, air pollution, heat-related flares, altered gut microbiome) • Discuss gut–brain interactions and consequences of stress on gastrointestinal diseases • Highlight climate-driven food and water quality issues and potential for infection	• Mitigate climate-driven gastrointestinal illnesses • Supports nutrition and safe food choices

Surgery and Anesthesiology [63,91]	• Make climate-informed decisions to support sustainable practice (eg, reduce waste, transition to lower-emission anesthesia)	• Reduces health care emissions to promote a healthier environment for children and families
Pulmonology [92]	• Educate families on using air quality monitoring tools • Create wildfire smoke respiratory health safety plans	• Empowers families to manage risks • Reduces exacerbations and hospitalizations related to environmental exposures
Allergy-Immunology [93,94]	• Discuss the effects of climate change on allergens, including longer seasons and greater potency and production	• Helps patients understand increases in severity of symptoms and prepare early for seasonal allergies
Dermatology [25,95]	• Provide anticipatory guidance to patients and families on the importance of skin protection from sun exposure, increased temperatures, air pollution, and humidity • Highlight products that can reduce or reverse environmental impacts (eg, thermally stable sunscreens)	• Prevents long-term consequences of climate exposure on children's skin

and engaging in climate change is a high priority for pediatric medical trainees. Many younger trainees have greater knowledge and experience with climate change and health topics and can leverage their expertise to help design curricula [26–28]. Pediatric clinicians should utilize opportunities to discuss climate with colleagues and patients to help link climate change to health and to highlight mutually beneficial changes. Climate change is top of mind for many pediatric patients; most youth are worried about climate change impacts [29,30]. Clinicians can also lead by example in everyday activities. For example, knowing when personal protective equipment (PPE) is needed, where to dispose of waste, how to optimize reuse and recycling. Personal transit and food choices offer health co-benefits when choosing active transit and plant-based foods.

Pediatric clinicians can also use their voices to speak out about climate change, its connection to health, and can advocate for changes. Media outlets offer a platform for pediatric clinicians to educate the public on the links between climate change and health to improve climate and health literacy. Social media can also be used to amplify clinical perspectives and combat misinformation by offering an expert perspective. For systems-level and policy change, joining an institution's sustainability committee can help drive changes within clinics, divisions/departments, and hospital systems more broadly. Participating in institutional clinical policy reviews can guide the creation of new policies or updates to existing policies that include sustainability considerations. Joining climate interest groups within national organizations (eg, Climate Psychiatry Alliance, Association of American Medical Colleges, American Academy of Pediatrics) can facilitate idea sharing, action planning, and advocacy for policy changes. There are several organizations and coalitions (eg, Physicians for Social Responsibility, 350, Citizen's Climate Lobby) that pediatric clinicians can partner with to testify for sustainable solutions in legislation at the local, state, federal, and global level.

The role of pediatric clinicians and systems as stewards of climate change, the environment, and children's health aligns with the *One Health* approach which recognizes that the health of people, animals, and our environment are inextricably linked [31]. Thus, experts across areas of human, animal, and environmental health must work together to support *climate adaptation*, adjusting to current and future climate impacts, and *climate mitigation*, tackling and reducing the scale of impacts, to achieve optimal health outcomes.

The role of health care systems

Unfortunately, health care systems contribute to climate change through all aspects of clinical care, thus sustainability should be embedded into all dimensions. The health care sector contributes a substantial proportion of greenhouse gas emissions, particularly in the United States. Estimates are that 8.5% of emissions come from the health care sector [32]. The U.S. health care industry represents 27% of emissions from health care worldwide [33] and is larger than most countries and would be the 13th largest contributor worldwide overall

[32,34]. As we seek to do no harm in medicine, we also must recognize our contributions to the problem of climate change, and how we can reduce impact. Health care is considered the most carbon-intensive US household service, 1692 kg CO_2e per capita in 2018–representing the highest among industrialized nations. Given such large emissions, a harm reduction approach may be considered worthwhile, with even 10% decreases representing substantial carbon emissions across the US International calls to reduce health care emissions are ongoing, with different levels of implementation across the globe [35,36].

The health care sector contributes to climate change through multiple forms of emissions, which are categorized as Scopes 1, 2, and 3, mostly from burning fossil fuels. These include the *direct energy emissions* from health care facilities and vehicles (Scope 1), *indirect energy emissions* through purchased energy sources (Scope 2), and *emissions from the health care supply chain* (Scope 3) to produce, transport, and dispose of goods and services in health care, including pharmaceuticals, medical devices, food, equipment, and other supplies [33]. In the U.S., as globally, the most emissions come from Scope 3 (82%), followed by Scope 2 (11%), and Scope 1 (7%) [35]. The biggest contributors within Scope 3 emissions are those from pharmaceuticals and chemicals (20%), with the U.S. health care sector being the second-largest industry contributing to global landfill waste. When described within health care entities, most emissions come from hospitals (36%), physician and clinical services (12%), and pharmaceuticals (10%) [37,38].

Health care systems globally, including those serving adults and children, should participate as leaders in education, advocacy and sustainability initiatives. Children's hospitals and providers are uniquely positioned to support climate advocacy within local communities. With significant reach and community investment, children's hospitals typically provide care across large geographic regions [39], offer educational and financial resources to benefit their communities [40], and are viewed as trusted institutions to address children's health needs and concerns [41]. Health care systems can support advocacy for climate-smart policies and drive internal climate action, considering climate change as a priority for clinical decision-making. For example, with rapid adoption of generative artificial intelligence in health care systems to optimize efficiency and workflow, climate concerns arise given the massive amount of energy, water, and land use for data centers. It will be critical to prioritize sustainable deployment of AI to reduce the environmental impact and include sustainability goals in internal policies [42].

Evidence-based changes must also be made to improve *health care sustainability*, considering both cost-efficient and environmentally conscious practices. Pediatric providers can partner with hospital administrators and sustainability experts to encourage health care sustainability solutions as well as *health care decarbonization* to reduce greenhouse gas emissions [43]. Some changes have already started, motivated out of necessity. For example, during the COVID-19 pandemic, the need for PPE added even higher volumes of health care waste to systems already relying largely on single-use, disposable equipment and supplies, inviting? Solutions to improve health care waste management systems to improve both human health and minimize environmental impact [44]. Health care systems are growing in their sustainability programs, promoting the responsible use of resources to improve sustainable practices in service of reducing health care contributions to greenhouse gas emissions [45].

Health care system levers of change

Many organizations provide guidance and resources to health care entities to address sustainability. These include Practice Green Health [46], American Hospital Association [47], and the American Society of Health Care Engineering [48]. Themes from all these guides include addressing the major contributors to health care emissions through a systematic approach, engaging clinicians in solutions, and contributing to research. Additional strategies include supporting societal transition to renewable energy to benefit population health and engaging in global and local policy implementation [49].

- Waste—Personal Protective Equipment, Procedures/Operating Room.
  - Across health care entities, medical waste is a large and growing problem for health care emissions and environmental pollution. PPE production, use, and disposal spiked rapidly in the COVID-19 global pandemic [50]. This has accelerated calls for renewable alternatives and reducing single use plastic in all forms in health care [44,51–54]. Many efforts to reduce single use PPE include adopting reusables in operating rooms [55], appropriate and evidence-based PPE policies such as the "Gloves Off" campaign [56,57], studying strictly necessary PPE to reduce infection, and reducing waste in ophthalmologic procedures.
- Food
  - Food in hospitals and health care facilities represents another area for progress. Consuming primarily plant-based foods and reducing beef, lamb, and pork consumption can provide higher benefits for both greenhouse gas reduction and for overall population health. Successful examples of food-system changes include hospital systems that have transitioned to plant-based foods and making plant-based meals the default option [58] and dissemination of the Cool Foods pledge [59].
- Chemicals/Pharmaceuticals
  - Chemicals represent a large portion of the supply chain (level 3) emissions, both for production and for emissions from use. These include anesthetic gases which are even more potent greenhouse gases [60], as well as propellants in aerosolized medications, such as metered dose inhalers used to treat asthma [61,62]. Very successful campaigns have been underway, often led by pediatric anesthesiologists [63], to reduce use of anesthetic gases that are highly potent greenhouse gases (eg, desflurane and nitrous oxide). In the United Kingdom and Europe, clinicians have made transitions to dry-powdered inhalers that are breath-actuated medications without propellants [61,64].
- Emerging high-resource technologies such as AI
  - AI technology is highly resource-intensive; however, there are conflicting data on whether overall impact may be positive or negative to greenhouse gas emissions, depending on use [65]. Review of health care use of AI

recommends that policy and governance are critical for responsible and sustainable AI and that collaboration can foster development of sustainable AI [42].

- Green buildings/energy/water
  - Health care buildings use energy and water; emissions from operating buildings, including energy to heat and cool, are part of Scope 1 emissions. Various strategies are available to make buildings more energy efficient. A major focus is renewable energy to reduce greenhouse gas emissions, which also benefits local air quality. LEED certification is an approach health care entities can use to achieve the "triple bottom line" of "people, planet and profit," where the benefits of energy efficiency over the lifetime of the building lower costs overall [66,67].
- Other supply chain purchasing
  - In addition to chemicals/pharmaceuticals and personal protective equipment, high impact products in the health care supply chain include medical devices and other equipment. Implementing medical waste treatment technologies (eg, autoclave, chemical disinfection) [68] or reusable versions of these products can substantially reduce waste and costs and efforts are underway in many facilities to offer more reusable alternatives [69–71].
- Transportation
  - Transportation as a sector represents the largest direct emissions contributor of US greenhouse gas emissions (28%) [72]. Patient transportation represents 6.5% of the US health care emissions, with less than 2% of patient transit occurring in electric vehicles as of 2022 [73]. Health care organizations can choose multiple approaches to reducing transportation related greenhouse gas emissions. These include switching to electric vehicle fleets, incentivizing staff to choose lower carbon transit options, updating infrastructure such as providing electric vehicle charging, and providing more telehealth options for patients [74]. Examples of transition include a successful pilot study to offer patient transit in electric vehicles [75].

FUTURE CONSIDERATIONS—HOW CAN WE CHANGE HEALTH CARE FOR THE FUTURE?

Prioritizing sustainability

Pediatric clinicians across disciplines are recognizing their roles in leading and prioritizing sustainability efforts. Given that Scope 3 emissions account for the largest percentage of health care emissions, climate-intensive divisions must be at the forefront for advocacy and change. This includes opportunities for change at the level of clinical care (eg, promote reusing and recycling materials), administrative operations (eg, sustainable purchasing), building management (eg, energy efficient appliances), personal lifestyle choices (eg, commuting, plant-based food choices), and organizational practices (eg, divesting from fossil fuel companies) [76].

Envision possibilities

There is so much opportunity to make current changes that will have long-term climate impacts to promote the health and safety of younger and future generations. Pediatric hospitals would benefit from establishing climate change committees including trainees, staff, and faculty to advance clinical care, advocacy, research, and education on the pediatric health effects of climate change [77]. Having cross-institutional collaboration ensures the representation of all voices and increases the capacity for this work to have impact. Taking climate action also directly benefits health care systems by lowering financial burdens through improved public health and reduced climate costs [78].

Bringing climate change impact into the equation

Health care decisions are often guided by bioethics through the principles of respecting patient autonomy, doing no harm, acting in the patient's best interest, and centering justice to ensure fair treatment and resource distribution. Traditional bioethics asks us only to consider the patient in front of us, with justice asking us to consider how this compares to medical care with others. This framework fails to consider collateral damage, such as the cost of procedures or climate impact, that in turn have effects on patient health and especially the most socially and economically vulnerable patients. The embedding of climate change considerations into all clinical decision making, with safety, is a radical paradigm shift. Assuming similar clinical effectiveness, medical interventions and clinical practices that have the lowest carbon footprint should be used. The primary method for measuring health care carbon footprint is the life-cycle assessment, a tool that quantifies the environmental impact of medical products or processes [79]. Understanding both clinical and carbon footprint data can inform treatment choices and promote more sustainable solutions.

Balancing risk with future harms of medical waste

An inherent conflict when addressing medical waste (eg, single use protective equipment, syringes, disposable instruments) is balancing the risk of infection control and safety with the environmental pollution and planetary harm that

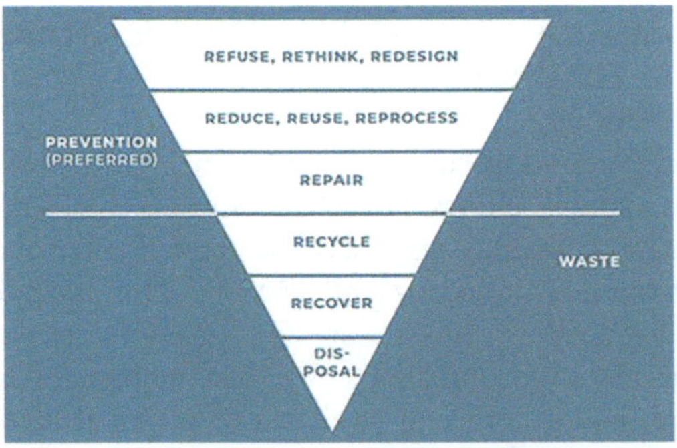

Fig. 2. Health care without harm reprocessing for a greener health care system diagram [94]. (© Health Care Without Harm Europe. Used with permission. Originally published Reprocessing as a vital component of a greener healthcare system in the EU: a focus on Denmark at https://europe.noharm.org/news/reprocessing-vital-component-greener-healthcare-system-eu-focus-denmark).

are a consequence of waste disposal. Navigating this ethical and practical dilemma requires innovative strategies and technological advances. For example, the treatment and disposal of used materials could be transformed to create new opportunities for *reprocessing* materials (Fig. 2), supporting *circularity* in waste management [70].

SUMMARY

Clinicians, especially pediatric clinicians, should understand their roles as leaders in climate stewardship. The interaction of climate change and children's health is an urgent challenge that must be actively addressed. Pediatric clinicians must recognize that the health and well-being of their patients is directly linked to the health of the planet. They must lead by example, prioritizing and advocating for changes that promote sustainable practices, divest from environmentally harmful industries, and advance climate education among trainees, colleagues, and patients' families. Climate stewardship is a win–win for people and the planet; it is synergistic with the triple aim of improving health care quality for individuals, populations, and reducing costs by providing high-value care [38]. By integrating climate change and environmental health into standard medical practice, institutional decision-making, and advocacy, pediatric clinicians affirm their commitment to the health of children. Bringing climate change into all aspects of health care will not only support the health outcomes of children today, but will ensure that the next-generation inherits a world where they can thrive.

CLINICS CARE POINTS

- Climate change has disproportionate consequences to pediatric health due to their physiologic and developmental vulnerabilities.
- Pediatric clinicians across specialties can directly incorporate climate change considerations into patient care, resident training, continuing education, and clinical policies.
- Scope 3 emissions (from production of goods and services) from the health care sector are the biggest contributors to global emissions.
- Health care systems can become more sustainable include reducing carbon emissions through use of renewable energy and electrification, adopting reusable products and reducing waste, especially single use plastic, and minimizing use of chemicals and products, such as anesthetic gases, that contribute to emissions.

Disclosures

The authors have nothing to disclose.

References

[1] What is climate change? - NASA science. 2022. Available at: https://science.nasa.gov/climate-change/what-is-climate-change/. Accessed October 13, 2025.

[2] *Fifth National Climate Assessment*, U.S. Global Change Research Program. In: Crimmins AR, Avery CW, Easterling DR, et al, editors 2023;. 2023. p. 1–1834. https://doi.org/10.7930/NCA5.2023; 2023.
[3] Quantifying the impact of climate change on human health. World Economic Forum. Available at: https://www.weforum.org/publications/quantifying-the-impact-of-climate-change-on-human-health/. Accessed October 13, 2025.
[4] Climate Change Overview: development news, research, data I World Bank. Available at: https://www.worldbank.org/en/topic/climatechange/overview. Accessed October 13, 2025.
[5] Pietras CJ. Rule-governed behavior and climate change: why climate warnings fail to motivate sufficient action. Behav Soc Issues 2022;31(1):373–417.
[6] Bolan S, Padhye LP, Jasemizad T, et al. Impacts of climate change on the fate of contaminants through extreme weather events. Sci Total Environ 2024;909:168388; https://doi.org/10.1016/j.scitotenv.2023.168388.
[7] Maslin M, Ramnath RD, Welsh GI, et al. Understanding the health impacts of the climate crisis. Future Healthc J 2025;12(1):100240; https://doi.org/10.1016/j.fhj.2025.100240.
[8] Economics C of B and, Watson K. Building resilient and responsible supply chains: insights from the healthcare industry. College of business and economics. 2025. Available at: https://www.boisestate.edu/cobe/blog/2025/04/building-resilient-and-responsible-supply-chains-insights-from-the-healthcare-industry/. Accessed October 13, 2025.
[9] Information (NCEI) NC for E. U.S. Billion-dollar Weather and Climate Disasters, 1980 - present (NCEI Accession 0209268). Available at: https://www.ncei.noaa.gov/access/metadata/landing-page/bin/iso?id=gov.noaa.nodc:0209268. Accessed October 13, 2025.
[10] Parnes MF, Bennett MB, Rao M, et al. The kids are not alright: the mental health toll of environmental injustice. Am J Bioeth 2024;24(3):40–4.
[11] Chen Z, Salam MT, Eckel SP, et al. Chronic effects of air pollution on respiratory health in Southern California children: findings from the Southern California Children's Health Study. J Thorac Dis 2015;7(1):46–58.
[12] US EPA O. Climate change and children's health. 2022. Available at: https://www.epa.gov/climateimpacts/climate-change-and-childrens-health. Accessed October 13, 2025.
[13] The climate crisis is a child rights crisis I UNICEF. Available at: https://www.unicef.org/reports/climate-crisis-child-rights-crisis. Accessed October 13, 2025.
[14] Kerr GH, van Donkelaar A, Martin RV, et al. Increasing racial and ethnic disparities in ambient air pollution-attributable morbidity and mortality in the United States. Environ Health Perspect 2024;132(3):37002; https://doi.org/10.1289/EHP11900.
[15] Climate Change and Children's Health I UNICEF USA. 2025. Available at: https://www.unicefusa.org/what-unicef-does/climate-change/childrens-health. Accessed October 13, 2025.
[16] Climate change is an urgent threat to pregnant women and children. Available at: https://www.who.int/news/item/21-11-2023-climate-change-is-an-urgent-threat-to-pregnant-women-and-children. Accessed October 13, 2025.
[17] Global climate change and child health: a review of pathways, impacts and measures to improve the evidence base. Available at: https://www.who.int/publications/m/item/global-climate-change-and-child-health. Accessed October 13, 2025.
[18] Global climate change and children's health: AAP recommendations. Available at: https://www.aap.org/en/patient-care/climate-change/global-climate-change-and-childrens-health-aap-recommendations/?srsltid=AfmBOoqQUBCS94ACYIOs0CjQ2y7jm-rXARtOKC1o_4luUDbBPIOVzsH8. Accessed October 13, 2025.
[19] A call to action: child health and the climate crisis I Health Care without Harm - europe. Available at: https://europe.noharm.org/news/call-action-child-health-and-climate-crisis. Accessed October 13, 2025.
[20] Pediatricians are essential supports for families – RAPID survey. Available at: https://rapidsurveyproject.com/article/pediatricians-are-essential-supports-for-families/. Accessed October 13, 2025.

[21] Bernhardt JM, Amiri A. Application of the socioecological model to mitigate risks of heat illness. Nurs Outlook 2024;72(3):102150; https://doi.org/10.1016/j.outlook.2024.102150.
[22] Philipsborn RP, Cowenhoven J, Bole A, et al. A pediatrician's guide to climate change-informed primary care. Curr Probl Pediatr Adolesc Health Care 2021;51(6):101027; https://doi.org/10.1016/j.cppeds.2021.101027.
[23] Lin E, Hussain MJ, Hunter K, et al. Addressing climate change concerns in pediatric health care settings: exploring parental and physician perspectives. Environ Int 2025;202:109661; https://doi.org/10.1016/j.envint.2025.109661.
[24] Parnes MF, Mosley L, Burris HH, et al. Climate change and environmental degradation: bioethical considerations and impact for neonatal care. Semin Perinatol 2025;49(6):152099; https://doi.org/10.1016/j.semperi.2025.152099.
[25] Schachtel A, Dyer JA, Boos MD. Climate change and pediatric skin health. Int J Womens Dermatol 2020;7(1):85–90.
[26] Cogen JD, Perkins A, Mockler B, et al. Pediatric resident and program director views on climate change and health curricula: a multi-institution study. Acad Med J Assoc Am Med Coll 2024;99(6):654–62.
[27] Philipsborn RP, Sheffield P, White A, et al. Climate change and the practice of medicine: essentials for resident education. Acad Med J Assoc Am Med Coll 2021;96(3):355–67.
[28] Mockler BK, Perkins A, Obremskey A, et al. Incorporating climate change action into pediatric residency training results in institutional change. J Grad Med Educ 2024;16(6 Suppl):161–2.
[29] Lewandowski RE, Clayton SD, Olbrich L, et al. Climate emotions, thoughts, and plans among US adolescents and young adults: a cross-sectional descriptive survey and analysis by political party identification and self-reported exposure to severe weather events. Lancet Planet Health 2024;0(0); https://doi.org/10.1016/S2542-5196(24)00229-8.
[30] Hickman C, Marks E, Pihkala P, et al. Climate anxiety in children and young people and their beliefs about government responses to climate change: a global survey. Lancet Planet Health 2021;5(12):e863–73.
[31] CDC. About one health. One Health 2025. Available at: https://www.cdc.gov/one-health/about/index.html. Accessed October 13, 2025.
[32] The health care leader's guide to sustainability and environmental stewardship I AHA. Available at: https://www.aha.org/sustainability/health-care-leaders-guide. Accessed October 13, 2025.
[33] Health Cares Climate Footprint, Available at: https://global.noharm.org/sites/default/files/documents-files/5961/HealthCaresClimateFootprint_092319.pdf (Accessed 13 October 2025), 2019.
[34] U.S. health system must come to terms with its environmental impact. American Medical Association. 2022. Available at: https://www.ama-assn.org/public-health/environmental-health/us-health-system-must-come-terms-its-environmental-impact. Accessed October 13, 2025.
[35] Eckelman MJ, Huang K, Lagasse R, et al. Health care pollution and public health damage in the United States: an update. Health Aff 2020;39(12):2071–9.
[36] Hough E, Cohen Tanugi-Carresse A. Supporting decarbonization of health systems—A review of international policy and practice on health care and climate change. Curr Environ Health Rep 2024;11(2):266–78.
[37] Seervai S, Gustafsson L, Abrams MK. *How the U.S. Health Care System Contributes to Climate Change,* Commonwealth Fund 2022. https://doi.org/10.26099/m2nn-gh13.
[38] Eckelman MJ, Sherman J. Environmental impacts of the U.S. health care system and effects on public health. PLoS One 2016;11(6):e0157014; https://doi.org/10.1371/journal.pone.0157014.
[39] Franz B, Cronin CE. Are children's hospitals unique in the community benefits they provide? Exploring decisions to prioritize community health needs among U.S. children's and general hospitals. Front Public Health 2020;8:47.

[40] Casimir G. Why children's hospitals are unique and So essential. Front Pediatr 2019;7: 305.
[41] Children's hospitals and pediatric healthcare. Jarrard Inc. Available at: https://jarrardinc.com/practices/childrens-hospitals-and-pediatric-healthcare/. Accessed October 13, 2025.
[42] Ueda D, Walston SL, Fujita S, et al. Climate change and artificial intelligence in healthcare: review and recommendations towards a sustainable future. Diagn Interv Imaging 2024;105 (11):453–9.
[43] Perera F, Nadeau K. Climate change, fossil-fuel pollution, and children's health. N Engl J Med 2022;386(24):2303–14.
[44] Global analysis of health care waste in the context of COVID-19. Available at: https://www.who.int/publications/i/item/9789240039612. Accessed October 13, 2025.
[45] Sustainability metrics and awards I Practice Greenhealth. Available at: https://practicegreenhealth.org/metrics-and-awards. Accessed October 13, 2025.
[46] Homepage I Practice Greenhealth. Available at: https://practicegreenhealth.org/. Accessed September 22, 2025.
[47] Sustainability for health care - achieving your sustainability goals I AHA. Available at: https://www.aha.org/sustainability. Accessed October 13, 2025.
[48] ASHE Sustainability Guide I ASHE. Available at: https://www.ashe.org/sustainability/guide. Accessed October 13, 2025.
[49] HealthCaresClimateFootprint_092319.pdf. Available at: https://global.noharm.org/sites/default/files/documents-files/5961/HealthCaresClimateFootprint_092319.pdf. Accessed September 22, 2025.
[50] Tonnes of COVID-19 health care waste expose urgent need to improve waste management systems. Available at: https://www.who.int/news/item/01-02-2022-tonnes-of-covid-19-health-care-waste-expose-urgent-need-to-improve-waste-management-systems. Accessed September 22, 2025.
[51] Smith M, Singh H, Sherman JD. Infection prevention, planetary health, and single-use plastics. JAMA 2023;330(20):1947–8.
[52] Sutjipto S, Aung AH, Soon MML, et al. Plastic waste and COVID-19 incidence among Hospital staff after deescalation in PPE use. JAMA Netw Open 2025;8(4):e255264; https://doi.org/10.1001/jamanetworkopen.2025.5264.
[53] Ong H, Thiel CL, Singh H. Health care actions for reducing plastic use and pollution. JAMA 2024;332(21):1783–4.
[54] Gadgil MA, Mehrotra P. Optimizing personal protective equipment for a sustainable future. JAMA Netw Open 2025;8(4):e255269; https://doi.org/10.1001/jamanetworkopen.2025.5269.
[55] Chang JH, Woo KP, Silva de Souza Lima Cano N, et al. Does reusable mean green? Comparison of the environmental impact of reusable operating room bed covers and lift sheets versus single-use. Surgeon 2024;22(4):236–41.
[56] Wilkie-Miskin T, Acosta MA, Browning S, et al. Gloves off!: environmental and financial impacts of an educational intervention to improve hand hygiene. A quality improvement study. Infect Dis Health 2025;31(1):100382.
[57] Lalakea ML, Noel JE, Meiklejohn DA. Reducing glove overuse in outpatient specialty clinics: cost reduction and environmental benefit. OTO Open 2025;9(1):e70103; https://doi.org/10.1002/oto2.70103.
[58] Morgenstern S, Redwood M, Herby A. An innovative program for hospital nutrition. Am J Lifestyle Med 2024;19(2):320–3.
[59] About coolfood: shaping the future of food - coolfood. Available at: https://coolfood.org/about/. Accessed October 13, 2025.
[60] The environmental impact of inhaled anesthetics. Available at: https://www.asahq.org/about-asa/governance-and-committees/asa-committees/environmental-sustainability/greening-the-operating-room/inhaled-anesthetics. Accessed October 13, 2025.

[61] Feldman WB, Furie G. The moral injury of inhaler prescribing. N Engl J Med 2025;392(9): 836–9.
[62] Feldman WB, Han J, Raymakers AJN, et al. Inhaler-related greenhouse gas emissions in the US: a serial cross-sectional analysis. JAMA 2025;334(18):1638–49.
[63] Hansen EE, Chiem JL, Righter-Foss K, et al. Project SPRUCE: saving our planet by reducing carbon emissions, a pediatric anesthesia sustainability quality improvement initiative. Anesth Analg 2023;137(1):98–107.
[64] Wilkinson A, Woodcock A. The environmental impact of inhalers for asthma: a green challenge and a golden opportunity. Br J Clin Pharmacol 2022;88(7):3016–22.
[65] CGEP C I. ICEF Artificial Intelligence for Climate Change Mitigation Roadmap (Second Edition). Center on Global Energy Policy at Columbia University SIPA I CGEP. 2024 Available at: https://www.energypolicy.columbia.edu/publications/icef-2024-roadmap-on-icef-artificial-intelligence-for-climate-change-mitigation-roadmap-second-edition/. Accessed October 13, 2025.
[66] Applying LEED to healthcare projects. U.S. Green Building Council. 2025. Available at: https://support.usgbc.org/hc/en-us/articles/12126333712659-Applying-LEED-to-healthcare-projects. Accessed October 13, 2025.
[67] Regulatory Agenda. Addressing greenhouse gas emissions from health care building energy use - NAM. Available at: https://nam.edu/perspectives/regulatory-agenda-addressing-greenhouse-gas-emissions-from-health-care-building-energy-use/. Accessed October 13, 2025.
[68] Sustainability, Available at: https://practicegreenhealth.org/sites/default/files/2024-01/2023-benchmark-data.pdf (Accessed 14 January 2026), 2023.
[69] Keil M, Viere T, Helms K, et al. The impact of switching from single-use to reusable healthcare products: a transparency checklist and systematic review of life-cycle assessments. Eur J Publ Health 2022;33(1):56–63.
[70] Hoveling T, Svindland Nijdam A, Monincx M, et al. Circular economy for medical devices: barriers, opportunities and best practices from a design perspective. Resour Conserv Recycl 2024;208:107719; https://doi.org/10.1016/j.resconrec.2024.107719.
[71] Goubil A, Lefèvre K, Couret C, et al. Understanding and quantifying the environmental impact of sterile medical devices: a carbon footprint study of single-use electrosurgical scalpels and their reusable alternatives. BMJ Surg Interv Health Technol 2025;7(1):e000348; https://doi.org/10.1136/bmjsit-2024-000348.
[72] US EPA O. Transportation sector emissions. 2025. Available at: https://www.epa.gov/ghgemissions/transportation-sector-emissions. Accessed October 13, 2025.
[73] Zurl H, Qian Z, Stelzl DR, et al. Carbon emissions from patient travel for health care. JAMA Netw Open 2025;8(3):e252513; https://doi.org/10.1001/jamanetworkopen.2025.2513.
[74] Kruger J. Decarbonizing Health Care: Low-Carbon Transportation Policies Can Reduce Health Care Emissions and Benefit Local Communities, *Georgetown Climate Center,* 1-38, 2024. Available at: https://www.georgetownclimate.org/files/report/Decarbonizing_Health_Care_Transportation_GCC_2024.pdf (Accessed 13 October 2025).
[75] Smolen KA, Luu J, Braunstein SE, et al. Shifting gears to green: a pilot study on decarbonizing patient transport. J Clim Change Health 2024;16:100297; https://doi.org/10.1016/j.joclim.2023.100297.
[76] Wooldridge G, Murthy S. Pediatric critical care and the climate emergency: our responsibilities and a call for change. Front Pediatr 2020;8; https://doi.org/10.3389/fped.2020.00472.
[77] One way to increase environmental sustainability across an Organization. Available at: https://www.childrenshospitals.org/news/childrens-hospitals-today/2024/04/one-way-to-increase-environmental-sustainability-across-an-organization. Accessed October 13, 2025.
[78] *Tackling climate change could be the greatest global health opportunity of the 21st century,* The Global Climate & Health Alliance. Available at: https://climateandhealthalliance.org/

wp-content/uploads/2023/05/GCHA-Climate-Change-paper.pdf (Accessed 13 October 2025).
[79] Nordberg L.B., Pohl H., Haavardsholm E.A., Lillegraven S., Bretthauer M. Carbon-Footprint Analyses in RCTs - Toward Sustainable Clinical Practice. *N Engl J Med.* 2024, 390(24), 2234-2236. doi:10.1056/NEJMp2402018C
[80] Ting J, Schweitzer D, Lansbury N. Practise as you preach: climate stewardship in healthcare integrating top-down and bottom-up approaches with clinician as positive role models for the community. Intern Med J 2025;55(4):547–9.
[81] Washington State Department of Health, Available at: https://doh.wa.gov/community-and-environment/climate-and-health/climate-justice (Accessed 13 October 2025).
[82] Decarbonization I AHA, Available at: https://www.aha.org/topics/decarbonization (Accessed 13 October 2025).
[83] Stanford V. Climate change adaptation: a guide for health and care professionals, Sustainable Healthcare, 2022. Available at: https://sustainablehealthcare.org.uk/blog-climate-change-adaptation/ (Accessed 13 October 2025).
[84] Ansah EW, Amoadu M, Obeng P, et al. Health systems response to climate change adaptation: a scoping review of global evidence. BMC Public Health 2024;24:2015.
[85] Circular economy introduction. Available at: https://www.ellenmacarthurfoundation.org/topics/circular-economy-introduction/overview. Accessed October 13, 2025.
[86] Nguyen MLT, Honcharov V, Ballard D, et al. Primary care physicians' experiences with and adaptations to time constraints. JAMA Netw Open 2024;7(4):e248827; https://doi.org/10.1001/jamanetworkopen.2024.8827.
[87] Sorensen CJ, Salas RN, Rublee C, et al. Clinical implications of climate change on US emergency medicine: challenges and opportunities. Ann Emerg Med 2020;76(2):168–78.
[88] Nicholas PK, Breakey S, McKinnon S, et al. A CLIMATE: a tool for assessment of climate-change-related health consequences in the emergency department. J Emerg Nurs 2021;47(4):532–42.e1.
[89] Clayton S, Parnes MF. Anxiety and activism in response to climate change. Curr Opin Psychol 2025;62:101996; https://doi.org/10.1016/j.copsyc.2025.101996.
[90] Wortzel JR, Guerrero APS, Aggarwal R, et al. Climate change and the professional obligation to socialize physicians and trainees into an environmentally sustainable medical culture. Acad Psychiatry 2022;46(5):556–61.
[91] Fitzpatrick CM, Muratore CS, Glick RD, et al. Why pediatric surgeons need to care about climate change. J Pediatr Surg 2025;60(8):162280; https://doi.org/10.1016/j.jpedsurg.2025.162280.
[92] Bignier C, Havet L, Brisoux M, et al. Climate change and children's respiratory health. Paediatr Respir Rev 2025;53:64–73.
[93] Sheffield PE, Weinberger KR, Kinney PL. Climate change, aeroallergens, and pediatric allergic disease. Mt Sinai J Med J Transl Pers Med 2011;78(1):78–84.
[94] What the practicing allergist can and should do regarding climate change - annals of allergy, asthma & immunology. Available at: https://www.annallergy.org/article/S1081-1206(23)00559-8/fulltext. Accessed October 13, 2025.
[95] Multani HK, Sraa KK, Abbas H, et al. Climate change and pediatric skin health: emerging threats, innovations, and equity gaps. Cureus 2025;17(9):e91397; https://doi.org/10.7759/cureus.91397.

9780443431883